Protein Engineering of Carcinoembryonic Antigen And their Receptors

Prof.Dr. Sami A. AL-Mudhaffar
Dr. Sahib A. AL-ATrakchi

PART (A)

Protein Engineering of Carcinoembryonic Antigen

Prof.Dr. Sami A. AL-Mudhaffar
Dr. Sahib A. AL-ATrakchi

List of Abbreviations

µci	Micro curie
µg	Microgram
ΔH*	Enthalpy of the excitation state
µl	Microliter
A_{235}	Absorbance at 235 nm
A_{260}	Absorbance at 260 nm
A_{280}	Absorbance at 280 nm
Ab	Antibody
AFP	Alpha-feto protein
Anti-CEA	Antibody against CEA
B	Bound
B_{max}	Maximal binding capacity
BSA	Bovine serum albumin
CA15-3	Carbohydrate antigen 15-3
CEA	Carcinoembryonic antigen
CPM	Counts per minute
CPS	Counts per second
DNA	Deoxy ribonucleic acid
EDTA	Ethylene diamine tetra acetic acid
ESR	Electron Spin Resonance
F	Free
FTIR	Fourier-transform infrared
IgA	Immunoglobulin A
IR	Infra-red
IRMA	Immunoradiometeric assay
IU	International unit
J	Joule
K	Kelvin
Ka	Affinity constant
KD	Kilo Dalton
Kd	Dissociation constant
KJ	Kilo Joule

KJ	Kilo Joule
M.wt	Molecular weight
Min	Minute
MRI	Magnetic resonance imaging
NMR	Nuclear Magnetic Resonance
NPS	Normal physiological saline
PAGE	Poly acrylamide gel electophoresis
PCR	Polymerase chain reaction
pI	Isoelectric Point
PSA	Phosphate Buffer Saline
r.p.m	Round per minute
RFLP	Restriction Fragment length polymorphism
RIA	Radioimmuno assay
RRA	Radioreceptor assay
SB%	Percent of specific binding
SDS	Sodium dodecyl sulfate
TB	Total binding
TED	Tris-EDTA-Diethotheritol
TEMED	N,N,N,N-tetra methyl ethylene diamine
TNM	Characteristic of the Primary Tumor (T), Regional Lymph nodes (N) and Distant Metastatic Deposits (M)
U.V	Ultraviolet
Ve	Elution Volume
Vo	Void Volume

Summary

This thesis included Biochemical and immunological properties of carcinoemberyonic antigen and their receptors in mammary adenocarcinoma and benign tissues. Also, this research is mainly designed to study the following sections and considered protein engineering main direction for these sections:

(1) Evaluation of the clinical value of preoperative serum tumor markers CA15-3 and carcinoembryonic antigen (CEA) in the diagnosis of breast cancer were carried out. These tumor markers were measured preoperatively in 122 patients. The results of both tumor markers were compared. The CA15-3 level was above normal (30 U/ml) in 54% of the patients with breast cancer. The CEA level was elevated in 44% of patients with breast cancer (more than 3 ng/ml). The CA15-3 was shown to be significantly positive in premenopausal status reaching 65.7% of premenopausal cases while CEA was 52%. Both tumor markers were insignificant in postmenopausal status and in relation to tumor T stage and tumor N State. CEA showed equal specificity and lower sensitivity compared with CA15-3. CEA was also less sensitive in differentiating between active and remission states of breast cancer.

(2) A method of immunoradiometric assay (IRMA) for cytosolic CEA was developed by using ^{125}I-anti-CEA antibody and found to be suitable for the assessment of those antigens fraction in mammary tumors. No correlation was found between cytosolic CEA and the histological grading.

(3) A method was developed for the purification and identification of human CEA from metastatic tumor using perchloric acid extraction, Ion exchange chromatography and column chromatography on sepharose 6B. The physiochemical properties of CEA preparation were investigated by different techniques. Sepctrophotometric studies were also performed to characterize the purified CEA. The effect of pH, solvent polarity and solvent perturbation was also studied.

(4) A new method of solid-phase radioimmunoassay was established according to the following that is to measure CEA in sera, it was characterize to be simple and suitable for automation:

(a) Highly purified CEA was labelled with radioiodine according to the chloramine-T-method. The specific activity of radioiodinated CEA is 15.2 µci/µg. Results showed that antigenic activity of CEA was stable after iodination reaction.
(b) Rabbit antiserum against CEA was produced and utilitized to develop a competitive RIA for CEA determination.
(c) The adsorption of a monospecific antibody to polymeric surface was used Incubation was performed in antibody-coated disposable tubes, washed-out with water and counted for quantitation of bound tracer.

(5) The characteristics of the binding of ^{125}I-CEA with their receptors in human breast cancer were investigated by using radioreceptor assay (RRA) technique. Different factors such as pH, protein concentration of the receptor, salt concentration, in addition to the effect of time and temperature affecting on this binding were extensively studied.

(6) Kinetic and thermodynamic studies were carried out for the binding ^{125}I-CEA with both cytosolic and nuclear receptor in mammary adenocarcinoma tissues. Time-course of the association of ^{125}I-CEA with their receptor at five different temperatures revealed the time and temperature dependency. Association kinetic studies indicated pseudo-first order kinetics for the binding. Time-course, Scatchard, Van't Hoffs and Arrhenius plots led to the theoretical determination of thermodynamic parameters of both the standard state (, i.e., $\Delta H°$, $\Delta G°$, $\Delta S°$) and transition state (, i.e., ΔH^*, ΔG^*, ΔS^*).

(7) CEA receptors were isolated and purified from cytosolic fractions of human malignant breast tumors homogenates by a series of purification techniques including: ammonium sulphate precipitation (50–90% saturation), ion exchange chromatography on DEAE-cellulose and CM-cellulose and on the gel filtration chromatography (sepharose 6B). The purified receptors were separated into two forms, anionic receptor and cationic receptor. The physicochemical properties, i.e., molecular weight, stock's radius, number of sub-units and pI, of cationic receptors were determined using several techniques such as SDS polyacrylamide gel electrophoresis, and isoelectric focusing. The results produced showed that activated CEA receptors were of two sub units of protein with identical M.W and pI.

(8) The biological activity of cationic receptor, unliganded CEA and CEA-receptor complex were evaluated by DNA-affinity column chromatography. The DNA used for the preparation of the column was isolated from whole blood of breast cancer patients and purified on sephadex G25 column. It was found that the ability of CEA-receptor complex to bind band was higher then unliganded CEA.

(9) A method was developed also for the preparation of DNA from normal and transformed cells (malignant cell) of the same patient and then the extracted crude DNA was purified by sephadex G25 spin-column. This method produced good yields of high molecular weight DNA as determined by agarose gel electrophoresis.

FTIR studies were performed to characterize the genetic alteration of transformed cells.

Table of Contents

Subject		Page No
	List of abbreviation	3
	Summary	5
Chapter one : introduction		16
1-1	Breast Cancer	17
1-2	Incidence at breast cancer	17
1-2-1	Worldwide incidence of breast cancer	17
1-2-2	Incidence of breast cancer in Iraq	18
1-3	Etiology and Risk Factor	19
1-4	Diagnosis of breast cancer	20
1-5	Tumor Markers	21
1-6	Carbohydrate Antigen 15-3	23
1-6-1	Physical and pathophysiological role	24
1-6-2	Alterations in malignant tumor tissue	24
1-7	Cancinoembryonic Antigen (CEA)	24
1-7-1	Molecular structure and chemistry of CEA	25
1-7-2	Role of CEA in immune response	28
1-7-3	CEA in breast cancer	29
1-8	Protein engineering	30
Chapter two : Clinical Role of CEA in Human Mammary		31
	Abstract	32
	Introduction	33
	Material and Methods	34
2-1	Chemical	34
2-2	Apparatus	34
2-3	Patients and clinical information	34
2-4	Blood samples	35
2-4-1	Estimation of serum CA15-3 Antigen levels	36
2-4-2	Estimation of serum CEA	38
2-5	Collection of specimens and preparation tissue homogenate	41
	Cytosol preparation	41
2-6	Statistical Analysis	41
	Result	42
	Serum determination of CA15-3 in breast cancer patients and controls	42

		Subject	Page No
		Normal control	42
		Benign breast disease	44
		Breast cancer	44
		Determination of CEA levels in sera of breast cancer Benign and control	47
		Normal control	47
		Benign breast disease	47
		Breast cancer	47
		Cytosol determination of CEA in Breast Cancer and Normal specimens	54
		Normal specimens	54
		Breast cancer tissue	54
		Discussion	58
		Chapter three : purification and physiochemical properties of CEA	60
		Abstract	61
		Introduction	62
		Material and Methods	63
3-1		Extraction and purification	63
	A	Extraction of CEA	63
	B	Purification of CEA	63
		Ion-exchange chromatography	63
		Preparation of the column	63
		Speration procedure	63
		Gel filtration chromatography	64
		1-preparation of the column	64
		2-purification procedure	64
		Calculation	65
3-2		Analysis of the purified fraction by slab Conventional polyacrylamide gel Electrophoresis solution used Solution used	66
		Procedure	67
3-3		Immunoelectrophoresis (IEP)	68
		Solution used	68
		Procedure	69
3-4		Determination of the molecular weight of purified CEA by gel filtration chromatography	70
3-5		Estimation of stocks radius of purified CEA	71

	Subject	Page No
3-6	Analysis of purified CEA by disc SDS-PAGE Stock solution used	71
	Procedure	72
3-7	Determination of isoelectric point of purified CEA	74
	Solution used	74
	Procedure	74
3-8	Carbohydrate content studies	75
	Calculation	76
3-9	Stability of CEA at -20 c	76
	Spectroscopic studies	77
3-10	Ultraviolet absorption	77
3-11	Factors affecting the absorption properties purified CEA	77
	1-PH effect on the spectrum of purified CEA	77
	2-polarity effect	78
	3-effect of urea, KCL and urea, KCL mixture on the spectrum of CEA	78
3-12	Structural studies of CEA	79
3-13	Estimation of absorption coefficient (a) of CEA	79
3-14	Fouler transform infrared spectroscopy	80
	Result and Discussion	81
	Isolation and purification of CEA	81
	Purity of CEA preparation	82
	Physiochemical properties of purified CEA	82
	Carbohydrate content	83
	Stability of crude and purified CEA	84
	Ultraviolet spectral results	84
	Factors effecting the absorption properties of purified CEA	85
	1-PH- effect	85
	2-Effect of solvent polarity on purified CEA U.V spectrum (solvent perturbation studies)	86
	3-The effect of urea on the CEA U.V spectrum	87
	Spectrophotometeric PH titration of purified CEA (structural studies)	88
	Estimation of absorption coefficient	89
	FTIR spectroscopic analysis	89

		Subject	Page No
Chapter four : preparation of CEA kit			107
		Abstract	108
		Introduction	109
		Material and Methods	110
	4-1	Preparation of purified CEA solution for immunization and standard immunization and antiserum generation	110
	4-2	Isolation of rabbit serum anti-CEA antibodies	111
	4-3	Ouchterlony double diffusion in gel	113
	4-4	Rabbit anti-CEA immunoglobulin purified	114
		A-Salt precipitation	
		B-Dialysis	
		C-Ion-Exchange chromatography	
		1-Preparation of chromatography column	
		2-Separation procedure	
	4-5	Methods used for identification of pure Anti-CEA immunoglobulins	116
		A-Cellulose acetate electrophoresis	116
		B-Immuno electrophoresis	117
	4-6	Preparation of radiolabelled CEA	117
		A-Radioiodination reaction	117
		B-Purification of radioiodinated using gel filtration	117
		C-Calculation	118
		D-Storage of radioiodinated tracer	118
	4-7	Immunochemical and physiochemical criteria of iodinated CEA clinical application	118
	4-8	Liquid phase competition RIA Assay condition	119
		A-Amount of anti-CEA	119
		B-The radioactive CEA amount	121
		C-Effect of temperature	121
		D-Effect of time	121
		E-Effect of PH	122
		F-Ionic strength effect	122
	4-9	The standard curve	123
		A-Solution	123
		B-Procedure	123
		C-Calculation	124

	Subject	Page No
4-10	Solid phase Radioimmunoassay	124
4-10-1	Preparation antibody coated tubes	124
	A-Activation of solid phase polyrene	124
	B-Binding of anti-CEA to solid phase	125
4-10-2	Assay condition	126
4-11	The standard curve for solid phase RIA	126
4-12	Evaluation of CEA RIA kit	127
4-13	The assessment of I-CEA concentration	127
	Result of Liquid – phase RIA	129
	Assay condition	129
	1-Amount of antibody	129
	2-The radioactive CEA	129
	3-Effect of temperature	130
	4-Time of reaction	130
	5-Effect of PH	130
	6-Ionic strength	130
	The preparation and properties of anti-CEA chemically attached to polystyrene tube	131
	Solid phase – Assay condition	133
	The standard curve	135
	Evaluation of CEA RIA kit preparation	135
	The determination of I-CEA concentration	136
		151
Chapter five : CEA Thermodynamic and Kinetic studies of CEA receptor – binding		
	Abstract	152
	Introduction	153
	Material and Methods	154
5-1	Chemicals	154
5-2	Apparatus	154
5-3	Buffers and reagents	154
5-4	Collection of specimens and preparation of tissue homogenate	155
5-5	Estimation of protein and DNA contents	156
5-6	Binding studies of I-CEA binding with its cytosolic and nuclear receptors in malignant	156

	Subject	Page No
5-6-1	Preliminary test of I-CEA binding with its cytosolic and nuclear receptors malignant mammary tissues	156
	A-Cytosolic CEA receptor	156
	B-Nuclear CEA receptor	157
5-6-2	Influence of I-CEA on the binding	158
5-6-3	Influence of receptor concentration on the binding with I-CEA	158
5-6-4	Temperature dependency of the binding	159
5-6-5	Time course of receptor binding	160
5-6-6	Effect of PH on the receptor binding	160
5-6-7	Effect of monovalent and divalent salt on the binding I-CEA to its receptor	161
5-6-8	Stability of CEA- receptor complex	162
5-7	Determination of affinity constant (Ka) and the maximal binding capacity (B max) of I-CEA associated with their cytosolic and nuclear receptor	162
5-8	Kinetic studies of receptor binding	164
5-9	Estimation of Hill coefficient (n) of receptor	165
5-10	Thermodynamic studies of CEA binding receptor	166
	Results and Discussion	168
	Preliminary test of I-CEA binding with its receptor in mammary carcinoma	168
	Influence of I-CEA concentration	169
	Effect of receptor concentration on the binding	169
	Effect of temperature	170
	Time course of receptor binding	170
	Effect of PH on the binding	171
	Effect of monovalent and divalent salts on the binding	171
	Stability of CEA receptor complex	172
	Scachard Analysis and Kinetic of CEA binding to their receptor	172

Subject	Page No
Estimation of Hillcoefficient (n) of nuclear and cytosolic receptor in Human Malignant breast tumors	175
The thermodynamic of receptor binding	176
Thermodynmic parameters of standard state	176
Thermodynmic parameters of transition state	176
Chapter six : Isolation and characterization CEA receptor in mammary tissues	197
Abstract	198
Introduction	198
Material and Methods	199
6-2 Patients and specimens	199
6-3 Preparation of cytosol	200
6-4 Purification of CEA receptor	200
6-4-1 Ammonium sulphate fractionation of crude cytosolic receptor	200
6-4-2 Ion exchange chromatography of cytosolic receptors	200
6-4-2-1 Anion exchange	201
6-4-2-2 Cation exchange	202
6-4-3 Gel filtration of cytosolic CEA receptor on sepharose CL-6B column	203
6-5 Characterization of purified CEA receptor and CEA receptor complex	204
6-5-1 Determination of molecular weight by gel filtration	204
6-5-2 Estimation of stock radius of purified receptor	204
6-5-3 Analysis of purified receptor by DISC SDS – PAGE	204
6-5-4 Determination of the isoelectric point (PI) of purified receptor	205
6-5-5 Carbohydrate content of purified CEA	205
6-6 U.V spectrum of the I-CEA receptor complex and purified cytosolic receptor	205
6-6-1 The U.V spectra of purified cytosolic CEA receptor	205
6-6-2 I-CEA receptor complex	205
Result and Discussion	207
Ammonium sulphate fractionation	207

	Subject	Page No
	Ion exchange chromatography	208
	Gel filtration step	209
	Physicochemcal properties of isolated receptor	210
	Carbohydrate content	211
	U.V spectrum analysis	211
Chapter seven : Evaluation of the Biological activity of CEA-cytosolic receptor		221
	Abstract	222
	Introduction	223
	Material and methods	225
7-1	Chemical	225
7-2	Equipment and Apparatus	226
7-3	Buffers and reagents	226
7-4	Collection of specimens	227
7-5	Isolation and purification of human DNA from whole blood of breast cancer patients	227
7-6	DNA coupling to CNBr activated sepharose	228
7-7	DNA affinity chromatography	229
7-8	Determination of organic phosphate	229
7-9	Isolation of DNA from tissue sample	230
7-10	Gel electrophoresis	232
7-11	Spectrophotometric studies by fourier transformed infrared spectra	232
	Results and Discussion	233
	Isolation and purification DNA from whole blood	233
	Coupling of DNA to CNBr activated sepharose	233
	Analysis of CEA receptor and CEA-receptor complex on affinity column	234
	Isolation of DNA from tumor cells	234
	Characterization of DNA structure by FTIR spectroscopy	235
Chapter eight : General Discussion		241
	Conclusion	246
	Future work	248
	References	249

Chapter one

INTRODUCTION

1-1 Breast Cancer

Breast cancer is a disease in which breast cells proliferate abnormally. The diagnosis of breast cancer is established histologically. Breast cancer may present as a breast lump, thickening, or skin change. Non-palpable cancers may be detected by mammography. A biopsy is necessary to confirm the diagnosis and determination the type of cancer present. [1]

When breast cancer cells metastasize from the original tumor and enter the blood stream or lymphatic system, they can form secondary tumors in other parts of the body.

Bilateral cancer is diagnosed when separate primary breast cancers arise in each breast; multifocal breast cancer is diagnosed when breast cancer presents in more than one site in the same breast. Breast cancer is staged from 0 to IV, where 0 is non-invasive tumor, stage I is a small locally invasive tumor without lymph node involvement, stage II is a medium-sized tumor with or without nodal metastases, stage III cancer is a locally advanced cancer, usually with axillary node metastases, and stage IV cancer has already metastasized to distant sites [2]. The survival rate is dependent upon the stage at which breast cancer is diagnosed.

1-2 Incidence at Breast Cancer

1-2.1 Worldwide Incidence of Breast Cancer:

World wide, there is a gradual increase in incidence of breast cancer at woman aged more than 25 years and reaches a peak at age of 50 years.

Some 50,000 woman in the United Kingdom and 250,000 woman in the United State are diagnosed as having breast cancer each year [3].

The highest incidence of the disease is encountered in North America, Northwest Europe, Australia, Newzeland. The lowest incidence is found in southeast Asia (Japan, Taiwan, and Singapore), although the incidence in Japan has increased in recent years, [3].

Breast cancer is the most common malignancy associated with pregnancy. With an increasing prevalence with increasing maternal age (Fig 1-1). [3]

Male breast cancer is rare. The ratio of male; female breast cancer is 1 to 125. [3]

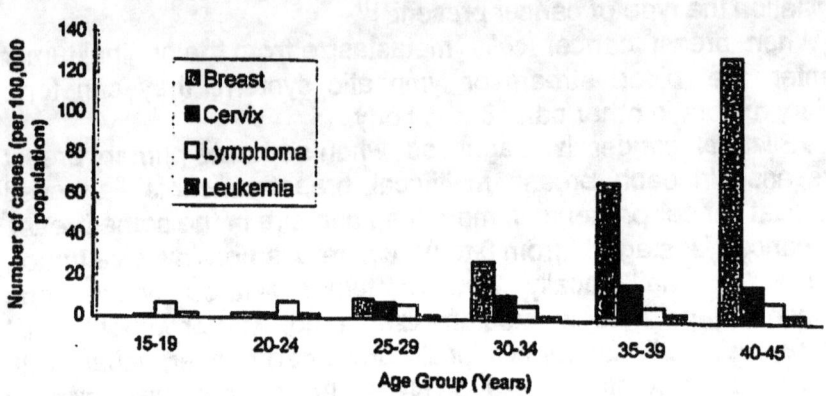

Fig. (1-1) Age-specific prevalence of malignancies in women of childbearing age [3].

1-2.2 Incidence of Breast Cancer in Iraq [4,5]

According to the data of Iraqi cancer Registry center collected during the period 1976-2000, there is a tendency toward an increase in the frequency of breast cancer incidence (Fig. 1-2).

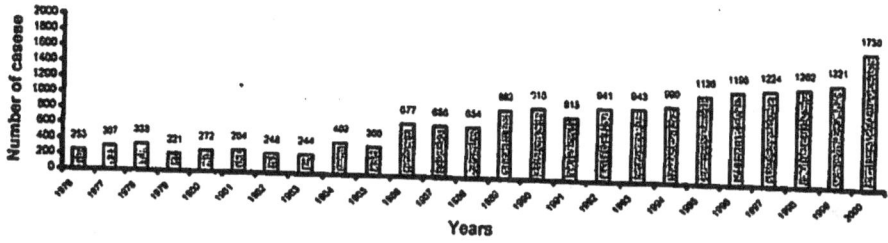

Fig. (1-2) the Annual number of Malignant Tumors of the Breast cases registered during the period 1976-2000 inclusive in Iraq [5].

Cancer of the breast is the commonest cancer in female and constitutes 31,87 % of all other cancers. A typical age – range of disease women is 30-60 years with a peak between 40 and 50 years of age. Patient under 30 years of age forms about 6% of the total cancer. The predominant histological typing is infiltrate duct carcinoma (60%); The rest is of special histological variants of carcinoma, lobular, medullar, comedo, cribriform, sirrhous and mucinous, paget,s disease and cystosarcoma phylloides .

The lobular carcinoma (in situ and infiltrative) constituted about 9.2% of all Iraqi incidence of breast cancer while is slightly higher than that reported from other countries.

1-3 Etiology and Risk Factors

Breast cancer is considered a multifactorial disorder caused by both non-genetic and genetic factor .A family history of breast cancer is an important contributor to breast cancer risk. [6]

Non-Genetic Factors:

Recognized contributors to breast cancer risk include menarche before age 12 years, [4] menopause after age 55 year, obesity, alcohol use, hormone replacement therapy, and excessive radiation exposure. Most of these risk factors produce less than a twofold increase in risk of breast cancer and thus may contribute relatively little to risk in women from high- risk families. Other potential risk factors include a diet that is high in fat and low in fiber, fruits, and vegetables, lack of exercise and induced abortion.

The relationship between these risk factors and genetic predisposition is not yet understood. [6,7,8]

Genetic factors: Genetic factors may be related to known mutation in dominant susceptibility gene such as $BRCA_1$ (on chromosome 17) and $BRCA_2$ (on chromosome 13) associated with hereditary breast cancer in younger age group. Mutation in the tumor suppressor gene P 53 is rare, found in about 1:10000 woman and contribute to an estimated 1% of breast cancer in woman diagnosed before age 40. [9,10,11]

1-4 Diagnosis of Breast Cancer

Early detection of breast cancer have led to the finding of tumor at earlier clinical stage, which has clearly been shown to reduce mortality.

The most common methods used for diagnosing of breast cancer are:

* Examination: include visual inspection (dimpling or swellings are worrisome signs). [12]
* X-Rays-radiology, computed topography, digital angiography [13]

- ❖ Radionuclides-single photon and positron emission tomography.
- ❖ Ultrasound: [14]
- ❖ Magnetic resonance-imaging and spectroscopy [15]
- ❖ The ermography [16]
- ❖ Transillumination [17]
- ❖ Biopsy techniques (Fine needle aspiration, core cutting needle biopsy, Excisional biopsy)
- ❖ Cytology [18]
- ❖ Clinical laboratory tests includes, blood picture and other test as tumor Marker tests [19]

1-5 Tumor Markers:

Tumor markers are molecules or substances that represent alterations from the normal state associated with the malignant process. Detecting and / or monitoring these changes might assist in evaluating cancer risk, diagnosis, prognosis, or response to treatment [20]. The absolute presence or the relative level of a marker differs between normal (or benign) and malignant states. Tumor markers can be assayed in the systemic circulation or examined in the tumor tissue and lymph nodes or bone marrow. Several circulating tumor markers have been investigated for one or more clinical uses in breast cancer (Table 1-1). [21]

Several criteria are used for characterization of an ideal tumor marker such as the following [21]:

1. It should be produced by or related to tumor cells.
2. It could be detectable in body fluids or tissues of cancer patients.
3. It should not be present in health or in benign diseases.
4. It could be present frequently early in the development in malignancies.
5. Its quantity reflects the bulk of malignancy.
6. It is detectable even when there is no clinical evidence of the tumor.
7. Its level could be correlated with the result of anticancer therapy.

There are two criteria that may be considered for investigation of a useful tumor marker. The first is that tumor marker would have a high degree of specificity, so there would be very few false positive. The second criterion is that tumor marker would be very sensitive and have few false negative results.

Table (1-1)
Tumor markers that have been investigated in breast cancer [21].

Tumor-associated antigens
    Carcinoembryonic antigen (CEA)
    Products of or related to products of the MUC-1 gene
        CA 15-3
        CA 27-29
        CA 549
        Breast cancer mucin (BCM)
        Mammary serum antigen (MSA)
        Mucinous carcinoma antigen (MCA)
    Tissue polypeptide antigen (TPA)
    Tissue polypeptide-specific antigen (TPS)
    Gross cystic disease protein (GCDP)
    Prostate-specific antigen (PSA)
Markers of tumor biology
    Extra-ceullular domain (ECD) of c-erb B-2/HER2/neu
    Molecules of adhesion and invasion
        E-selection
        Soluble urokinase plasminogen activator receptor (SuPAR)
        Intercellular adhesion molecule-1 (ICAM-1)
    Molecules associated with angiogenesis
        Vascular endothelial growth factor (VEGF)
        Basic fibroblast growth factor (bFGF)
        Hepatocyte growth factor (HGF)
        HUVEC assay
Antibody response against TAAs
    c-erb B-2/HER2/neu
    p 53

1-6 Carbohydrate Antigen 15-3 (CA 15-3)

CA15-3 is abreast-associated antigen defined by reactivity with two monoclonal antibodies, namely, DF_3 and $115D_8$, in a double- determinant or sandwich-type immuno- assay. The $115D_8$ antibody was prepared against human milk-fat globulin membrane [22] while the DF_3 antibody was raised against a membrane-enriched fraction of human breast carcinoma [23]. Now it is known that the CA 15-3molecule is a mucin, being a product of the MUCI gene, other names for this mucin include (polymorphic epithelial mucin PEM), epithelial membrane antigen EMB or episalin.

The MUCI antigen is a trans membrane glycoprotein containing a large extracellular domain of 31 amino acids and a cytoplasm domain of 69 amino acids. [24]

The extracellular domain includes a region of nearly identical repeats of 20 amino acids. The number of repeats varies from about 25 to over 125 because of genetic polymorphism. The repeat units are rich in serine, threonine and proline residues and are extensively O-glycosylated. The deduced amino acid sequence also contains potential N-glycosyl sites. [24]

Although the core protein of MUCI appears identical in different tissues, the extent of glycosylation can vary from organ to organ [24]. Thus, in the mammary gland. MUCI has a relative molecular mass (M.wt) of 250-500 Kd and contains approximately 50% carbohydrate by weight, while in the pancreas it has a M.wt of more than 1000 Kd and about 50% carbohydrate. In colonic cancer cells, the mucin has a M.wt of 600-800 Kd, 80-90% being carbohydrate [24]. These differences in amount of glycosylation may depend on the activity level of glycosyltransferases and glycosidases in different tissue [24]. There is, however, no evidence that these differences in glycosylation confer organ specificity on the CA15-3 assay.

Recently, the epitops reacting with one of the antibodies used to define CA 15-3 was identified. The DF_3 antibody was shown [25] to directed to a region in the Thr-Arg-Pro-Ala-Pro-Gly-Ser sequence of the tandem repeat.

Whether the number of tandem repeats affects reactivity with the DF₃ antibody is unknown. The epitope interacting with the 115D₈ antibody remains to be determined.

1-6.1 Physiological and Pathophysiological role

The physiological function of mucins is thought to be cell protection and lubrication. Although the precise function of the MUCI protein is unknown, recent evidence suggests that it may play a role in cell adhesion. In that it appears to reduce both cell-cell and cell - extra cellular matrix interaction[25]. In particular, the MUCI protein has been shown to override cadherin E-mediated cell–cell adhesion[26]. As loss of cadherin E is involved in cancer metastasis [27]. MUCI may indirectly contribute to this process.

MUCI may also contribute to cancer progression by inhibiting tumor cell cytolysis by either cytotoxic T-cells or lymphokin-activated (LAK) cells. MUCI also causes apoptosis of T-cells [28] and inhibits proliferation of these cells. [29]

1-6.2 Alterations in malignant tumor tissue

In comparison with normal breast tissue, the MUCI gene in frequently overexpressed in malignant breast tumors.

This has been shown at the mRNA level by use of an hybridization and at the protein level by immunhistochemistry[24]. In addition to this overexpression aberrant glycosylation can occur in malignancy[24]. This altered glycosylation may expose epitope sites, which are not present in the mucin from normal cells. Furthermore, in normal tissue, MUCI expression is confined in the apical of glandular epithelial cells. Whereas in cancerous tissue expression can be detected over the entire cell membrane [30].

1-7 Carcino Embryonic Antigen (CEA)

During the development in mammals, products termed " embryo antigens or fetal antigens . " are products at various stages of embryonic, fetal life [31]. These antigens are present in high concentration in sera and decrease to low levels or disappear after birth. In cancer cases, these antigens originate within tumor cells and enter the circulation as a result of secretion by tumor or as breakdown of product of tumor cells [32].

CEA is an emybro antigen that appears during embryonic development or in cases of malignant neoplasm's [33]. CEA has been one of the most popular and most frequently used tumor Markers in clinical practice. It has been first described by Gold and Freeman in 1960 and is reported to be highly specific and sensitive for colorectal carcinoma [34]. Elevations of CEA have also been observed in breast, pancreatic, lung, thyroid and uterine cervical cancers [35].

1-7.1 Molecular Structure and Chemistry of CEA

CEA is heterogeneous group of glycoprotein with a molecular mass of 150 to 200 Kd [36,37]. The primary structure of CEA deduced from cDNA sequence, demonstrating that CEA is synthesized as a precursor with a single polypeptide chain of 668 amino acids that can be divided in five domains, an N-terminal of 109 amino acid with lysine in the N-terminal position, for the most part is free of glycosylation sites. Three repeating loop domains, each held together by two disulfide bridges (these loop domains carrying the bulk of the sites of N-linked glycosylation), these three are very homologous repetitive domains of 178 residues each and mostly hydrophobic residues at C-terminal, which are suggested to comprise a membrane anchor [38,39].

CEA contains (50-60)% carbohydrate, consisting of hexose, hexosamine, sialic acid [40,41]. Biosynthesis of the carbohydrate moiety of a glycoprotein is believed to be a post-ribosomal event in which the enzymatic assembly of the saccharide chains takes place after the protein has been completed [42]. Glycoprotein structure is therefore only partly under genetic control and considerable variation in structure is possible. This variation often takes the form of micro-heterogeneity of the intermediate and peripheral sugar residues whereas the innermost carbohydrate residues are relatively homogeneous in structure. The enzymatic activity for the biosynthesis and possible breakdown or modification of glycoprotein may vary in different individuals and the malignant state [43]. It is not surprising to find variation in the carbohydrate content and composition between different CEA preparation. The principal carbohydrate constituent of CEA, is N-acetylglucosamin, which usually constitutes approximately 40% of the total carbohydrate content. In contrast, N-acetylgalactosamine is either absent or present only in very low concentration, other carbohydrate constituent of CEA are mannose, galactose, fucose and variable amount of sialic acid [44]. It has been shown that the N-linked attachment of carbohydrate units to polypeptide chain that takes place at the sequence Asn-X-Thr or Asn-X-Ser [45]. The general structural feature of CEA shown in Figure (1-3).

The circles represent unknown numbers of sugar residues. It is known however that the carbohydrate moiety of CEA exists as multiple side chains attached through asparagine linkages to glucosamine residues. It is also likely that the side chains are distributed asymmetrically although on average there appears to be about seven residues per side chain and a maximum of about 80 chains. Fucose and sialic acid are present at non-reducing ends and the latter residues are attached to the 3-position in galactose. Galactose and mannose constitute the intermediate portion of the carbohydrate moiety where branching occurs. Six disulfide bonds stabilize the protein moiety of CEA. The available evidence suggests that the antigenic site in CEA is situated in the innermost carbohydrate chains or in the protein and activity is abolished if the three-dimensional structure of the protein is destabilized by cleavage of the disulfide bonds. [44]

The physical properties of CEA are summarized as follows [44-48].

1. Soluble in water
2. Soluble in perchloric acid
3. Soluble in 50% saturated ammonium sulfate
4. Insoluble in ethanol
5. Heat stable
6. Sedimentation coefficient of 7-8 s
7. Mobility on agar electrophoresis at pH 8.6
8. Single polydisperse band on polyacrylamide gel electrophoresis
9. Molecular weight of 200000 ± 20000
10. Isoelectric points of < 3 and 3.75 ± 0.25

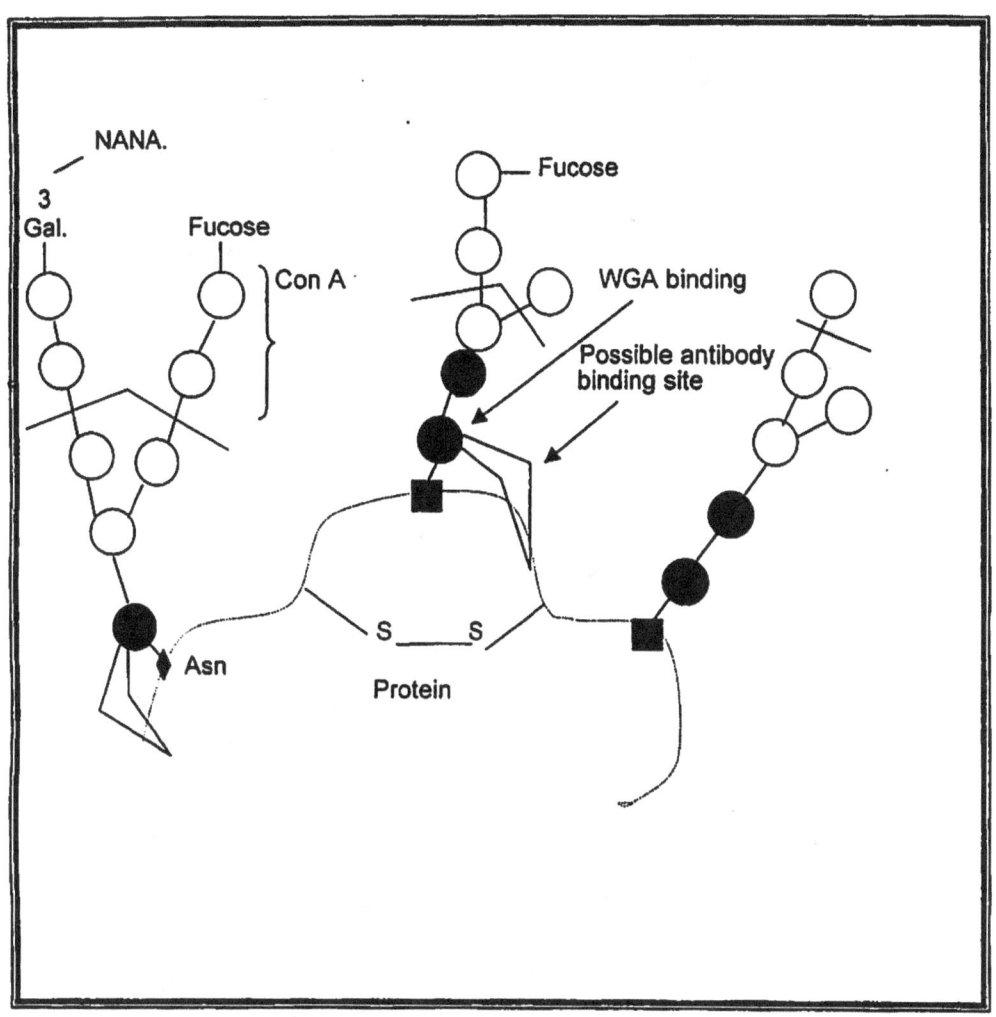

Fig. (1-3):(Schematic model of the general structural features of CEA)

○ Intermediate chains mainly MANNOSE and GALACTOSE
● N-ACETYLGLUCOSAMINE
■ Asparagine
(WGA) Wheat germ agglutinin

(All details are explained in the text).

1-7.2 Role of CEA IN Immune Response

CEA is localized in the apical portion of normal cells. The protective role of CEA for these cells has been supposed to based on its carbohydrate content and binding to some bacterial[49]. Cancers of epithelial origin, adenocarcinoma mass express CEA at high frequency and change its localization from apical portion to intracytoplasm, then basolateral membrane and finally outside the cell, i.e., into the stroma. The dedifferent of these cells reflect by such changes in the localization of cellular CEA, i.e., the loss of polar distribution of surface CEA in cells, may trigger the immunosurveillance system against the initiation of malignant processes that take place by cell-mediated immunity which involve the following cells, cytoxic T-cell (CTL), non—cytotoxic (delayed type hypersensitivity, DTH), Macrophages, natural killer cell (NK) and lymphocyte secreting cytotoxic factors like lymphokines activated killer (LAK). Each of these effects employs different lytic mechanism so that the tumor cell may show susceptibility to a spectrum of killer cells. In addition many of these effected cells secrete proteins which are themselves lytic for trasformed cells such as tumor necrosis factor (TNF)[50-53]. This is immunoreactive role for CEA. On the other hand, CEA is immunosuppressive, it induces suppressor lymphocytes, Inhibits natural killer cells activity, and suppresses the humoral immune response[50-58]. Many studies indicated the activity and number of NK cells in various breast carcinomas was found to be low and natural cytotoxicity did not seem to play a significant role[50-54]. Other studies showed that CEA could promote metastasis by several mechanisms, e.g., modulation of Immune responses[59], facilitation of intracellular adhesion[60], and cellular migration[61]. On the other hand, CEA may act as growth factor attachment factor. It may enhance the binding of tumor cells to normal cells as they pass through the microcirculation of distant organs[50-61].

1-7.3 CEA in Breast Cancer

Recent investigations have revealed that many tumors can produce CEA. Breast cancer is the most common among these tumors[32-35]. Vidan et.al[34,35] reported that the first case of breast cancer with hepatic metastasis, show high serum CEA, and then several case reports followed. Most of these cases were associated with liver and bone metastasis[48,49].

A considerable number of articles on CEA production on the colorectal tumors are available, but little work has been done on CEA in the management of patients with breast cancer. Many hypothesis have been formulated in attempt to explain the mechanism of CEA secretion by breast cancer, suggesting that CEA may be secreted by primary or metastasis tumor cells, or by perimetastic and regenerative hepatic reactions[37,38].

The exact mechanisms by which CEA is secreted in adult tumor cell and why it is present in greater quantities in the secondary rather than primary cancer are still unclear[42]. However in some cases, there was no evidence of hepatic metastasis and CEA level declined after resection of breast cancer, indicating production of CEA by breast cancer itself. Many cases of CEA producing breast cancer were subsequently reported, and some of the author's clinicopathologically investigated this cancer[47,48].

The breast cancer, CEA localization in cancer cells classified into three types, CEA located along apical surface, CEA located in the cytoplasm and CEA located in the surrounding stroma of tumor cells.

These types are classified according to immunocytohist-ochemical studies[47,48]. There have been several reports of CEA associated with breast cancer, with and without metastasis to the liver or bone[47,48].

In general, it was showed a trend of increasing CEA level in breast carcinoma, although their incidence and correlation with clinical stage, site and histomorphology of the disease were not clear[49,50].

1-8 Protein Engineering

There are various methods used to alter the amino acid sequence of a protein (primary structure), and then secondary, tertiary and quaternary structures are affected. Specific parameters, such as stability kinetics and biological are used to follow these modifications. Accordingly carcinoembryonic antigen was selected as model for this type of protein engineering. However, such protein engineering is much more complex than it might appear at first sight. Before rational changes can be made in a CEA and its receptor it was extremely useful to know it's three-dimensional structure and what residues are important in the maintenance of this structure. Since CEA has special activity (antigenic), it is important to know which amino acid residues have antigenic activity that the modification of that amino acid will change the antigenicity of CEA[263-265]. This information is lacking for most proteins. Even where such information is available it was difficult to predict what specific changes will produce. Despite the fact that there is still a large degree of concepts in protein engineering, a number of successes have been achieved in the following areas:
1. Stability: Increased thermo stability.
    Increased stability at low, high pH value.
    Resistance to oxidation.
2. Altering the kinetic properties of protein.
3. Monoclonal antibody (MAb) Engineering for immunotherapy.
4. Production of pure therapeutic protein in a foreign host such as a bacterium or yeast.

The goal of protein engineering is to mutate the structure of a protein in a predictable manner as well as to change its structure in vitro so as to generate a protein molecule of chosen affinity or activity.

CHAPTER TWO

CLINICAL ROLE OF CEA IN HUMAN MAMMARY CARCINOMA

ABSTRACT

Single measurement of the two-biochemical tumor markers (CA 15-3) and CEA were carried out in serum samples obtained from 40 healthy donors, 22 breast benign patients and 122 breast cancer patients. Mean values of these tumor markers in breast cancer patients were significantly higher ($P<0.05$) than that found in healthy normal or patients with benign breast tumors.

CA15-3 shows the best sensitivity (54%) for detecting preoperative breast cancer patients, than CEA, which gave (44%) sensitivity. Also, CA15-3 gave the highest specificity (100%) for discriminating non-malignant patients while CEA had specificity of (77%).

The cytosolic CEA concentration was determined in the tumor, benign and normal tissue of breast cancer patients. Significant differences between values from the tumor and normal specimens were found. There was no correlation between the preoperative levels of serum CEA and cytosol level of CEA in the patients with carcinoma. Also, CEA in cytosols did not correlate with either stage or histology. It was concluded that the test might provide calculable information for the evaluation and planning of treatment.

INTRODUCTION

The role of breast cancer tumor markers is to enhance the clinic ability to provide more effective management of the disease, CEA was among the earliest circulation tumor markers proposed for evaluation of breast cancer, but its clinical utility was limited by lack of sensitivity and specificity [62]. In adult life, high circulating levels of CEA are found in a variety of metastatic cancers including breast cancer, in contrast to metastatic breast cancer, CEA level are rarely elevated in sera from patient with primary breast cancer [63,64]. The reasons for this are unknown, but it raises the question, does CEA exist in primary tumors and if so what factors effect its concentration.

The objective of present study was to evaluate the clinical application of biochemical tumor markers CA 15-3 and CEA in the diagnosis and monitoring of breast cancer. Also, this study investigates the distribution of CEA in breast tumor cytosols and correlates its levels with a variety of biochemical pathologic parameters.

MATERIALS AND METHODS

2.1 CHEMICAL:
All laboratory chemicals and reagents were of annalar grade. Tris (hydroxymethylamino methane) was obtained from BDH.

All buffer solutions were prepared by dissolving the appropriate amount of salts in distilled water and the required pH was adjusted.

2.2 APPARATUS:
The apparatus used during this study were, LKB gamma Counter type 1270 Rack, Backman Model-25 spectrophotometer, cooling centrifuge type Hettsch, Pye-Unicam pH meter.

2.3 PATIENTS AND CLINICAL INFORMATIONS:
Inclusion in this series required the following condition:
(1) Untreated primary breast carcinoma
(2) No evidence of liver disease;
(3) No anemia (Hb ≥ 12 g/dl);
(4) No Iron overload
(5) No heavy smoking habit (≥15 cigarettes/day) [65]

Three groups of breast cancer patients and one group with benign breast tumors were included in this study. Group 1 contained 38 premenopausal patients with breast cancer. Group 2 consisted of 82 postmenopausal patients with breast cancer. Group 3 consisted of 25 patients with known metastatic (metastatic group). Group 4 comprised 22 patients with benign breast tumors. In addition 4 groups of age matched healthy subjects were also included.

All patients were admitted for treatment to Baghdad Medical city, AL–Husaney, AL-Arabia, and AL-Saddoon Hospitals. They were histologically proven, newly diagnosed and not underwent any type of therapy. Clinical information was recorded at the times were entered into the study by proper investigations and include age, menopausal status, tumor size, type of carcinoma. Characteristics of all patients are summarized in table (2-1):

Table (2.1) Characteristics of 122 patients

Patients characteristics	No of patients	%
MENOPAUSAL STATUS		
Pre-	38	31.14
Post-	84	68.85
Tumor size		
T1 (Primary tumor up to 2 cm diameter)	10	8.19
T2 (2-5 cm ± skin tethering)	40	32.78
T3 (5-10 cm, infiltration or ulceration of skin, fixation to underlying muscle)	47	38.52
T4 (More 10 cm, skin over whole breast involved, or invasion of chest)	25	20.49
Nodal status		
N0 (No palpable nodes)	56	62.22
N1 (Mobile homolateral nodes)	34	30.6
Metastasis		
M0 (No clinically detectable metastatic deposits)	47	65.27
M1 (metastatic deposits detected in other than regional lymph nodes)	25	27.7
Tumor type		
ductal	73	59.8
lobular	19	13.1
Special types	30	24.5

2.4 BLOOD SAMPLES:

Blood samples for measurement of CEA and CA 15-3 were obtained from healthy donors (40 woman aged 18 to 55 years with no any disease) and all details are explained in the text patients with breast cancer. 5ml blood were withdrawn from every patient one day before mastectomy or biopsy. The diagnosis was confirmed postoperatively by histological examination. All serum were separated and stored frozen (-20 C°) until the determination of biochemical markers was performed.

2.4.1 ESTIMATION OF CA 15-3 ANTIGEN LEVELS:

IRMA–CA15-3 is a solid phase two sites immunoradiometeric assay, utilizes two monoclonal antibodies (MAB) which were prepared against antigenic sites on the CA15-3 molecule. The first antibody is MAB115D8 which is directed against antigen of human milk fat globule membrane and the second one MAB DF3 which is directed against a membrane fraction of human breast cancer. The 115D8 antibody is coated on the polystyrene tube (Solid phase) ; while the DF3 antibody is used as a tracer after being raidiolabelled with iodine 125. The CA15-3 antigen molecules present in the standards or the samples to be test are "sandwiched" between the two antibodies. Following the formation of the coated antibody / antigen / iodinated antibody sandwich, the unbound tracer is easily remove by a washing step. The radioactivity bound to the solid phase is proportional to the concentration of CA15-3 present in the sample.

Reagent:

The reagents IRMA CA15-3 kit was provided by Byksangetec Diagostica GmbH & Co. KG/France.
1. ^{125}I-anti CA15-3 monoclonal (mouse), radioactivity content 10µCi (370Kβq).
2. Six standards bovine serum albumin in phosphate buffer. 0, 15, 50, 125 and 250 U.ml^{-1}. Of CA15-3 antigen.
3. Diluent (0.0 U.ml^{-1}), bovine serum albumin in phosphate buffer.

Patient sera and control were diluted prior to assaying (1:100) by adding 20µl of control serum or sample to 2000µl of diluent into uncoated tubes and mixed thoroughly.

Procedure:

The assay protocol is described in table (2-2)

Table (2-2) IRMA assays protocol of serum CA 15-3 U.ml $^{-1}$

	CA15-3, standards (U/ml)					Control		Unknown samples	
	0	15	50	125	250	Level I	Level II	1	2.etc
Coated tube no.	1,2	3,4	5,6	7,8	9,10	11,12	13,14	15,16	17...
Standards, Control, Patient samples (µl.)	←──────────── 100µl ────────────→								
^{125}I-anti CA 15-3 (µl.)	←──────────── 100µl ────────────→								
	Incubated for 2h. at 25°c in horizontal shaker,								
	Aspirate, wash three times with 1 ml of distilled water								
	Measurement of the radioactivity bound in gamma counter								

Calculations:

1. The mean net count for each group of tubes was counted in gamma counter for 1 min.
2. The (B / B max)% ratio was computed for each standard and unknown samples as follows:

$$(B/B_{max})\% = \frac{\text{Standard or samples mean count}}{\text{Mean counts of the 250 U.ml}^{-1} \text{ standard}} \times 100$$

3. The standard curve was drawn by plotting the (B/B $_{max}$)% value for each standard against the corresponding concentration U.ml $^{-1}$ on log-log graph paper figure (2-1).
4. The resulting concentration of the patient samples and controls can be directly interpolated from the standard curve by the use of their (B/B $_{max}$)% values.

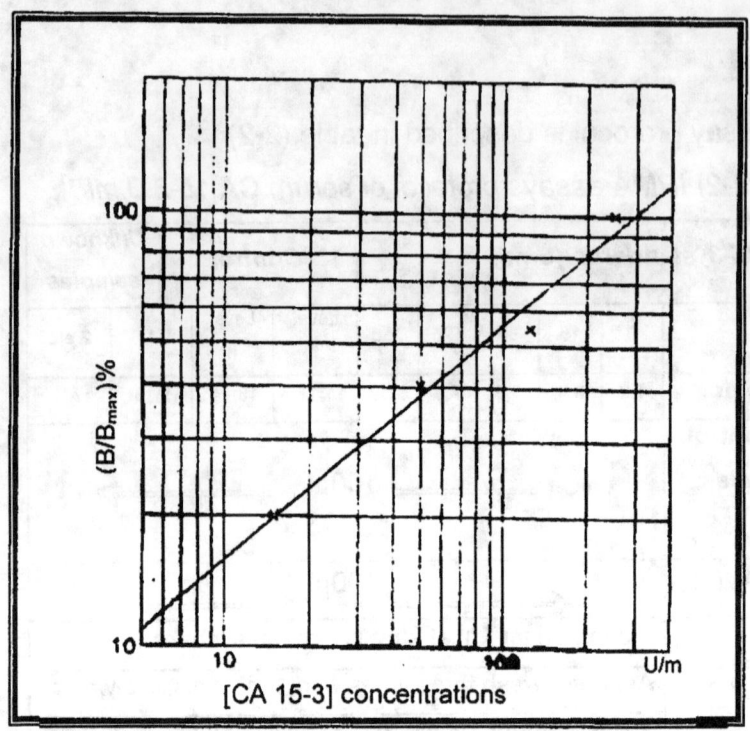

Fig (2-1) The standard curve CA15-3 IRMA (logarithmic plot)

(All details are explained in the text)

2.4.2 ESTIMATION OF SERUM CEA:

Serum CEA level was analyzed immunoradiometrically using CEA kit provided by Byksangetec Diagostica GmbH & Co. KG/France.

Principle of Assay:
As described in section (2.4.1).

Reagent:
1 - ^{125}I-Labeled-anti CEA antibody:
   This reagent served as the tracer which was diluted in buffer mixture.
2 - Anti-CEA monoclonal antibody coated tubes:
   Ready for use.
3 - Standard: 5 vials (0-5 ml) and 1 vial of zero standards (6-ml); ready for use.

The standard vials contain CEA in buffer, in concentration ranging from 0 to 400 ng/ml.
4 - Washing solution concentrate (20X); 1 vial.
The concentrate was diluted with distill water before use to obtain a diluted washing solution
5 - Control samples:
It contained cell culture CEA antigen (human) at a fixed concentration.

Procedure:

The assay protocol is described in table (2-3):

Table (2-3)

IRMA assays protocol of serum CEA ng/ml

	CEA standard (ng. ml^{-1})						Control		Unknown samples	
	0	1	5	20	100	400	Level I	Level II	1	2-etc
Coated tube no.	1,2	3,4	5,6	7,8	9,10	11,12	13,14	15,16	17,18	19,etc.
Standards (μl)	100	100	100	100	100	100	–	–	–	–
Control serum or samples (μl)	–	–	–	–	–	–	100	100	100	100
Incubation buffer (μl)	100	100	100	100	100	100	100	100	100	100

Then the mixtures were gently mixed then incubated for 2h. at 37°C in water bath, aspirated, and rinsed twice with 1.0 ml deionized water.
- Then two hundred µl of ^{125}I-anti CEA antibody were added to all tubes.
- Two additional ordinary tubes were prepared for total activity computation containing only 200 µl ^{125}I-anti CEA antibody.

- The assay tubes were incubated for 2h. at 37°C, then, aspirated the free tracer and washed twice with 1.0 ml de-ionized water.
- The radioactivity of tubes was then measured.

Calculations:

1. The mean net count for each group of tubes was counted in gamma counter for 1.0 minute.
2. The (B/T)% ratio was computed for each standard and unknown samples as follow:

$$(B/T)\% = \frac{\text{Standard or samples mean count}}{\text{Total activity means count}} \times 100$$

3. A standard curve was drawn by plotting the percent value for each standard (vertical axis) versus CEA concentration (horizontal axis) on log-logarithmic graph paper. Fig 2-2
4. CEA concentrations of unknown were calculated from the standard curve using the mean of their duplicate counts.

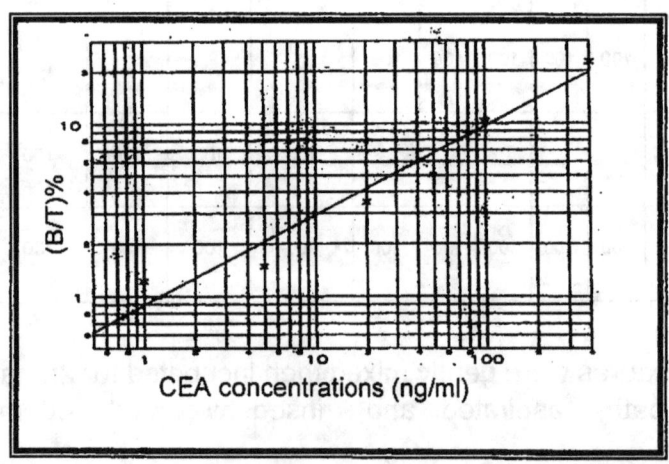

Fig (2-2) The standard curve of CEA IRMA (logarithmic plot)
(All detail are explained in text)

2.5 COLLECTION OF SPECIMENS AND PREPARATION OF TISSUE HOMOGENATE:

The source of tissue in this series of experiments was human breast. The specimens removed surgically from primary adenocarcinoma of the breast were taken only the central, obviously cancerous portion was used as tumor tissue for extraction.

Normal tissue extract was prepared from section of breast more than 7cm distant from the visible edges of the tumor. In this way the problem of individual-specific antigenic differences between normal and tumor tissue was overcome. All tissues were placed in labeled clean polystyrene container in normal saline and kept at -20°C until use, some times the specimens were processed immediately. Only pathologically confirmed benign and tumor tissue specimens were taken into the study.

Cytosol preparation:

Samples were trimned of fat, weight, minced, in four volumes of homogenization buffer, (10% glycerol, 10-mM dithiotheritol, 10 mM Tris, 1.5 mM EDTA). The homogenization was done on an ice bath.

The homogenate was filtered through a nylon mesh sieve to eliminate fibers of connective tissues, then centrifuged at 2000 xg for 10 min at 4°C. The pellet was neglected and the supernatant was centrifuged at 2000 xg for 30 min at 4°C.

After removing the upper layer of fat, an appropriate volume of cytosolic (500-µl) was diluted to 2.5 ml with homogenization buffer and treated with an equal volume of 1.2 mole/liter perchloric acid. After 30 min, the mixture centrifuge at 2000 xg for 10 min and the supernatant was dialyzed for 12 hours against distilled water [66].

CEA was determined in an aliquot of perchloric acid extract by the solid phase sandwich (IRMA) as described in section (2.4.2).

Protein Assay:

The total protein in the cytosol was measured by the method of Lowry.

Aliquots were taken from the cytosol for each test.

2.6 STATISTICAL ANALYSIS

The results of serum and tissues determination of CEA and CA15-3 were analyzed statistically and the values were expressed as mean ±SD. The levels of significance were determined by Analysis of variance (ANOVA). [67]

Results

Serum Determination of CA15-3 in Breast Cancer Patients and Controls

The determination of CA_{15-3} antigen in breast cancer patients was performed on single blood sample which was taken either preoperatively, post operatively (pretherapeuticaly, or post therapeutically or from metastatic group).

The data of CA15-3 measurements in normal healthy individuals, benign breast tumors and malignant breast tumor will be presented separately.

Normal Controls:

Low levels of CA_{15-3} were observed in the sera of 40 apparently healthy woman used as a Control (Fig 2-3). The mean CA_{15-3} levels (±SD) in these woman was (15.7±1.24 u/ml) with an upper normal value of 30 u/ml (Table 2-4).

Table 2-4

Serum determination of CA 15-3 antigen in cancer patients and controls

(All details are explained in the text)

Women clinically diagnosed	No of cases	Serum level of CA 15-3 unit/ml		
		Mean	±SD	F-Value
Normal controls	40	15.7	1.24	
Benign breast tumors	22	16.40	1.64	P>0.05 (N.S)
Breast cancer				
Collectively	200	40.28	1.46	P<0.05
Preoperative	122	43.8	5.43	P<0.05
Postoperative	25	26.76	1.42	P<0.05
Postheropeutic	28	17.6	6.27	P>0.05
Metastatic group	25	56.12	22.18	P<0.05

P – value ≤ 0.05 is considerd significant

N.s = Not significant

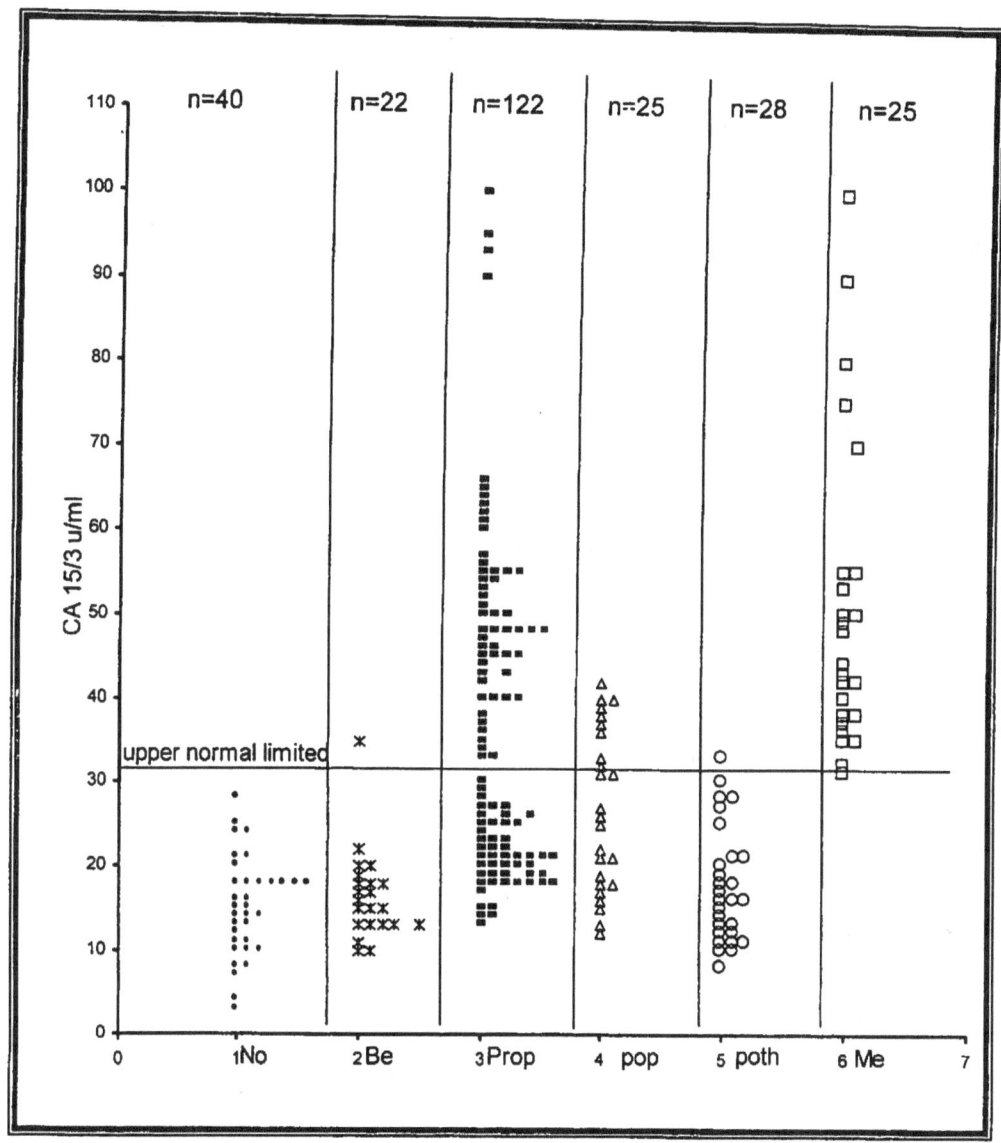

Fig. (2-3): Distribution of CA 15-3 value over different groups of patients
(n)=Number of patients, (No)=Normal, (Be)=Benign,
(prop)=Preoperative, (pop)=Postoperative
(poth)=Postherapy, (Me)=Metastatic

A positive scoring or an abnormal level was indicated by those values of CA15-3 which exceede the 30 u/ml limited. All normal controls had CA15-3 concentration lower than 30 u/ml (Fig 2-3), suggesting a test specificity of 100% for the ability of this marker to exclude normal individuals.

Benign Breast Cases:

Of the 22 sample from patients with histologically confirmed benign breast cases, none had level of CA15-3 above 30 u/ml (Table2-4), The mean level of CA_{15-3} antigen observed in these patients (16.4±1.64 lm) was not significantly different from normal controls (P>0.05) (Table 2-4). Our data are in good agreement with the literature [68-69].

Breast Cancer:

The data of table (2-4) show that the mean serum value ±SD (43.8 ± 5.48 u/ml) of CA 15-3 for breast cancer patients, is significantly higher than that in normal controls (P < 0.05).

Also the percentage sensitivity of patients with abnormal value of CA 15-3 is 54%, which is quite different from that of patients with benign breast disease (Table 2-5). These results are in agreement with some investigators[70]. The results in Table (2-6) indicate that the rate of positive scoring of CA 15-3 increased as the grade of breast cancer raised from stage I to IV. These findings are in good agreement with earlier report [71].

Table 2-5

Incidence of elevated serum CA 15-3 in-patients with benign and malignant breast tumors (All details are explained in the text).

Cases	No. patients	No. of elevated CA 15-3 level	% Patients with elevated CA15-3 level
Benign breast tumors	22	0	0%
Breast cancers collectively	200	102	51%
Preoperative	122	65	54%
Post operative	25	11	44%
Post therapeutic	28	1	3.57%
Metastatic group	25	25	100%

Table 2-6

Correlation of elevated CA 15-3 levels (% sensitivity) with the TNM stage of breast cancer (All details are explained in the text).

Disease stage	No. patient	No. elevated CA_{15-3} level	%
I	10	2	20
II	40	12	30
III	47	22	46.8
IV	25	25	100

The correlation between the histological classification of human malignant mammary carcinomas and percentage sensitivity of CA 15-3 antigen was also examined. As can be seen in table (2-7) high antigen values are associated with the invasive pure forms of breast malignancy. These results confirmed analogues findings by others[68-70].

In table (2-8) the percentage of positive scoring of CA 15-3 is presented in relation to menopausal status of breast cancer in women. The postmenopausal patients gave the lowest percentage (44%) of CA15-3 positive scoring, in comparison to the premenopausal patients with (65%) sensitivity.

The post therapeutic patients who had a good prognosis (i.e. good response to therapy) gave the lowest percentage (3.57) of CA15-3 positive scoring, in comparison to postoperative (pretherapeutic) patients with 44% sensitivity or the preoperative patients with 54% sensitivity and the Metastatic group with 100% sensitivity. The later group was at active stage of the disease and had metastases either to the skin, lung, and bone or lymph nodes subsequent to their therapy. The present sensitivity of CA15-3 for preoperative patients agree well with similar percentage of sensitivity observed by others [68-70].

Table 2-7 Incidence of elevated CA15-3 level in-patients with malignant breast tumor of different histology
(All details are explained in the text).

Histological classification of breast cancer	No. patients	No. elevated CA 15-3 level	% patients with elevated serum CA15-3 level
A- Noninvasive			
Intraductal or comedo carcinoma	5	2	40
Lobular carcinoma in situ	-	-	-
B- Invasive pure form			
Infiltrating duct	65	36	55.38
Medullary	3	3	100
Infiltration lobular	19	2	10.5
Adenocystic	4	1	25
Tubular	4	2	50
Papillary	-	-	-
mucinous	1	0	-
Carcino-sarcoma (ex. Cystosar-coma phylloides)	1	1	100
C- Paget's disease	-	-	-
Mixed histologies	-	-	-

Table 2-8 Positivity of CA15-3 in relation to menopausal status
(All details are explained in the text).

Menopausal state	No. patients	No. elevated CA 15-3 level	% patients with elevated CA15-3
premenopausal	38	25	65.7
postmenopausal	84	37	44

DETERMINATION OF CEA LEVELS IN SERA OF BREAST CANCER, BENIGN AND CONTROLS

Normal controls:

Low levels of serum CEA were observed in normal women (n=40) (Fig 2-4) who had a mean value (±SD) 1.57 ± 0.99 ng/ml, (Table 2-9) with the cut off value of 3 ng/ml, and a percentage specificity of 88%. These values are close to those obtained by others [68-71].

Benign Breast Tumor:

Of 22 samples from patients with histologically confirmed benign breast disease, five of them had CEA > 3 ng/ml. The other 17 patients gave CEA value 2.25 ±1.5, which is not significantly different from normal controls (P > 0.05) (Table 2-9). The present studies also show that the mean values of CEA in benign Patients and Control individuals are close to each other.

Breast Cancer:

A mean serum value of CEA (6.8 ± 3.7) for breast cancer patients is shown in Table 2-9 which is significantly higher than normal controls (P < 0.05).

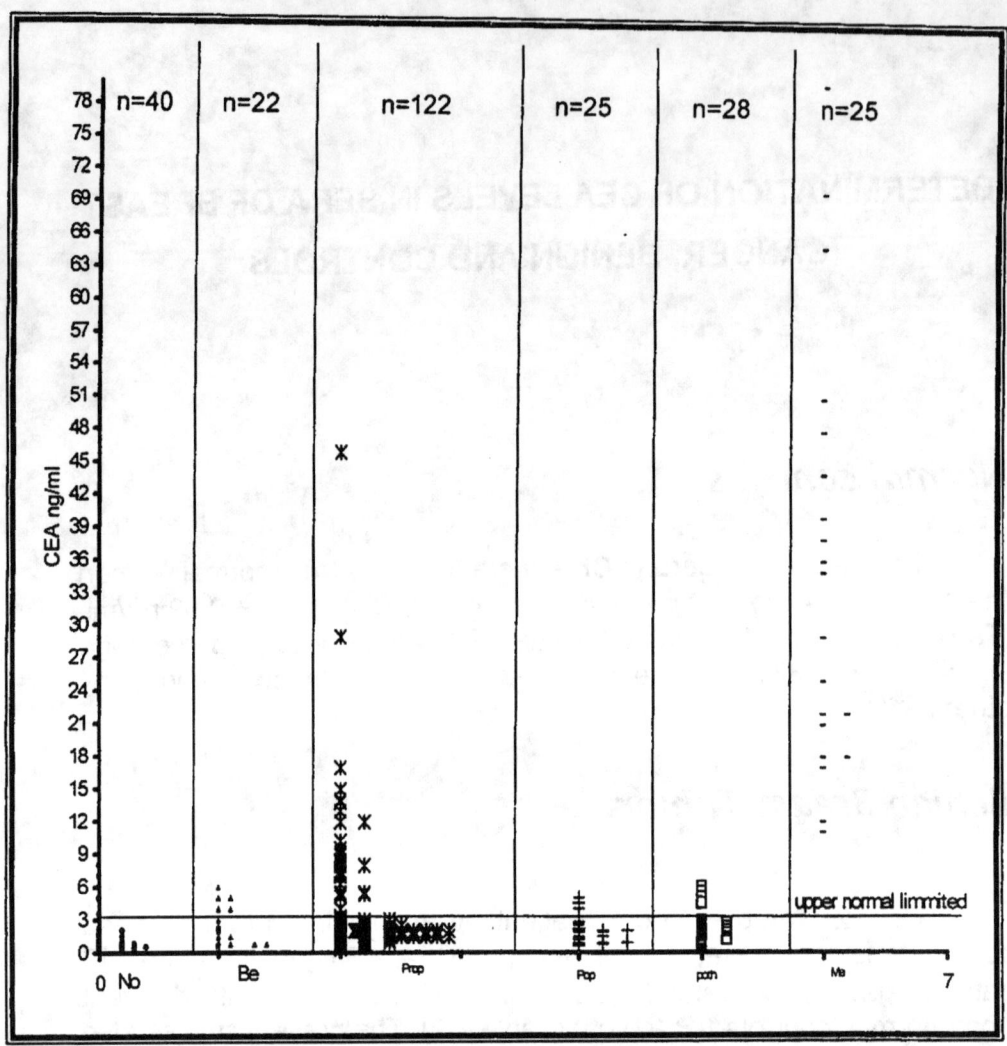

Fig .(2-4):-Distribution of CEA value over different groups of patients (n)=Number of patients, (No)=normal, (Be)=benign, (prop)=Preoperative, (pop)= postoperative, (poth)= posttherapy, (Me)=Metastatic

Also the percentage sensitivity of CEA is 29.5% in preoperative breast cancer (Table 2-10), compared with 22% sensitivity for benign breast patients. The data reported by Heinze. et al[71], showed about 41% sensitivity of CEA for breast cancer patients by using a similar cut off limit of normal value.

It seems from the results of table (2-11) that there is no significant correlation between the increased concentration of serum CEA and the grade and staging of breast cancer patients especially at stages I, II and III, of the disease. However good correlation was observed between CEA sensitivity and patients at stage IV (Metastases), since a positive scoring of CEA was detected in 20 out of 25 cancer (80% sensitivity) these results confirm an earlier study reported by Heinze et. al[71]. Concerning the histological classification of human breast tumors, table 2-12 indicates high CEA level found invasive pure form of tumors. The percentage of CEA values was distributed as 75%, 54% and 75% for the tumors, medullar carcinoma, infiltrating duct carcinoma, and tubular carcinoma respectively. A lower CEA was observed in other breast malignancies such as infiltrating lobular carcinoma (42%), adenocystic carcinoma (25%) and intraductal noninvasive type (20%).

There was no positive scoring of CEA levels in post therapeutic breast cancer patients (Table 2-10). However, about 12% of all postoperative breast cancer patients gave abnormal high CEA level compared to 29.5 sensitivity of CEA for preoperative breast cancer patient and 100% positive scoring of CEA level for metastatic group. This result is similar to that reported in the literature [70-72].

The serum level of CEA was markedly affected by menopausal status. High rate of positive scoring was found in premenopausal 52% table (2-13). Compared with 19% sensitivity for postmenopausal.

Table (2-9)
Serum determination of CEA in cancer patients and controls
(All details are explained in the text).

Woman clinically diagnosed	No. of cases	Serum level of CEA ng/ml		
		Mean	±SD	F value
Serum control	40	1.57	0.99	
Benign breast tumors	22	2.25	1.5	P>.05 N.S
Breast cancers (collectively)	200	10.5	2.63	P<.05
Preoperative	122	6.8	3.7	P<.05
Postoperative	25	2.28	1.57	P>.05
Post therapeutic	28	2.09	1.8	P>.05
Metastatic group	25	46.24	5.84	P<.05

Table (2-10)
Incidence of elevated levels of serum CEA in malignant and benign patients (All details are explained in the text).

Cases	No. patients	No. elevated CEA level	% Patient with elevated CEA
Benign breast tumor	22	5	22.72
Breast cancer (collectively)	200	67	33.5
Preoperative	122	36	29.5
Postoperative	25	3	12
Post therapeutic	28	3	10.7
Metastatic group	25	25	100

Table (2-11)

Incidence of elevated levels of serum CEA (% sensitivity) in breast cancer patients according to TNM staging

(All details are explained in the text).

Disease stage	No. patients	No. elevated CEA level	% Patient with elevated CEA
I	10	6	60
II	40	14	35
III	47	26	55
IV	25	20	80

Table (2-12)

Incidence of elevated CEA level in patients with malignant breast tumors of different histology (All details are explained in the text).

Histological classification of breast cancer	No. patients	No. elevated CEA level	% patients with elevated serum CEA
A- Noninvasive			
Intraductal or comedo carcinoma	5	1	20
Lobular carcinoma in situ	-	-	-
B- Invasive pure forms			
Infiltrating duct	65	35	54
Medullary	4	3	75
Infiltrating	19	8	42
Mucinous	1	0	-
Adenocystic	4	1	25
Tubular	4	3	75
Papillary	-	-	-
Carcino-sarcoma (ex. Cystosarcoma phylloides)	1	1	100
C- Paget's disease	-	-	-
Mixed histologies	-	-	-

Table (2-13)

Positivity of CEA in relation to menopausal status

(All details are explained in the text)

Menopausal state	No. patients	No. elevated CEA level	% patient with elevated CEA
Premenopausal	38	20	52.6
postmenopausal	84	16	19

DETERMINATION OF CYTOSOLIC CEA IN BREAST CANCER AND NORMAL SPECIMENS

Normal Specimens:

Cytosolic CEA was assayed in 32 specimens of normal individuals (Fig 2-5). The normal level of this glycoprotein is presented in table (2–14) indicating a mean value of 2.2 ± 0.81 ng/mg cytosol protein (cp) and range of 0-3.7 ng CEA/mg protein. The specificity of CEA in cytosol for excluding normal individuals was 93%, by regarding the normal/abnormal cutoff value of 3.0 ng/mg cytosol protein. At present no report is available in the literature on the cutoff value of CEA in cytosol.

Benign Breast Tumor:

When the assay was performed on 12 patients with benign breast tumors, supernormal levels (concentration > 3ng/mg cytosol protein) of CEA were observed in 4 of these patients, suggesting a specificity of 67% (Table 2-15) and mean value of 2.8 ± 0.05 ng/mg cytosol protein. (Table 2-14) which is not significantly different from that of normal ($p>0.05$). There have been no previous reports on the CEA level in cytosol with breast benign tumors.

Breast Cancer Tissue:

The distribution of CEA in breast carcinoma tissue is shown in (Fig 2-5). CEA concentration > 3 ng/mg protein was found in 51/62 primary carcinoma.

The percentage sensitivity of CEA for cancer specimens is about 82% (Table 2-15), compared with 6% for normal specimens. The mean value of CEA in cancer specimens is 17.25 ± 3.4 which is significantly higher ($P<0.05$) than in benign and normal (Table 2-14). One female case shows very high levels of CEA (117 ng/mg protein) died within 3 months after surgery.

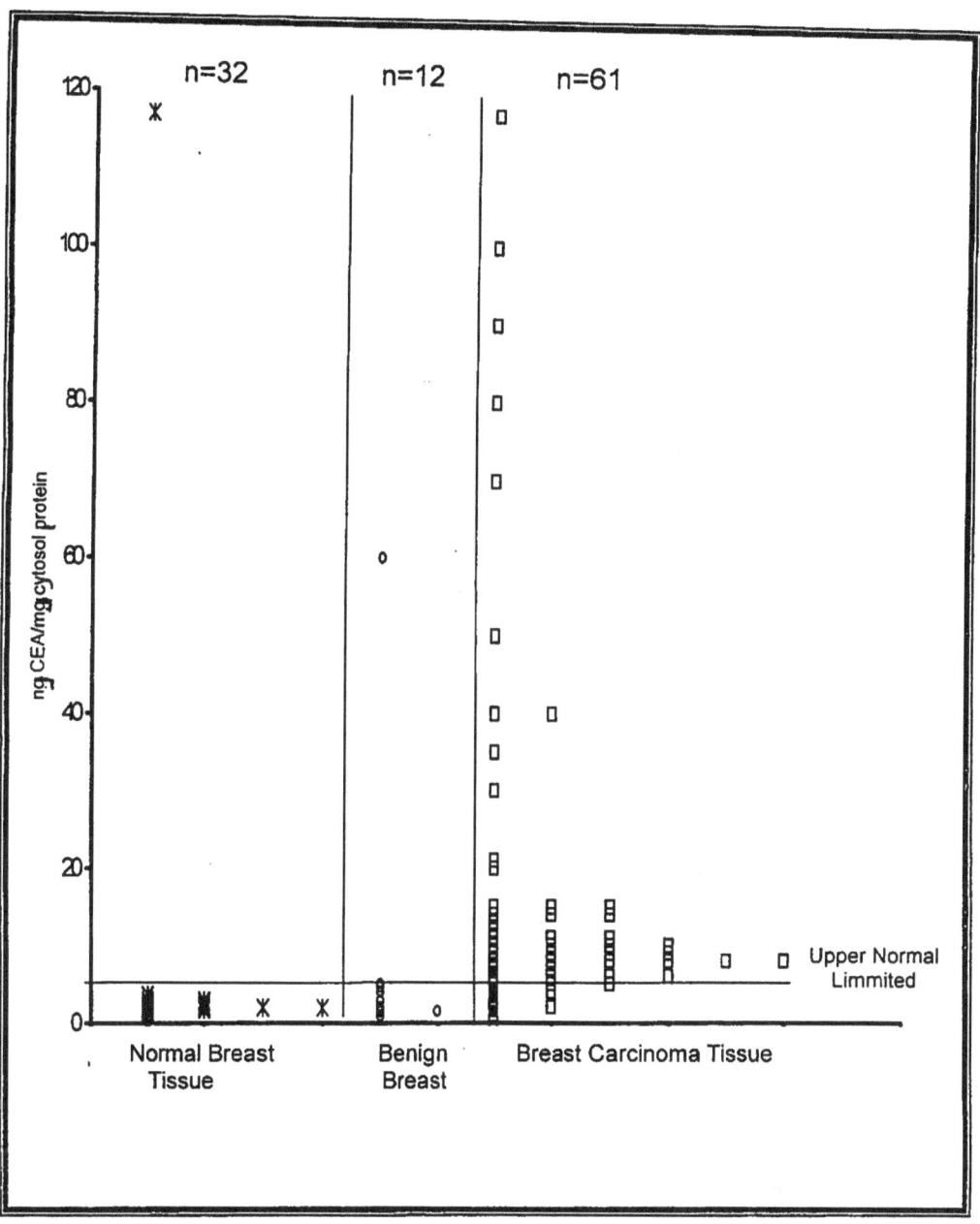

Fig (2-5): Distribution of sytosolic CEA value in human breast carcinomas, benign breast tumors, and normal breast tissues . (n)=Number of patients cut off value = 3 ng CEA/mg protein

It seems from the results that there is no significant correlation between preoperative level of serum CEA and cytosol level of CEA. Also cytosolic CEA didn't correlate with either carcinoma stage or histological classification.

Table (2-14)

Cytosolic CEA determination in cancer, benign, and normal, human breast tissue (All details are explained in the text)

Source of tissue	No. sample	Cytosol level of CEA (ng/mg protein)		F value
		Mean	±SD	
Normal	32	2.2	0.08	
Benign	12	2.8	0.05	P>0.05 N.S
Primary carcinomas	62	17.25	3.4	P<.05

Table (2-15)

Sensitivities and specificity's of CEA in normal, benign, and human breast carcinoma tissue.

(All details are explained in the text)

Source of tissue	No. specimens	No. Positive cases	% Positive	No. Negative cases	% Negative
Normal	32	2	6	30	93.75
Benign	12	4	33	8	66.6
Primary carcinoma	62	51	82	11	17.7

Positive > 3ng CEA/mg protein

Negative < 3ng CEA/ mg protein

Most research on CEA has concentrated on measurement of this glycoprotein in sera from patients with cancer. However, a logical first step in the study of tumor markers would be examination of the tumor tissue for the presence of particular marker of interest. Primary breast cancer in contrast to metastatic disease rarely causes elevation of circulating levels of CEA. Our work shows that this is not due to the absence of CEA from primary tumors. It could however relate to the tumor bulk which may not be sufficiently large to produce elevate serum level at the localized stage, The prognostic value of CEA in the tissue is not yet defined. Some authors reported a correlation between presence of CEA in the tissue and a worse prognosis[73]; other authors found such a relationship only in tumors of 3 cm or smaller [74/75]; others deny any relation between CEA and prognosis [76] or do not take into account this problem [77,78/79]. Furthermore, CEA in the tissue does not appear to be related to the degree of differentiation of tissue [77,79].

Analysis of CEA in the cytosol may prove to be helpful in evaluating plasma CEA as marker for recurrence subsequently in tumors with low CEA cytosol values must produce bulky metastases before blood CEA concentration increases measurably. Also, the clinical utility of the tests may lie in providing additional information on the tumor proliferation rate in term of planning the treatment for woman with early stage breast cancer.

Discussion

The comparative study was carried out in an attempt to overcome the limitation of specificity and, sensitivity of single tumor marker determination. Hence a combination of two Markers that could complement each other in function, were used.

CA15-3 showed the best sensitivity (54%) for detecting preoperative breast cancer patients (Table 2-16) and CEA gave 29.5% sensitivities. However the low specificity (77%) of CEA for discriminating benign from cancerous patients, as well as its general elevation in other type of cancer puts some doubt on clinical detecting breast cancer patients. Therefore, a combination of CEA and CA 15-3 (with %100 specificity), though not tested as such but it can be better to be choice as a diagnostic tool for preoperative patients with breast cancer.

According to the initial determination, the groups free of metastases showed normal CEA serum level below 3ng/ml in 78.68%, where as only 29.5% were in the intermediate pathological range (exceeding 3ng/ml). A significantly different distribution ($P< 0.05$) was found in the patient group with metastases. Thus it may be concluded that CEA test recognized all cases with proven metastases, but does not recognize all cases without metastases.

Owing to lack of a understanding of the pathophysiological behavior of the CEA produced by malignant tumors, no body can explain why high CEA – concentration in tumors are not in all cases to be found in the serum. A reason for this finding may be, that the CEA may be masked by naturally occuring substances after leaving the tumor, giving rise to negative or unreasonably low results.

From 53 follow - up cases with 5 –15 serial determinations over 3–12 months, 25 cases had constantly normal CEA levels or values not exceeding 3ng/ml. All these patients were free of metastases, This associate with a regression of the disease.

From the 28 cases (52.8%) with increased CEA levels, 25 had proven metastases. In 3 further patients, no metastases were found; one of these patients had CEA levels between 14 and 40 ng/ml over a period of 12 months, the other patient had rather constant levels between 7 and 13 ng/ml over an observation period of 10 months. The patients with metastases and elevated CEA levels in direction to higher values. Most of these patients developed clinical progression of disease during the observation period.

In conclusion, the present results lead to the following:
1. In mastectomized patients without metastases, CEA serum levels remain within the normal or low pathological range.
2. Most of mastectomized patient with metastatic breast cancer shows slightly to obviously pathological serum CEA levels. The percentage of pathological values is less with isolated lymph node involvement and gradually from skin to liver, lung, bone up to significantly higher percentage with multiple organ manifestation.
3. Follow – up studies during drug or radio therapy show a correlation of increasing CEA concentration with progression, decreasing values with remission and persistent or slightly fluctuating levels with stationary disease.
4. The CEA test may not be recommended for screening of breast cancer, but as a valuable adjuvant of monitoring metastatic disease and the response to therapy.

The reported results are essentially consistent with the finding of several other investigators [68-72].

Table (2-16)

Comparison of the sensitivity and specificity of the two marker

(All details are explained in the text)

Tumor marker	% sensitivity for preoperative detection of breast cancer patient	% specificity for discriminating normal and benign patient	
		Normal	benign
CA 15-3	54	100	100
CEA	29.5	73	77

CHAPTER THREE

PURIFICATION AND PHYSICOCHEMICAL PROPERTIES OF CEA

Abstract

A procedure has been described for the purification of the CEA of the human mammary carcinoma. Tumor tissue extraction in (0.6) M perchloric acid followed by Ion exchange and column chromatography on Sepharose CL–6B column resulted in highly purified CEA preparation as determined by both immunological and physico-chemical criteria. Such as, immunoelectrophoresis, stocks radius, isoelectric point, M.wt., stability and carbohydrate content. The collected data suggest that CEAs of mammary adenocarcinoma tissues with stocks radius (53 A°), pI (4) and the M.wt. have been found to be 175 KD.

Finally purified CEA preparation gave rise to single band by disc SDS – polyacrylamide gel electrophoresis and a single preciptin arc against corresponding monoclonal anti–CEA on immunoelectrophoresis. The purified CEA contained approximately 40% carbohydrate through determination by phenol – sulfuric acid method.

Also, the characterization was carried out through spectroscopic studies using ultraviolet absorption molecules. Factor affecting the absorption properties of purified CEA such as, pH, polarity, effect of solvent perturbation and pH titration have been studied, the results indicates that there are different effects of these factors on the CEA spectrum. The pH titration of purified CEA shows that the amino acid tyrosine is located on the surface of the CEA.

Fourier transform infrared (FTIR) spectroscopy in the 4000–250 cm^{-1} region was used to characterize the CEA structure of mammary carcinoma and standard individual. A set of IR bands characteristic of CEA conformation were obtained.

INTRODUCTION

Carcinoembryonic antigen (CEA) is the name given by Gold and Freedman to a tumor – specific antigen found in adenocarcinoma of the digestive system [77].

That the CEA is a glycoprotein was evident from its solubility and apparent stability in perchloric acid [78]. In view of the heterogeneous nature of the glycoprotein it is impossible to define CEA precisely in terms of physical and chemical properties. A definition of CEA at the present time has to be based on its specific immunological reaction with a monospecific anti – CEA antiserum, which has been shown to be identical in specificity to the original antiserum prepared by Gold and Freedman [41]. This is important since it has been clearly established that CEA possesses at least two different immunogenic groups; a unique group, which defines CEA – likes molecules and second is common to CEA and the normal glycoprotein (NGP) that is also found in normal and tumor tissues [79,80,81,82].

There are several procedures available for the isolation and purification of CEA from different sources [83,84,85]. Most of these depends on routine methods by perchloric acid extraction and then using gel–filtration however, other methods such as affinity chromatography was used for purification of CEA from liver affected by metastasis of colon carcinoma [86].

The best spectroscopic methods for characterization of CEA are the solvent perturbation technique [87]. In the solvent perturbation method of probing the surface of protein molecules, advantage is taken from the fact that the spectra of chromophoric residue coming freely in contact with the solvent is sensitive to change in the physical properties of the solvent, such as refractive index, dielectric constant, and solvent-solute interaction, in the immediate vicinity of chromophores [88]. There are several studies on the application of solvent perturbation technique of different spectroscopy such as those related to studying the location of chromophoric side chains in globular proteins (milk proteins, α- lacta albumin, ... etc) dissolved in aqueous media [89-92].

The objective of this part of the thesis was the preparation of a pure sample of CEA from mammary carcinoma (CEA) for immunological and physicochemical studies.

Also this chapter deals with the structural studies of CEA using spectroscopic techniques, UV and FTIR.

Materials and methods

3-1 Extraction & Purification:

A – Extraction of CEA:

The preparation of tissue specimen was carried out as described previously in section (2-5). The complete isolation was carried at 4°C. The PCA supernatant adjusted to pH 7.2 with 14N NH_4OH and then lyophilized.

B – Purification of CEA:

1. Ion Exchange chromatography

a. Preparation of the column

A column of 1.8x20 cm was used and packed with the weak anion exchanger DEAE-Sephadex A-50. For the preparation of the gel, DEAE- Sephadex A-50 powder was swelled in Tris buffer 0.02 M pH 7.4 (40 ml/g of powder) for 48 hr at room temperature without stirring. During the swelling period the supernatant was removed and replaced with fresh buffer several times.

The gel was poured into the column down a glass rod with bed volume of 37 ml. Two bed volumes of Tris buffer pH 7.2 were run at flow rate of 60 ml/h through the column in order to reach equilibrium.

b. Separation procedure:

An aliquot of the lyophilized powder of the perchloric acid extracted from tumor tissue dissolved in 10 ml Tris buffer was loaded on the column. After an initial pre wash with 60 ml of Tris buffer pH 7.2 at flow rate of 60 ml/h. CEA was eluted with 400 ml linear gradient of sodium chloride, 0.0 M to 0.3 M, in Tris buffer. Fractions of 2 ml were collected. The eluate was constantly monitored for its spectrophotometric absorption at 280nm, and CEA activity was preformed as described in section (2.4.2). The specific binding of each fraction was calculated and plotted against the elution volume. Selected Fractions containing most of CEA were pooled, dialyzed against de-ionized water at 4°C for 48 hr and then concentrated to 5 ml with dialysis against sucrose. The protein content was determined using Lowry, et. al method[93]. CEA content was determined by IRMA method to carry out next experiments.

2. Gel filtration chromatography

a. Preparation of the column:

The dimensions of the column were chosen according to the following equation [94]:

$$\text{Diameter} = \sqrt[3]{m/10} \text{ cm}$$

Where (m) is the amount of protein in mg.
The length = 30×diameter. In view of such calculation, a 2×85 cm column was used.

The gel was prepared by allowing the pre-swollen gel to swell again in Tris buffer pH 7.4, then settled and excess buffer was decanted. This step was repeated several times. The gel slurry was degassed by suction and left for 24 h at 4°C to equilibrate with the buffer. The swollen gel was suspended and carefully poured into the column (2×85 cm) down the wall. After the gel has settled the column outlet was opened, continuing packing till the gel reached a bed height of 85 cm then equilibrated with Tris buffer pH 7.2 . The void volume of the column was estimated using blue dextran 2000 then, elution was carried out with the same buffer using a flow rate of 20 ml/hr. Fractions of 5ml were collected and their absorbance were measured at 600 nm. The volume of the buffer that required eluting the blue dextran represents the void volume (~90ml) of the column.

b. Purification procedure

The concentrated fractions obtained from DEAE-sephadex ion exchange, containing the CEA activity were loaded to a 6B-Sepharose column. Fractions of 4ml were obtained by elution with Tris buffer 0.2 M pH 7.2 at flow rate 20 ml/h. For each fraction, constant monitoring for its spectrophotometric absorption at 280 nm and CEA activity was performed as described in section 2.4.2. The total binding of each fraction was calculated and plotted against the elution volume.

C- Calculations:

1. In each fraction, the protein concentration was determined according to Lowry et al. [93].
2. Total activity of binding CEA was estimated by the double antibody method (IRMA) as described in section 2.4.2. (Total concentration mg/ml).
3. The specific binding activity was estimated from the following formula:

$$\text{Specific binding activity} = \frac{\text{Total binding - activity } (\mu g)}{\text{Total protein (mg)}}$$

4. The purification fold for CEA was determined using the following formula:

$$\text{Purification fold of CEA} = \frac{\text{Specific binding activity of purified CEA } (\mu g/mg \text{ protein})}{\text{Specific binding activity of crude CEA } (\mu g/mg \text{ protein})}$$

5. (yield)% was determined as follow:

$$\text{Yield \%} = \frac{\text{Total binding activity of purified CEA } (\mu g/ml)}{\text{Total binding activity of crude CEA } (\mu g/ml)} \times 100$$

3-2 Analysis of the purified fraction by slab conventional polyacrylamide gel electrophoresis (PAGE):

PAGE technique was used to specify the purity of the CEA.

Solutions used:

(A) Tris-glycine solution (pH 8.9):
22.84 gms of Glycine was dissolved in one litter of distilled water. The pH of the solution was adjusted to 8.9 with tris-hydroxyaminomethane. The volume was then completed to 2 liters with distilled water.

(B) Electrode buffer: This was prepared by the 1:1 (v:v) dilution of solution (A).

(C) Polyacrylamide solution:
22.2 gms of acrylamide and 0.6 gm. of N,N-methylene bisacrylamide were dissolved in 60 ml. of distilled water. The solution completed to a final volume of 100 ml. with distilled water.

(D) TEMD

(E) Ammonium persulphate (15 mg/ml)
150 mgs. Ammonium persulphate were dissolved in 10 mls. of distilled water (freshly prepared before used).

(F) Bromophenol blue solution 0.25 % (W/V).

(G) Fixing solution:
This solution prepared by dissolving 57 gms. of trichloroacetic acid and 17 gms. of sulphosalicylic acid in 150 mls. of ethanol (95%), then the volume was completed to 500 mls. with distilled water.

(H) Staining solution:
1.25 gms. of coomassie Brilliant Blue R-250 were dissolved in a mixture of exactly 227 mls. ethanol and 46 ml. glacial acetic acid. The volume of the solution completed to 500 mls. with distilled water.

(I) Destaining solution:
Volumes of 300 mls. ethanol and 100 mls. glacial acetic acid were thoroughly mixed. The solution was then completed to a final volume of 1 litter with distilled water.

(J) Preserving solution:
This solution was prepared by mixing 300 mls. of ethanol with 100 mls. glacial acetic and 100 mls. glycerol. Distilled water was then added to a final volume of 1 L.

(K) Four protein solutions were used at concentration of 1300 µg/ml.

1. Homogenate protein. (fig. (3-2-A)).
2. Protein fraction I: partially purified CEA by PCA. (Fig. (3-2-B)).
3. Protein fraction II: purified by ion exchange. (Fig. (3-2-C)).
4. Protein fraction III: purified by gel filtration. (Fig. (3-2-D)).

The above two purified protein fractions were concentrated to the optimum concentration (1300 µg/ml.) by dialysis against sucrose.

Procedure:

1. Polyacrylamide gel (conc. 7.5 %) was prepared by mixing the following solution respectively (According to the application Note 306 issued by LKB Company).
   7.5 mls. distilled water
   33.0 mls. solution (A)
   22.2 mls. solution (C)
   3.2 mls. solution (D)
   0.1 mls. solution (E)
2. The gel slab was prepared and fixed in an electrophoresis Apparatus type LKB. The optimum conditions fixed in the application Note 306 were exactly followed.
3. The electrophoretic migration continued until the blue stain of Bromophenol blue reached the gel margin.
4. The gel was then divided into two parts. Part one was sliced to 0.5 cm segments, each segment was placed in 500 µl of TED buffer pH 7.2, then sliced and cracked softly and left for 24 hr. at 4°C. then the CEA binding activity evaluated by IRAM Method as described in section (2.4.2).
5. Part two of the gel slab was immersed in the fixing solution (solution H) for 1 hr., then transferred to the staining solution (solution I) for 2 hrs. in order to stain all the proteins separated by electrophoresis. Excess staining was removed by soaking the gel with destaining solution (solution J). It is preferable to replace the destaining solution twice or thrice in order to secure a complete and fast removal of the excess stain and hence getting more clear bands.
6. The gel slab was kept in the preserving solution (solution L) for 1 hr. to preserve it from dryness and tears.

3-3 Immunoelectrophoresis (IEP) [95-97]

IEP technique was used for immunochemical identity of the purified CEA preparation and standard CEA.

Solutions used:

(A) Barbital/barbital – Na buffer, (pH 8.6)
- 5,5 – diethyl barbituric acid (barbital) 30g.
- 5,5 diethyl – sodium barbiturate (barbital – Na) = 155g.
- Sodium azide 10g.
- Calcium lactate 3g.
- Distilled water to make 10 liters.

The barbital dissolves after a few minutes in 1 litter of boiling distilled water under magnetic stirring. Heating is then discontinued and the barbital – Na is added. When this has dissolved, sodium azide and calcium lactate were added. Finally, distilled water was added to a final volume of 10 liters[98].

(B) 1% agarose in Barbital / barbital – Na buffer, pH 8.6

Two grams of agarose were added to 200 ml of the diluted buffer and dissolved by gentle heating on a magnetic stirrer. The solution was boiled for 5-6 min to ensure that the agarose is completely dissolved. The solution was kept fluid at 56°C in water bath and ready for use after temperature equilibration.

(C) Staining solution, ponceus S
- Trichloro acetic acid (TCA)   30 grams
- Ponceus S   2 grams
- Distilled water   100 grams

The dye dissolved by heating to 60°C followed by cooling at room temperature and filtering through filter paper.

(D) Destaining solution:
    10 % glacial acetic acid.

(E) Fixing solution:
    Picric acid   14 g
    Distilled water   1000 ml
    Glacial acetic acid   200 ml

The picric acid added to water, which is then heated to 60°C. the warm solution is filtered through filter paper and finally the glacial acetic acid is added.

(H) Washing solutions:
1. 0.1 M NaCl
2. distilled water

(I) Two samples of CEA solutions were prepared at concentration of 1300 µg/ml
1. CEA provided by CEA IRMA Kit / Byksangetes Diagostic GmbH&Co. KG / France.
2. The purified CEA preparation.

(J) The anti – CEA monoclonal solution provided by Byksangetes Diagostic GmbH&Co. KG / France).

Procedure:

1. An agarose – coated microscope slide (25x75 mm) was used as support for the gel then placed on a horizontal surface, and about 2 ml of buffer 1% agarose was poured onto the slide.
2. Holes of 1 mm and trough of 2 mm wide were made by means of gel puncher, the gel in the hole was removed by a Pasteur pipette.
3. The upper well was loaded with standard CEA and other one was loaded with purified CEA preparation.
4. The slide was then placed in electrophoresis chamber and connected to buffer vessels by filter paper wicks.
5. Electrophoresis was performed with a potential gradient of 3-6 V/cm, corresponding to total of 70 – 200 v. Initial current was 50 mA/plate. At 4°C for 80 min.
6. After termination of electrophoresis, the agarose gel was removed from the trough and 100µl of monoclonal anti–CEA was introduced into trough.
7. Incubation of the plate was performed in a humid chamber for 24h.
8. Fixing 30 min in fixing solution.
9. **Washing**: This is done by washing it twice in 0.1 M NaCl and once with distilled water.
10. **Drying**: Cover the gel with 3 layers of filter paper and place a glass plate and a weight (1 to 2 kg) over them. Remove after 10 min and finish drying in a stream of hot air in front of a heating fan.

11. **Staining**: 10 min in staining solution.
12. **Destaining**: 10% glacial acetic acid till the background become clear.
13. **Drying**: in a stream of hot air in front of a heating fan.

3-4 Determination of the Molecular Weight of Purified CEA by Gel Filtration Chromatography [98]

Sepharose 6B column (2x90 cm) was used for this purpose as described in section 3-1. The gel was prepared by allowing the powder to swell in excess of Tris buffer pH 7.2 (40 ml/g of powder). The mixture was left to stand for three days at room temperature without stirring, then the slurry was processed and packed as mentioned in section 3 – 1. The column was calibrated by a gel filtration calibration kit, purchased from pharmacy Fine Chemicals which contain six standard proteins. Standard protein solutions were prepared according to the manufacturer instruction, then applied through three portions (1-ml portion), proteins 1 and 3 in the first, proteins 2 and 5 in the second and 4 and 6 in the third portion. Elution was carried out with Tris buffer pH 7.4 at a flow rate of 20 ml/h. The absorbencies of the fractions collected were measured at 280 nm to evaluate the elution volume (Ve) of the standard proteins. CEA protein was applied to the calibrated 6B Sepharose column and elution was as described in section 3-1 B (gel filtration). The partition coefficients (Kav) of the proteins eluted were determined using the following formula:

$$K_{av} = \frac{V_e - V_o}{V_t - V_o}$$

Where; V_o : void volume, V_e : elution volume V_t : the volume of the bed gel. The values of Kav were plotted vs. the values of log M. wt of the proteins eluted. The M. wt. of CEA was calculated from the standard curve obtained.

Standard proteins:

Pharmacy electrophoresis calibration kit for determination of M. wt by gel filtration was used. The kit comprises six highly purified proteins individually packed. Each protein was reconstituted in 1 ml Tris buffer pH 7.4. The six proteins and their M. wt as detailed below:

Protein	M. wt(kD)
Thyroglobulin	669
Ferritin	440
Catalase	232
Aldolase	158
BSA	67
Ovalbumin	43

3-5 Estimation of Stock's Radius of Purified CEA [98]

The gel filtration procedure was run on 6B-sepharose column exactly as mentioned in section 3-4 using Pharmacia calibration kit of six standard proteins, the partition coefficients (Kav) were determined and the values of (- log Kav) ½ were calculated, then plotted against the stock's radius of standard proteins eluted. The stock's radius of CEA was calculated from the straight line obtained.

3-6 Analysis of Purified CEA by Disc SDS - PAGE [95-98]

Disk SDS–PAGE technique was used to assess the homogeneity of purified CEA and for the estimation of molecular weights.

Stock solutions used:

(A) Staking gel buffer (Tris – HCl at pH 6.8)
6.0 gram of Tris in 40 ml titrated to pH 6.8 with 1 M HCl; bring to 100 ml by distilled water.

(B) Resolving gel buffer (Tris – HCl at pH 8.8)
36.3 g of Tris and 48.0 ml of 1M HCl brought to 100 ml; titrate to pH 8.8 with HCl, if necessary.

(C) Reservoir buffer (Tris – glycine at pH 8.3)
3 g of Tris and 14.4 g of glycine in 1 litter.

(D) Acrylamide – Bisacrylamide
30 g of acrylamide, 0.8 g of bisacrylamide per 100 ml distilled water.

(E) Ammonium persulphate (APS) 1.5 % w/v, freshly prepared before use.

(H) TEMED (N,N,N,N – tetramethyl – ethylenene diamine): was used as supplied.
(I) SDS, 10 %, w/v: 10 grams in 100 ml D.W; filter through watman No 1 paper befor use.
(J) Bromophenol blue 0.25%.
(K) Coomassi Brilliant blue R-250: as described in section 3–2.
(L) Destaining solution: as described in section 3 – 2.
(M) Stock sample buffer: prepared by mixing 4.8 ml distilled water, 12 ml staking gel buffer, 2 ml of SDS 10 % w/v solution, 2 gm sucrose, 0.5 ml of bromophenol blue 0.25%.

Procedure:

(1) **Resolving gel preparation:** The gel was prepared by mixing the following materials:
- Distilled water   4.85 ml
- Resolving gel buffer   2.50 ml
- Acrylamide – Bisacrylamid 2.50 ml
- 10% (w/v) SDS solution   0.10 ml

Then, Degassing for minutes followed by 50 µl of APS and 5µl TEMED, were added and mixed carefully. The tubes stood vertically to ensure a horizontal meniscus and the prepared resolving gel mixture was carefully introduced into the tubes, up to the 2ml mark, by means of a pasteur pipette.

Immediately, 3 drops of butanol were layered above the gel to avoid introduction of oxygen.

The gel needed 10 – 15 minutes to set.

(2) **Staking gel preparation:**
The gel was prepared by mixing the following materials:
- Distilled water   0.1 ml
- Stacking gel buffer (Tris – HCl, pH 6.8)   2.5 ml
- Acrylamide – Bisacrylamid   1.3 ml
- 10% (w/v) SDS solution   0.1 ml

Mixed well, then degassed for 10 minutes followed by the addition of 50µl of 10% APS and 5µl TEMED mixed carefully, the prepared gel mixture was carefully introduced into tubes. Immediately 3 – 4 drops of butanol were layered above the gel.

The gel was left at room temperature for 12 h. to set.

(3) Sample preparation:

The samples were prepared by mixing 300 µl of stock sample buffer with 200 µl sample solution (0.2 mg/ml) followed by 50 µl 2–mercaptoethanol. Heating samples can be accomplished by inserting the vial of sample into a larger test tube and placing the test tube in boling water bath.

Standard proteins were treated exactly as described for sample preparation.

(4) The electrophoretic run:

Prior to electrophoresis, the lower caps were removed and the tubes placed in position in the electrophoresis apparatus. Hundred µl of samples were layered on top of each gel below a layer of electrode buffer and electrophoresis was performed at 60 volts until the sample runs into the stacking gel, then 120 volts until the dye front migrates to within 1 cm of the bottom of gel. Under these conditions the required total time was 5h.

The gel was removed from their glass tubes by gentle rimming with a fine needle attached to a syringe, slowly ejecting water at the same time while rotating the tube [99].

The gels were introduced into 10cm glass tubes containing fixation solution for 1h, the process for protein staining and destaining as described in section (3-2).

The relative mobility (Rm) of each standard protein and sample was measured as follows:

$$Rm = \frac{\text{Distance moved by the protein}}{\text{Distance moved by the bromophenol blue}}$$

The log M.wt of the standard proteins was plotted against the Rm value and the molecular weight of CEA was calculated from straight line.

3-7 Determination of Isoelectric Point (PI) of Purified CEA [95-97,99,100]

Isoelectric focusing technique was used to determine the PI of CEA protein according to Wringley method [99].

Solution used:

(A) Ampholine carrier (LKB) pH range (3.5 – 10)
(B) Acrylamide – Bisacrylamide
As described in section 3-6
(C) APS 1.5% (w/v): as described in section 3-6
(D) Anode solution : 0.5 M H_2So_4
(E) Cathode solution : 0.5 M NaOH
(I) Protective solution: This was prepared by mixing 1% Ampholine carrier with 5% sucrose.

Procedure:

The anode and cathode solutions were placed in their reservoirs. The electric circuit was connected and the sample (100 µl) were loaded on top of each gel below layer of protective solution, then the LKB instruction conditions were used by application of 1500 volts and a current of 50 mA for 3 hr. after electrophoresis, the gel was divided into three parts. Part one was sliced to 0.5 cm segments and each segment was put in 500 µl of TED buffer pH 7.2, then cracked softly and left over night at 4°C.

The binding activity was evaluated for the mixture as described in section (2-4-2). Part two of the gels was processed for coomassie blue staining of proteins. Part three of the gels was sliced to 0.5 cm segment and each segment was placed in 2 ml of de-ionized water, then cracked softly and left overnight at 4°C. the pH of the segment solution was measured. A calibration curve was plotted between pH and the number of gel segments. The pH of the segment that has the highest specific binding of CEA equal to its isoelectric point.

3-8 Carbohydrate Content Studies

Solution used:

1. Phenol solution   5%
2. H_2SO_4 98% concentration
3. Standard glucose: The standard glucose solution with different concentrations (0,8,24,40,56,80) µg/ml were prepared by serial dilution from a stock solution of glucose (80 µg/ml) (Table 3-1)

Procedure:

The method of phenol-sulfuric acid which was described by Dubois[101], used to determined the total carbohydrate of CEA in the sample.

The assay protocol was described in table (3-1)

Table (3 -1): Concentration of Standard glucose solution
(All details are explained in the text)

Tube No	Stock solution of glucose volume ml	Distilled water volume added ml	Concentration of glucose µg
1	0	1.0	0
2	0.1	0.9	8
3	0.3	0.7	24
4	0.5	0.5	40
5	0.7	0.3	56
6	1	0	80

Then 1ml of 5% phenol solution was added to 5ml of concentration H_2SO_4 for each test tube mixed well and left at room temperature until cooling.

The absorbencies of tubes were read at 490 nm.

The sample was treated exactly as described for standard carbohydrate.

Calculation:

The standard curve was obtained by plotting the absorbance at 490 nm against the corresponding concentrations of standard glucose solution, used to determine carbohydrate in sample, as shown in figure (3-1).

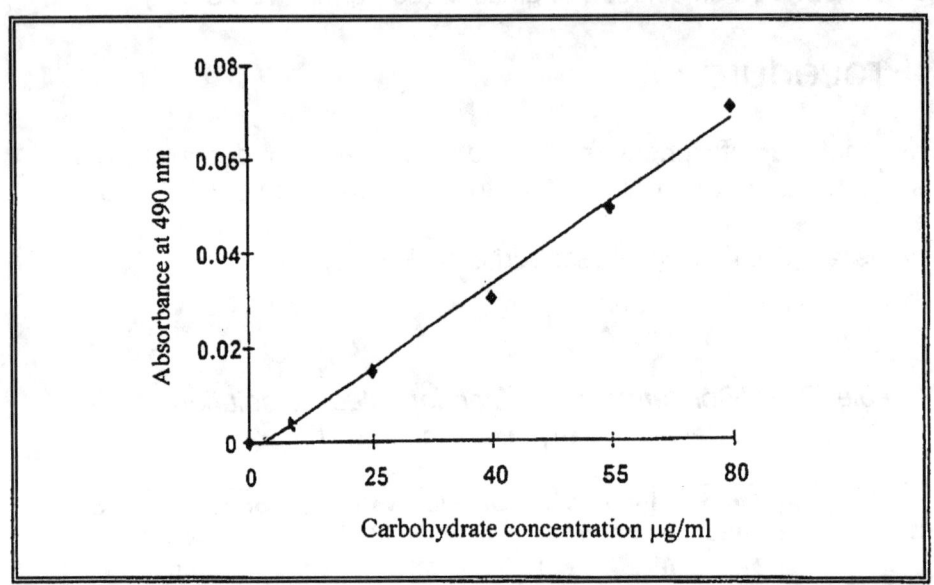

Fig (3-1): Standard curve of carbohydrate determination
(All details are explained in the text)

3-9 Stability of CEA at -20°C

Crude and purified CEA prepared were stored at -20°C for several time intervals. The frozen specimen was thawed in each interval and the binding activity was measured as described in section (2-4-2).

The remaining activity was calculated and plotted against the storage periods.

Spectroscopic Studies

This study was aimed to elucidate the spectroscopic properties of purified CEA.

3-10 Ultraviolet Absorption: (UV)

The ultraviolet absorption of the purified human CEA and CEA provided (CEA IRMA Kit / Byksangetes Diagostic GmbH&Co. KG / France) were continuously scanned from 200 – 350 nm by a Shimadzu UV.

A volume of 50 μl of CEA (1.3 mg/ml) was completed to 1 ml with tris buffer pH 7.2, then the absorption spectrum was measured against the same buffer in reference beam.

3-11 Factors Affecting the Absorption Properties of Purified CEA

1. pH Effect on the spectrum of purified CEA:

Solutions:

1. 0.01 M tris hydroxyl methyl amino ethan buffer of pH 7.2 was prepared by dissolving 0.302 gm of the tris in 250 ml distilled water and required pH was adjusted by addition of 0.1 N HCl.
2. Citrate buffer (pH 3) was prepared as follows:
    Solution A: Citric acid (0.1 M); 10.50 gm citric acid was dissolved in 500 ml distilled water.
    Solution B: Sodium citrate (0.1 M); 14.7050 gm sodium citrate was dissolved in 500 ml distill water.
    Citrate buffer pH 3 were prepared by mixing 46.5 ml of solution A with an appropriate amount (3.5 ml) of solution B to obtain the required pH.
3. Phosphate buffer (pH 11) was prepared as follows:
    Solution A: Dibasic sodium phosphate (0.1 M); 4.4497 gm $Na_2HpO_4 \cdot 2H_2O$ was dissolved in 250 ml distilled water.
    Solution B: Sodium hydroxide (0.1 M); 0.4 gm NaOH was dissolved in 100 ml distilled water.

Phosphate buffer (pH 11) was prepared by mixing 60 ml of solution A with an appropriate amounts of solution B to obtain the required pH.

Procedure:

Fifty microliter of human purified CEA preparation (1.3 mg/ml) was completed to 1 ml with different buffer at different pH values (3 to 11). The samples were then transferred to 0.5 cm cuvette in the sample beam and the buffer at the adjusted pH in reference beam, the absorption spectrum was scanned.

2. Polarity effect:

The CEA was studied spectrophotometerically by the addition of different solvents:

Ethanol, ethylene glycol, glycerol and poly ethylene glycol in a percent of 20% prepared in tris buffer pH 7.2 for example, CEA in 20% ethanol:

A volume of 50µl of purified CEA solution (1.3 mg/ml) was completed to 1 ml with tris buffer pH 7.2 in the presence of 20% ethanol. Each of these mixtures was placed in test cell against 20% ethanol prepared in the same buffer in the reference beam. The absorption spectrum was measured in the area of (200 – 350 nm).

The experiment was repeated by using other solvents individually.

3. Effect of urea, KCl. and urea, KCl mixture on the spectrum of CEA :

Solutions used:

1. Eight molar of urea was prepared by dissolving 24.02 gm of urea in 50 ml of tris buffer at pH 7.2
2. 0.03 M KCl was prepared by dissolving 0.2737 gm of the salt in 50 ml of corresponding buffer.
3. Tris buffer solution was prepared as described in section (3-11-1)

Procedure:

Fifty μl of CEA was pipetted in a set of three tubes. The volume was completed to 1 ml with tris buffer pH 7.2 contains 0.03 M KCl, 8M urea and mixture 1:1 of both 8 urea and 0.03 M KCl respectively then each of which was placed in 1.0 cm cuvette in the sample beam and the buffer at the same pH in the presence of the same salt in the reference beam.
The absorption spectrum was scanned.

3-12 Structural Studies of CEA

Solution used:

Preparation of buffers used in these experiments was described in section (3 – 11):

Procedure

A series of the samples were prepared at pH ranged from 6 to 11 using different buffers.
The maximum absorbance of each sample was measured at wavelength of 295 nm, the absorbance of λ_{max} at each pH value was plotted versus the corresponding pH.
Another series of samples were prepared at pH ranging from 3 to 8 using different buffer.
The maximum absorbance of each sample was measured at wavelength of 211.0 nm. The absorbance of λ_{max} at each pH value was plotted versus in the corresponding pH.

3-13 Estimation of Absorption Coefficient (a_s) of CEA

The standard CEA solution with different concentrations (0.15, 0.3, 0.5, 0.6, 0.8, 0.9, 1) mg/ml were prepared by serial dilution from a stock solution 2 (mg/ml) with tris buffer pH 7.2. The maximum absorbance of each sample was measured at wavelength of 280 nm, the absorbance value for each sample was plotted versus the corresponding concentration.

Calculation:

Specific absorption coefficient (a_s) of human CEA at $\lambda_{max} = 280$ was calculated using Lambert Beer's law [102]:

$$A = a_s c \ell$$

Where
A: Absorbance
C: Human CEA concentration (mg/ml)
ℓ: Length of light path in (cm)
a_s: Specific absorption coefficient in (ml.mg^{-1}.cm^{-1}) at 280 nm

$$(a_s)_{280} = \frac{A}{c\ell} = \frac{\text{slope of stander curve}}{\text{length of light path in cm}} = (ml).(mg^{-1}).(cm^{-1})$$

3-14 Fouler Transform Infrared Spectroscopy (FTIR)

Bach of purified CEA sample with concentration (1mg/ml) for Human Mammary carcinoma and CEA standard were lyophoilized. FTIR absorption spectra of CEA were obtained by KBr films with approximately a 1:100 weight ratio of CEA sample to KBr. The water content was rigorously controlled, as this parameter is essntial to stabilize the structure.

All FTIR spectra were measured from 4000 to 250 cm^{-1} by spectrophotometer (FTIR – 8300) SHIMADZU.

Results and Discussion

Isolation and Purification of CEA

The results of a representative purification of CEA are shown in Table (3 - 2), Fig (3 - 2, 3 - 3).

CEA has been purified by different techniques. In this study metastases tumor lesions was used whenever possible in order to obtain large quantities of cancer from single sources. Purification has been achieved by a sequence of procedures including perchloric acid extraction, Ion exchange and molecular sieve on sepharose 6B. Recent modification in this purification procedure has included the order of chromatographic steps, the gel filtration step of the purification protocol as the final. This protocol is more convenient than other methods of CEA purification that have been reported [41,78,83-85,103-165]. The final product (CEA) show a high degree of purity as determined by both phyiscochemical and immunochemical criteria (Fig 3-4,3-5), Also good yield and activity of CEA were obtained.

The purification by PCA was a chivied by denaturating and precipitating most of the tissue proteins while has a few effects on CEA, which remain in the solution [106]. CEA is generally considered to be stable in acid because it is soluble and its immunological properties are not destroyed. Table (3–2) shows that this step gives nearly 2.5 fold purification and complete recovery of CEA.

Upon DEAE – sephadex, the PCA of the tumor homogenate resolved into a number of components (Fig 3–2 (A&B)). The elution was performed with linear gradient of sodium chloride, 0.0 M to 0.3 M in Tris buffer then selected fraction containing CEA (Fig 3–2) were pooled, dialyzed, and then concentrated as described in section (3–1–B–2).

Ion exchange fractionation increased the specific binding activity 7.7 folds with a yield of 28% when this preparation was applied on gel filtration column, results obtained were depicted in greater details in (Fig 3–3) reveate(d three peaks. The second one was found to have binding activity, whereas the other were not. The resultant fraction that contained the binding activity of the second peak represents the finally purified CEA.

The purification fold by gel filtration step was 66.3 with 22.3% yield. The data suggested that the CEA proteins in mammary carcinoma are one form identical in molecular parameters.

Purity of CEA Preparation

The purity of isolated CEA was analyzed and confirmed by conventional polyacrylamide gel electrophoresis by using binding activity and coomasie blue stain as marker for detection of the CEA (Fig 3 – 4).

Immuoelectrophoresis of the CEA against its corresponding monoclonal anti – CEA gave rise to a single precipitin arc, corroborating that the CEA preparation contained no other cross – reacting substance contaminants Fig (3 – 5).

An important considration in comparing the CEA isolated with CEA provided by Byksangetec Diagostic Gmbh&Co. France in it's degree of immunochemical identity, both CEA gave a single preceptin arc in the same position when reacted with anti – CEA monoclonal antibody provided by Byksangetec Diagostic Gmbh&Co. France. As can be seen in Fig (3 – 5) essentially similar arcs were obtained with both materials in beta globulin region.

Physicochemical Properties of Purified CEA

The physicochemical properties of purified CEA were investigated using different techniques. The molecular weight was determined by gel filtration and Disc–SDS– polyocrylamide gel electrophoresis (SDS – PAGE). The stock's radius of purified CEA was estimated by gel filtration technique. The isoelectric point was evaluated using Disc gel of Ampholine PAGE.

Determination of molecular weight and stock's radius by gel filtration was carried out using standard proteins of known molecular weights and stock's radius. These proteins were applied to the column and eluted with Tris buffer (Fig 3 – 6, 3 – 7). The elution volume (Ve) of each protein was estimated then Kav value was calculated as described in section (3–4). The application of the Kav value to the calibration curve (Fig 3 – 8 and 3 – 9) was led to the determination of the two molecular parameters. The purification of CEA by different techniques yielded finally purified CEA. The molecular weight and stock's radius of this protein was 175 KD and 53 A°.

The molecular weight of purified CEA also was determined by disc SDS–PAGE, (Fig 3–10) illustrated the calibration curve that was obtained in the presence of 1% SDS. The relative mobility's (Rm) of the CEA protein was determined by segmentation of the gel into 0.5 cm slices after removing the SDS by washing and dialysis against Tris buffer the fraction was tested for the binding activity. Application of Rm value for CEA protein to the calibration curve yielded the molecular weight. (Fig 3 – 11) shows the disc SDS – PAGE profile for purified CEA. The results indicated a single band for CEA. The M.wt of CEA found to be 155 KD. The collected data of disc SDS – PAGE and those obtained from gel filtration chromatography suggested that the activated form of CEA were monomeric proteins. The molecular weight of activated CEA is 169 KD. These results are in agreement with studies revealed that CEA prepared from tissue and cells were M.wt 150 – 300 KD [107-112].

Isolectric focusing technique was used for the estimation of isoelectric points (pI) of purified CEA.

Disc polyacrylamide gel was used containing ampholine with pH range 3.5 – 10.5, the gel then sliced and the binding activity of each segment with its pH was measured and coomasie blue as described in section (3 – 7). (Fig 3 – 12) was used to obtain the pI of CEA.

The results showed that the pI of purified CEA was (4). Many investigators have observed the CEA with isoelectric points of 3.5, 4.0, 4.25 and 4.5[112-115]. On the other hand, observations of CEA preparation with single isoelectric points of 4.8 [115] and 4.7 [113] has been reported.

Isoelectric focusing of crude tumor extracts yielded peaks of CEA activity at pH 2.4, 3 and 4.5 through 6.4 [114]. In addition to that, Almudaffar and Al-Rubaee [112] isolated CEA from oral cancer tissue by gel filtration chromatography using sepharose CL-6B and sephadex G-50, and concluded that they were two types of CEA one with m.wt 1000 KD and pI value 6.3 while the second protein from the same tumor appeared to be (158 KD) and 8 as pI value.

Carbohydrate Content

The quantities of carbohydrate in finally purified CEA were approximately 40% as was determined by phenol–sulfuric acid method. These results are in good agreement with those reported previously.

The most marked variation between different CEA preparations is the content of carbohydrate, which can vary between about 80% for purified CEA of gastric origin to about 40% for CEA, derived from colonic metastases [44].

The principal carbohydrate constituent of purified CEA preparation is N-acetylglucosamine, which was usually, constitutes approximatly 25% of total carbohydrate content of each preparation [116].

In contrast, N-acetylglucosamine is either absent or present only in very low concentrations in purified CEA preparations. Some degree of variation is usually noted in the fucose, mannose, galactose and sialic acid content of preparation of CEA derived from colonic tumor's [116].

Stability of Crude and Purified CEA at -20°C

The crude and purified fractions of CEA were stored at -20°C during the experiment. It was carried out in order to study the stability of CEA and to check their efficiencies of binding through out the storage period. The results showed that CEA of crude fraction was more stable than this of purified fraction (Fig 3 – 13).

The Ultraviolet Spectral Results

(Fig 3–14) shows UV spectra (200–350 nm) for two types of CEA molecules. Standard and purified CEA from human mammary carcinoma at pH 7.2.

The parameters, which are usually measured, at absorbance and wavelength corresponding to a peak of maximum absorption (λ_{max}) consist of multiple peaks, at 280 nm, 235 nm for purified CEA and 275 nm, 230 nm for standard CEA. As a result, purified CEA has characteristic spectra and can be identified by its peaks, the first peak (at 235 nm) is due to amide group in the polypeptide bond of purified CEA molecule with contribution of the histidyl residues, [117]. While the second peak (at 280) is assigned to the side chain chromophor of tryrosin and phenylalanine [88].

The spectrum curve had a shape like a shoulder at near by 290 nm from that tryptophan that gives an ultraviolet absorption spectrum with a maximum at 290 nm. It was suggested that CEA may contain tryptophan as amino acid component [118].

Factors Effecting the Absorption Properties of Purified CEA

The absorption spectrum of purified CEA is primarily determined by the chemical structure of the molecule. However, a large number environmental factors produce defectable change in λ_{max}.

Environmental factor consists of pH, the polarity of solvent or neighboring molecule[117]. These environmental factors effect provide the basis for the use of absorption spectroscopy in characterizing CEA. The general features of these environmental effects on the spectrum of molecule are the following.

1. pH Effect

The pH of the solvent determines the Ionization State of ionizable chromophore in the protein molecule [117].

The UV spectrum of purified CEA was determined at four pH's (1.6, 3, 9, 11) (Fig 3 – 15) shows these spectra.

It seems that in acid region (1.6, 3) there were a blue shift in λ_{max} for the peptide bond, as shown in Fig (3 – 15) in pH 1.6 shifted to 215 nm while in pH3 shifted to 225.

The blue shift is due to the increasing of hydrogen bond formed in the presence of highly positively charged state [97]. The result is in agreement with Al-kazzaz observation [119].

Also the decrease associated with dispersed λ_{max} 280 nm of tyrosine and phenylalanine due to the conformational changes and the chromophore in native molecule were buried in the interior of their molecules [120,121].

When the pH was increased from neutral to basic region (pH 9,11) There were a significant shift to a longer wavelength (red shift) in λ_{max2} from 280 to near 300 nm, while no significant changes in λ_{max1} value was observed as shown in Fig (3-14).

The red shift is due to the slightly increase in the energies of electronic transition of the aromatic rings from the formation of the electron - with drowning ammonium groups [122].

It is known that in the acidic region the phenolic OH groups are not ionized; so there is no $n \rightarrow \pi^*$ or $\pi \rightarrow \pi^*$ transition.

In the neutral pH region, the native organization of CEA is fairly compacting, rigid, and has a remarkably hydrophilic exposed molecular surface. Conformational changes occur in CEA in acid and alkaline pH regions; extensive hydrophobic areas in CEA are exposed by both acid and alkaline transition [121-122].

2. Effect of Solvent Polarity on Purified CEA UV. Spectrum (Solvent Perturbation Studies)

The determination of whether an amino acid is internal or external is carried out by measuring the spectra of a protein in a polar and non-polar solvent. In fact, protein is rarely studied in completely non-polar solvents because most proteins are either insoluble or denatured in these solvents.

The table (3-3) and (Fig 3-16) shows, the effect of different solvents on purified CEA at neutral pH 7.2.

When comparing values of λ_{max} of purified CEA in presence of 20% ethanol, or other solvents with that obtained in the absence of these solvents, (λ_{max1} = 235.0 nm obtained in pervious experiment), (Fig 3-16) shows that there is a shift towards longer wavelength at 240, 241.6 nm in the presence ethylene glycol and polyethylene glycol respectively. These alterations in the position at λ_{max1} are all due to the inter molecular hydrogen bonding between amide bond in CEA molecule with EG and PEG. The intermolecular hydrogen bonding increase as the concentration of solution increase and additional band started to appear at longer or shorter wavelength [122].

There was a significant blue shift (~ 12, 10 nm) in the λ_{max1} for CEA in the presence of 20% of ethanol and glycerol respectively. This blue shift indicated that the protein was defolded (rigid) and the exposed histidyl residues were buried interior the molecule in presence of ethanol and glycerol.

Unfortunately, it will be difficult to detect histidyl difference spectra in protein because of it's high absorbency occurred in the low wavelength region which contributed with peptide bond absorbance, there for high difference of spectrum is caused by tyrosine, tyrptophan and phenylalanin [87].

When comparing the effect of the different solvents that were used in this study, on the shift of λ_{max2} which is due to tyrosyl residues in the purified CEA spectrum. A red shift was noticed from 280 nm to 300 nm, which were assigned to new chromophore (tryptophyl residues) appeared on the surface of CEA molecule. These were embedded in an interior region of the protein in the absence of the polyhydroxyl solvent [123].

The effect of 20% chloroform, ether, and DMSO at pH 7.2 are shown in table (3 – 3). The absence of any λ_{max} was observed, this indicates the proteins were denaturated due to change in the secondary and tertiary structures of the protein [88].

3. The Effect of Urea, KCl and Urea - KCl Mixture on the CEA UV. Spectrum

Table (3–4) and Fig (3–17) show the effect of 8M urea, 0.03 KCl and a mixture of (1:1) of 8M Urea, 0.03 KCl on λ_{max} of the CEA UV. spectrum at pH 7.2. Comparing the values of λ_{max} of this molecule obtained in absence of urea or KCl with those obtained in presence of 8M urea in table (3 – 4), it seems that there was a significant red shift in λ_{max1} of the poly peptide bond, for purified CEA spectrum while λ_{max2} of aromatic amino acid i.e tyrosyl residues in CEA was disappeared.

These results indicate that the molecules solvated with urea (dipole-dipole interaction) produce a red–shift and new chromophore come to the surface. The red shift is due to the intermolecular hydrogen bonding between the oxygen of the amide group and the solvent [87].

When 0.03 MKCl was used, there was a slight blue shift (4 nm) in the λ_{max1} of the polypeptide bond as shown in Fig (3–17), and a new absorption peak appeared in the spectrum near 300 nm which could be assigned to the $n \rightarrow \pi^*$ transition in the aromatic ring of the tryptophyl residues.

Such a blue or a red shift can arise by introducing positive (K^+) or negative (Cl^-) charge near the chromophore (the amide group) which might interact directly with the π electron system of the amide group [124].

When 8M urea was mixed with 0.03M KCl, the same shift in λ_{max1} was observed when 8M urea was used alone with CEA. This means that the shift caused by mixture may be due to the effect of urea, but not to 0.03 M KCl.

As was seen, the changes occurred in absorption were near 230 nm and near 280 nm. This was also observed by Glazer who noted that solvent perturbation or denaturation of protein produces many changes in absorption near 230 nm and 280 nm. Some of this change in absorption may be produced by change in the $n \rightarrow \pi^*$ absorption of polypeptide bonds in the protein either because of a change in their geometrical arrangement, or because of an environmental changes[125].

Spectrophotometric pH Titration of Purified CEA (Structural Studies)

Spectrophotometric pH titration is followed the changes in absorbance of the chromophore with increasing pH. Many studies of protein structure require the determination of pka values for proton dissociation from ionizable amino acid side chains, because these values give an indication of the location of the amino acid in the protein. This can often be done spectrophotometrically because dissociation often changes the spectrum of one of the chromophores, the observation of tyrosine dissociation was performed by measuring the absorption at 295 nm (λ_{max} for the ionized form of tyrosine), and the observation of histidine dissociation was carried out by measuring the absorption at 211 nm [198].

(Fig 3–18) shows the pH titration curves of CEA for tyrosine and histidine respectively. (A) Curve show that the pka values for tyrosine is 9.02, while the pka values for histidine in (B) Curve was equal to 5.5

In (Fig 3–18), the spectral changes as a function of pH for ionizable groups (i.e., the OH of tyrosin, imidazol of histidine) have the same pka as it would be if they were free in solution then the amino acid tyrosine and histidine in CEA are located on the surface of the protein [88].

From the same fig it was found:
(1) About 53% of tyrosine are located on the surface of purified human CEA molecule.
(2) About 47% of tyrosine residues are buried interior the folded structure of purified CEA.
(3) About 67% of histidine residues are located on the surface of purified human CEA molecule.
(4) About 33% of histidine residues are embedded in the interior region of purified CEA molecule.

The internal tyrosine residues are in strongly non-polar environment. On the other hand, the histidine residues present on the molecule surface of purified CEA and internal histidine residues are likely to be in strongly polar environment.

Estimation of Absorption Coefficient (a_s)

Fig (3 – 19) show standard curve of purified CEA at (λ_{max} 280 nm. The specific absorption coefficient (a_s) $_{280}$ was found to be 4.16 ml.mg^{-1}.cm^{-1} according to Lamber Beer's Law as described in section (3 – 13).

This is not very high absorption coefficient; its sensitivity would have been detected as more than one- percent.

FTIR Spectroscopic Results [122,126,127]

FTIR spectroscopy serves as another qualitative tool to characterize nondestructively the principal classes of chemical groups that compose the CEAs under study and complements the information obtained from UV spectroscopy.

Comparison of the FTIR spectra of standard CEA and purified CEA in (Fig 3–20,3–21), show that both of them exhibit a similar series of bands indicating that the major types of chemical groups present in each of these samples are similar. The frequency positions of the bands remain remarkably constant for all two types of CEA (Table 3–5).

In this section highlight the most obvious distinctions in the two spectra and related them to the information obtained by UV spectroscopy.

Few groups constitute the major portion of these proteins and thus produce relatively strong absorption in the IR spectra. These groups include alkyl moieties, both methyl (-CH_3) and methylene (-CH_2-); amides (-NH-(-C=O)-; aromatic ring; carbonyls (-C=O); alkoxy (-C-O-); and hydroxyl (-OH) (Table 3 – 5 and Fig 3 – 20, 3 – 21). The spectra indicate that one other important constituent group, sulfhydral (-SH-), are also present, but, based on their relatively lower intensities, they probably occur in somewhat smaller quantities. For they're no marked distinction among the two type of CEA studied with respect to the identity of the major categories of functional groups present in the samples.

FTIR spectroscopy offers several advantages over older dispersive techniques. Among these are enhanced signal – to – noise ratios and higher frequency accuracy and reproducibility. These advantages are particularly important when one wishes to search for relatively small changes in a complex system [126-127].

Table (3-2): Purification steps of CEA from malignant breast tumor
(All details are explained in the text)

Purification step	Total protein (mg)	Total activity (CEA.con.) µg	Specific binding activity µg/mg	Yield (%)	Purification (fold)
1. crude extract	215	2795	13	100	1
2. PCA extract	85	2800	33	100	2.5
3. Ion Exchange Chromatography DEAE-Sephadex	8	800	100	28.6	7.7
4. Gel-filtration Sepharose CL-6B	0.725	625	862	22.36	66.3

Table (3-3): The effect of solvent polarity on λ_{max} value of purified CEA UV spectrum at pH 7
(All details are explained in the text)

solvent	λ_{max1} (nm)	λ_{max2} (nm)
Tris buffer (H$_2$O)	235	280
20% ethanol	222.4	300
20% EG	240	300.8
20% glycerol	225	300
20% PEG	241.6	300.6
20% chloroform	-	-
20% DMSo	-	-
20% Ether	-	-

Table (3-4): The effect of 8M urea, 0.03 M KCl and mixture of urea+KCl on the λ_{max} of CEA Spectra at neutral pH (7.2)
(All details are explained in the text)

solvent	λ_{max1} (nm)	λ_{max2} (nm)
Tris buffer (pH 7.2)	235	280
8 urea	249.6	-
0.03 KCl	230.4	297
Urea+KCl mix(1:1)	241	-

Table (3-5): infrared band of CEA
(All details are explained in the text)

Band cm^{-1}	Proposed assignment [122]	Relative intensity*
3300 br	-OH stretch (hydrogen-bonded hydroxyl)	vs
3068	-CH- stretch (aromatic; olefinic)	w
2930	-CH$_2$-asym stretch	w
2380	-CH$_3$-asym stretch	vw
2340	-CH$_2$-asym stretch	vw
1658	Amide I (hydrogen-bonded-C=O stretch	vs
1539	Amide II (hydrogen-bonded-NH bend)	s
1450	-CH$_3$ asy bend, -CH$_3$ sym bend (methoxy); aromatic ring stretch (ortho-di substituted)	ms
1394	CH$_3$ sym stretch at 2 or 3° carbon	s
1247	-C-O-stretch (aromatic ether, AOR; acid dimers with electron with drawing group); amide III (-C-N-Stretch)	ms
1168	Aromatic ring bending (para-and ortho- disubstituted); C-O-C Stretch (alky / ether)	s
1118	-C-O-Stretch (hydrated polyols and carbohydrates)	ms
933	-OH- bend carboxylic acid dimer	ms
700	?	
621	?	
528	Ring bend caromatic, para disubstituted	mw

*Relative peak intensity: vs, very strong; s, strong; ms, medium strong; m, medium; mw, medium weak; w, weak; vw, very weak.

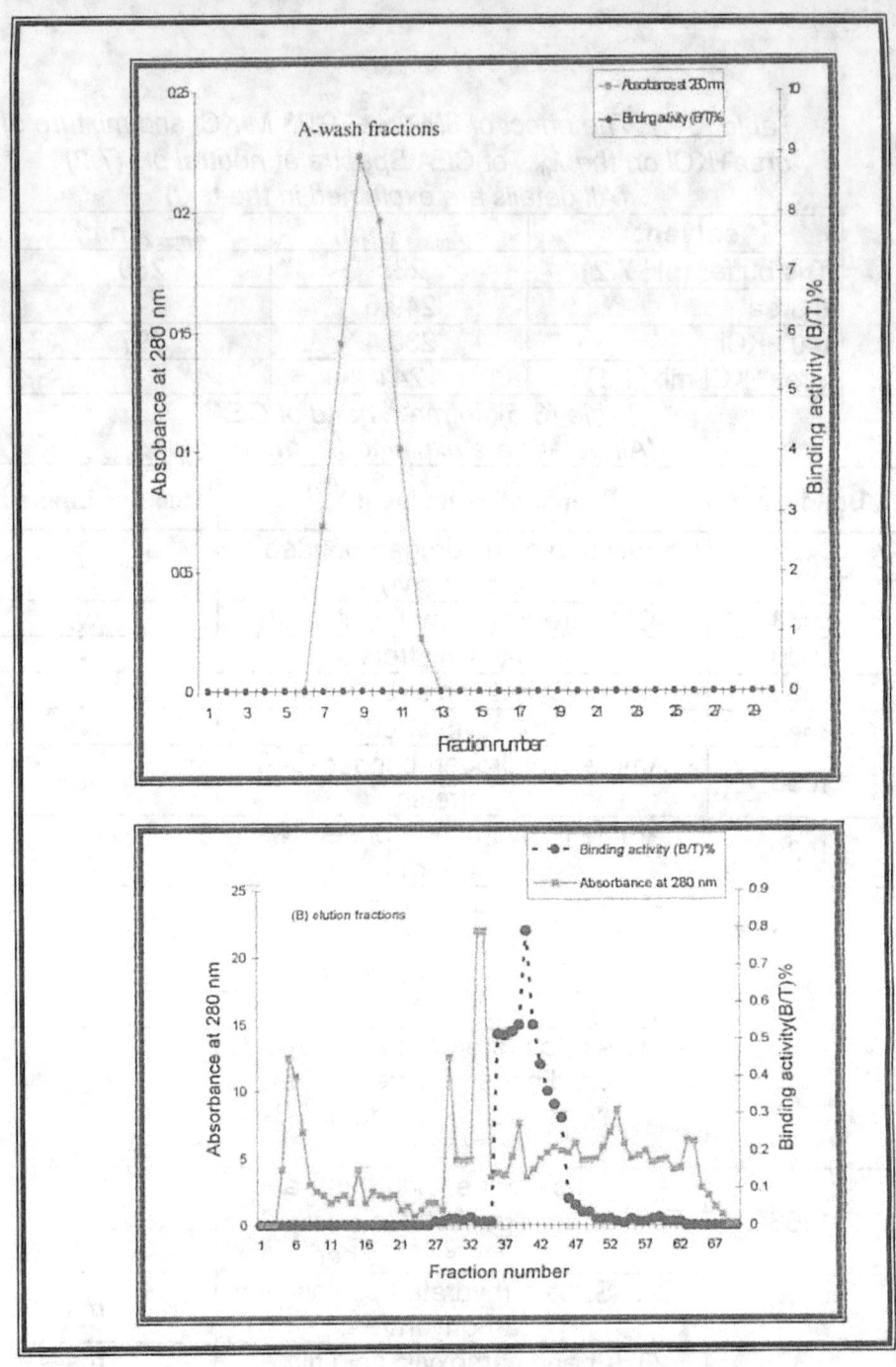

Fig. (3-2): Ion exchange chromatography of CEA Isolation on DEAE-Sephadex A50-column equlibirated with 0.02 Moler tris buffer . 2ml fraction were collected After washing with 60 ml of tris buffer (A-Fractions wash) .The column was developed with linear gradient of Sodium chloride ,0.00 - 0.3 M in tris buffer (B-elution fractions) .
(All details are explained in the text)

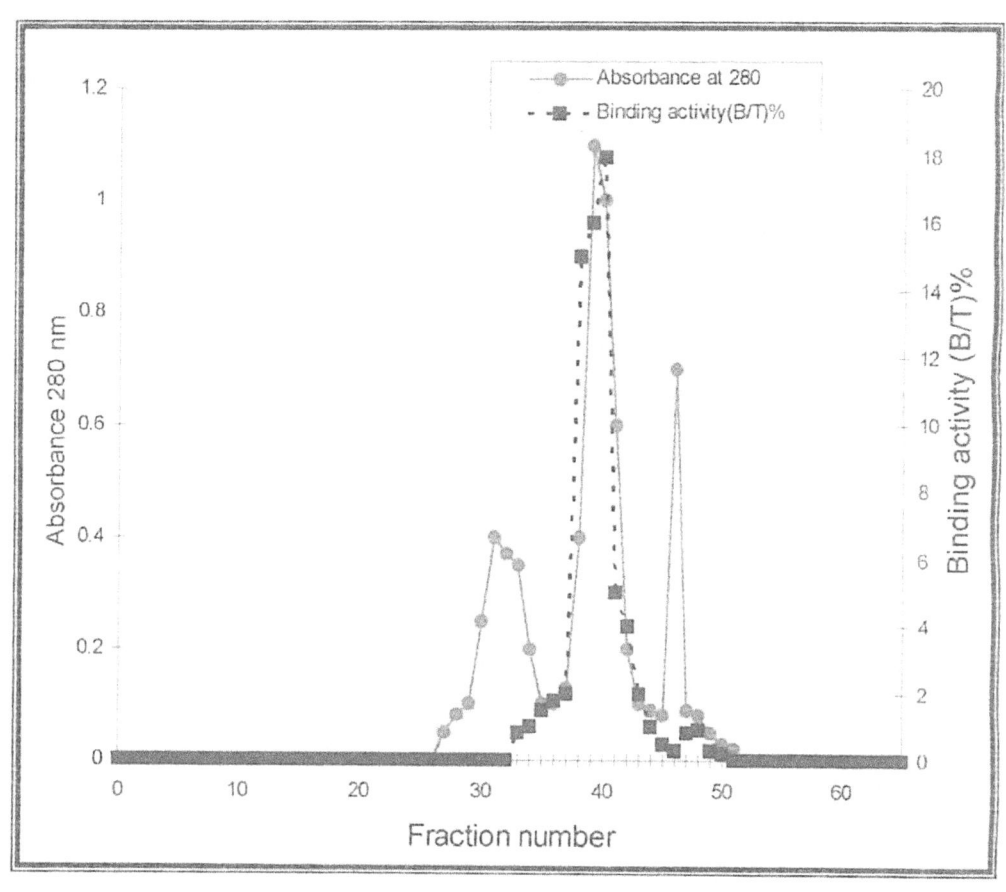

*Fig (3-3): Gel filtration profile of CEA on sepharose CL – 6B column
(All details are explained in the text)*

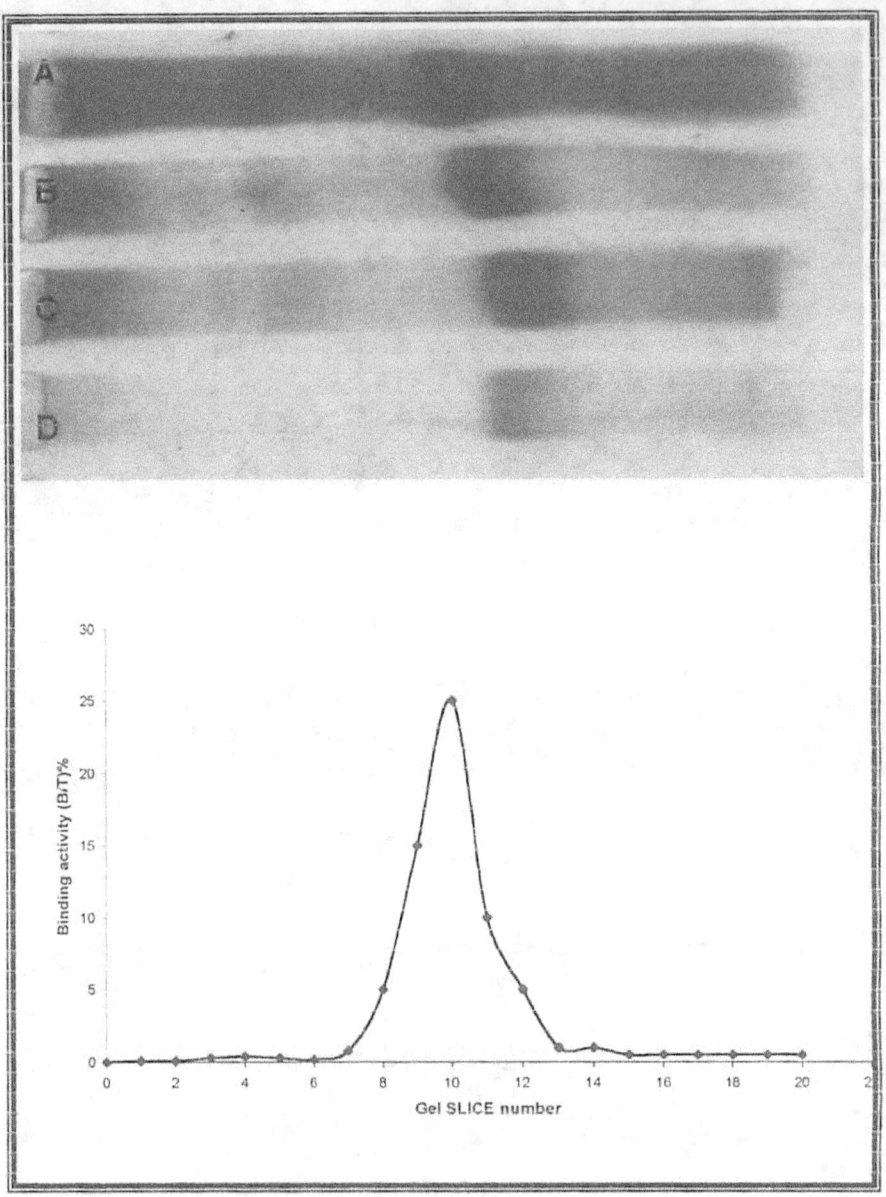

*Fig. (3-4): Conventional – PAGE profile of CEA purification.
Fraction, A-D products of purification steps 1-4 as
described in table (3-3), and the binding activity in each
0.5 cm gel slice
(A)= Crude extract
(B)= Partially purified CEA by PCA
(C)= CEA purified by Ion exchange step
(D)= Finally purified CEA
(All details are explained in the text)*

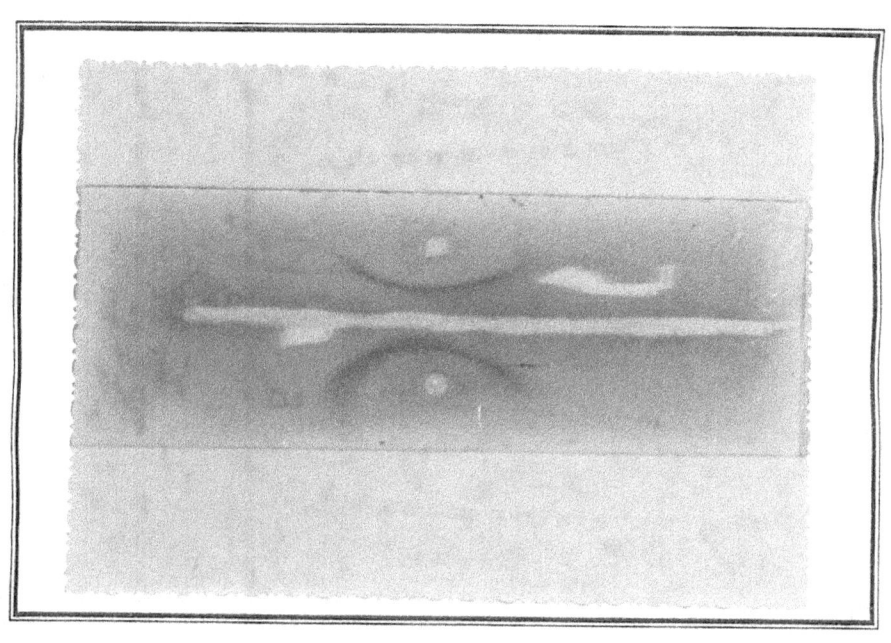

Fig. (3 – 5): Immunoelectrophoretic pattern of purified CEA preparation. The upper well contains CEA standard, and lower well contains purified CEA of human mammary carcinoma.

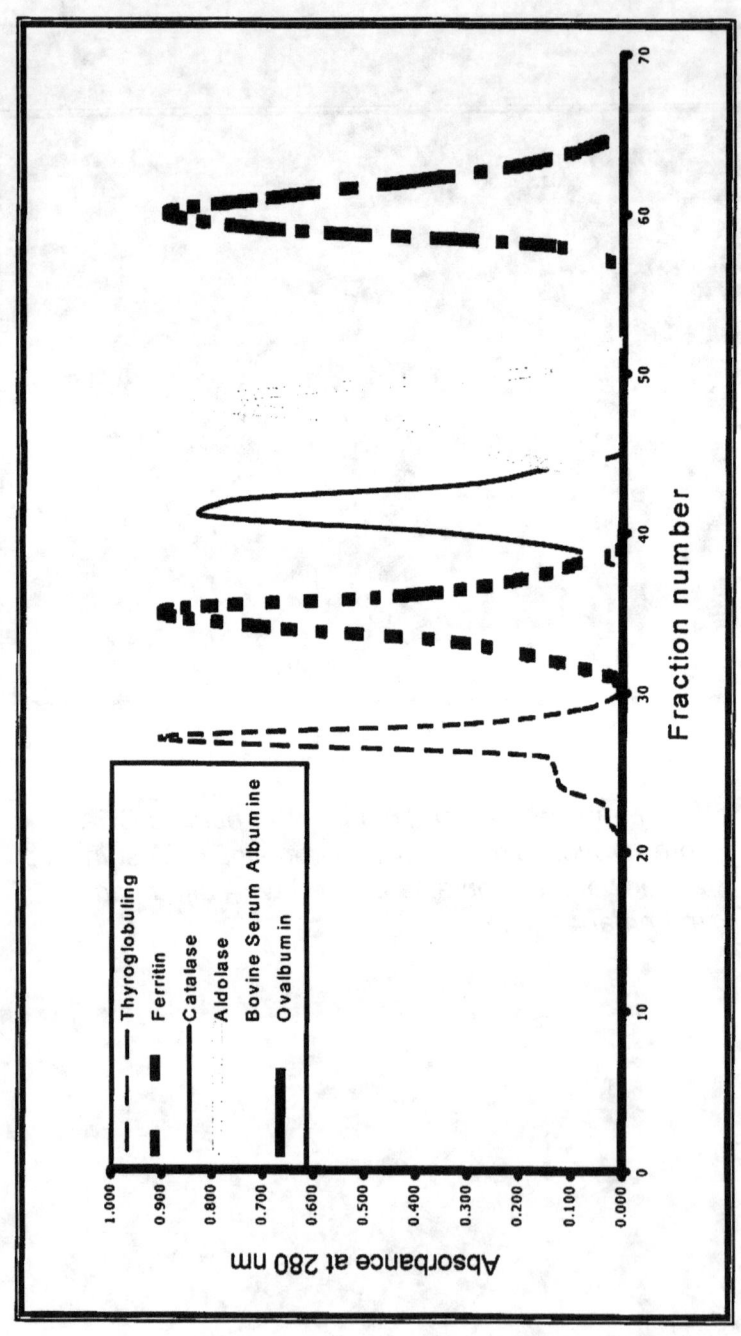

Fig (3-6) Sepharose CL-6B Chromatography of standard proteins of Pharmacia gel filteration kit
(All details are explained in the text)

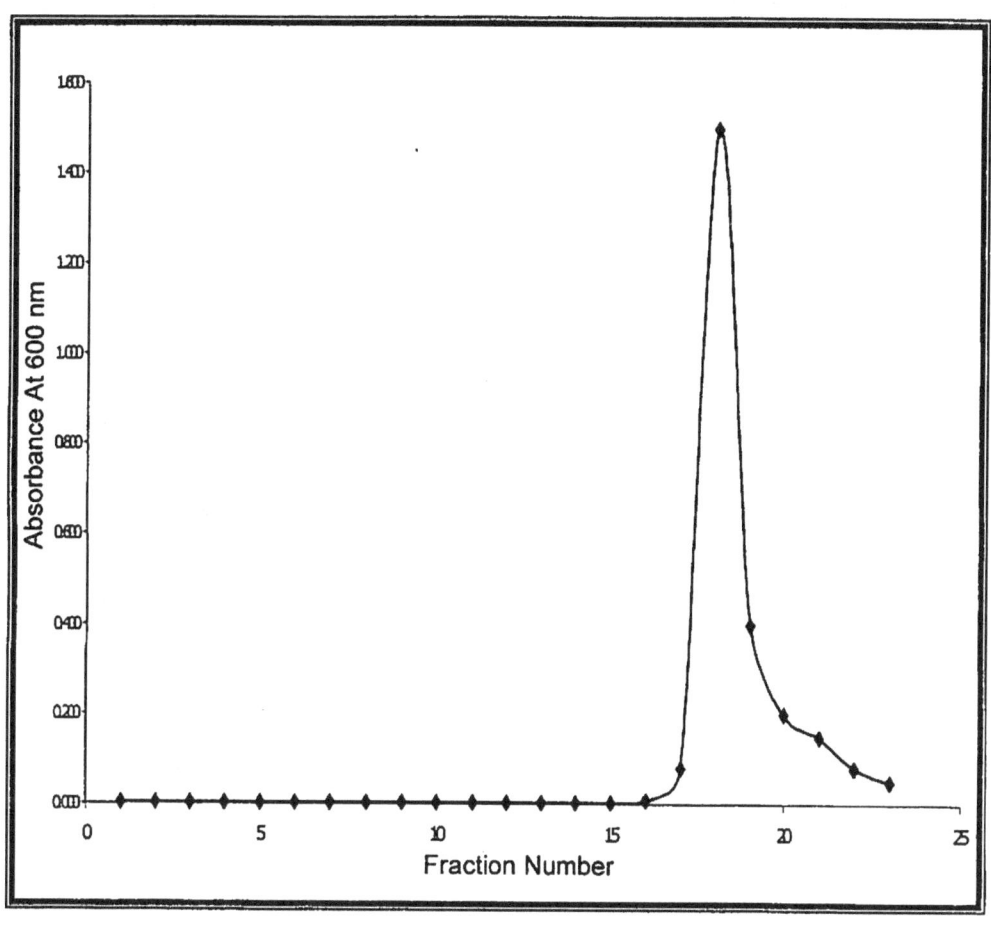

*Fig (3-7) Sepharose 6B-CL Chromatography of Blue Dextran 2000
(All details are explained in the text)*

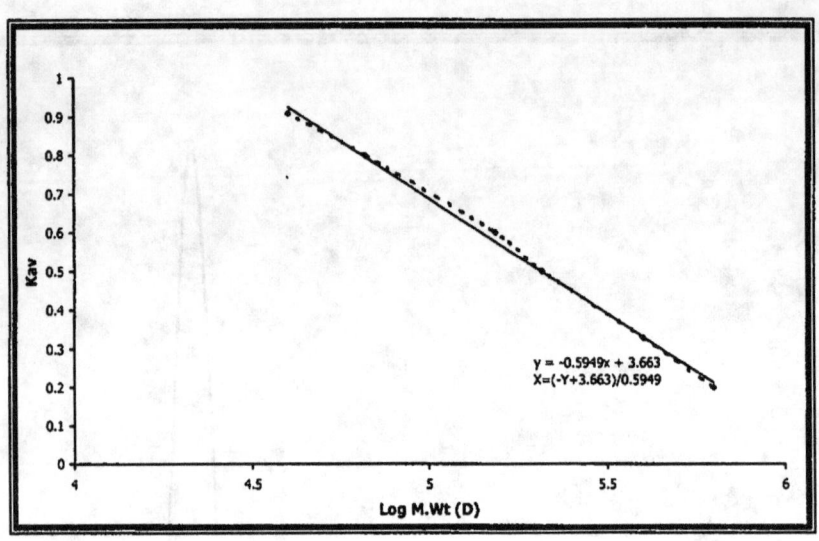

Fig. (3-8): Calibration Curve for Determination of M.wt by gel filtration Chromatography
(All details are explained in the text)

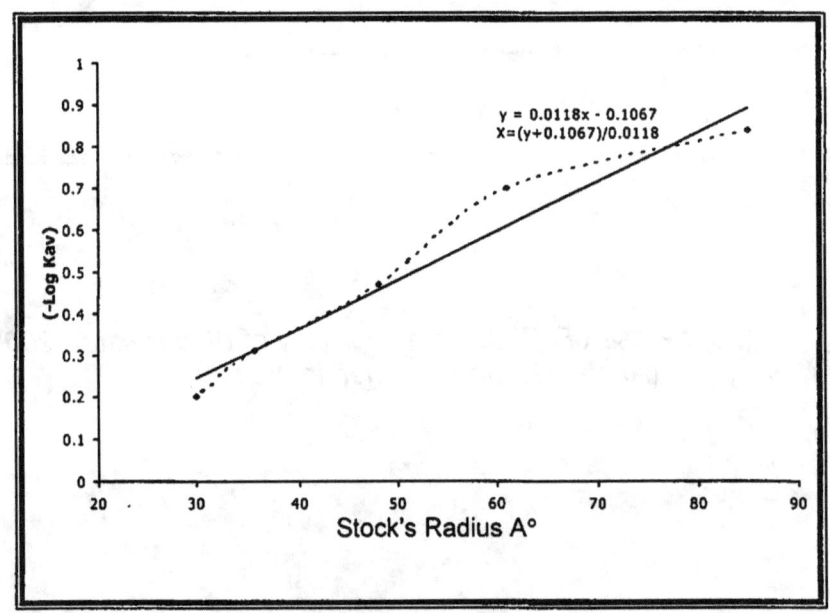

Fig 3-9 Calibration Curve for estimation of stock's radius by gel filtration
(All details are explained in the text)

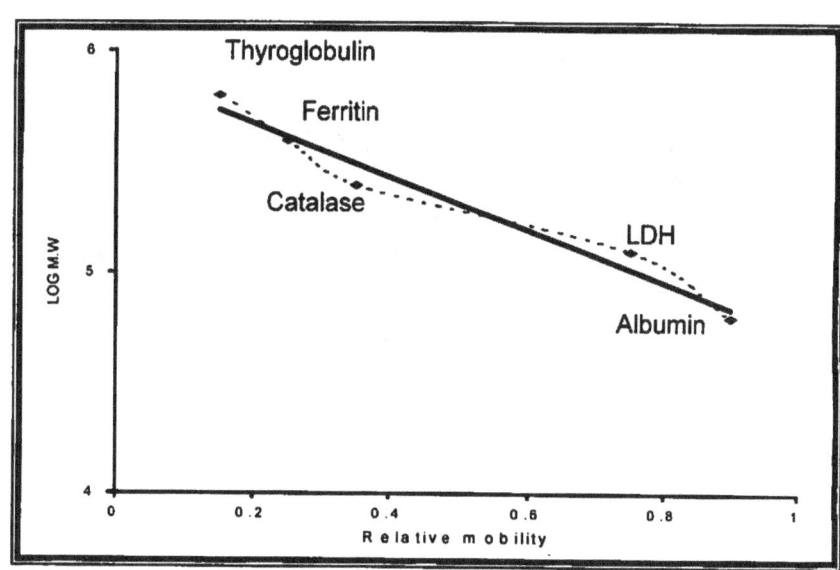

Fig. (3-10): calibration Curve for determination of M.wt by SDS – polyacrylamide gel disc electrophoresis. (All details are explained in the text)

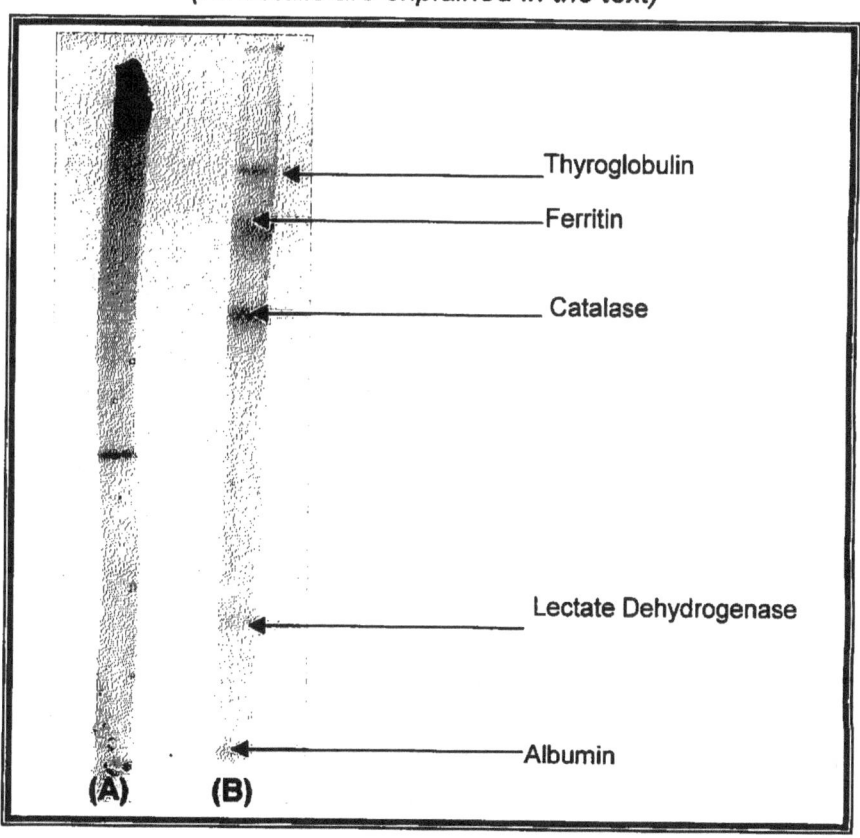

Fig. (3-11):SDS-PAGE disc electrophoresis. illustrate the electophoretic profile of finally purified CEA (A) and high M.wt standard protein (B). the anode is to the buttom (All details are explained in the text)

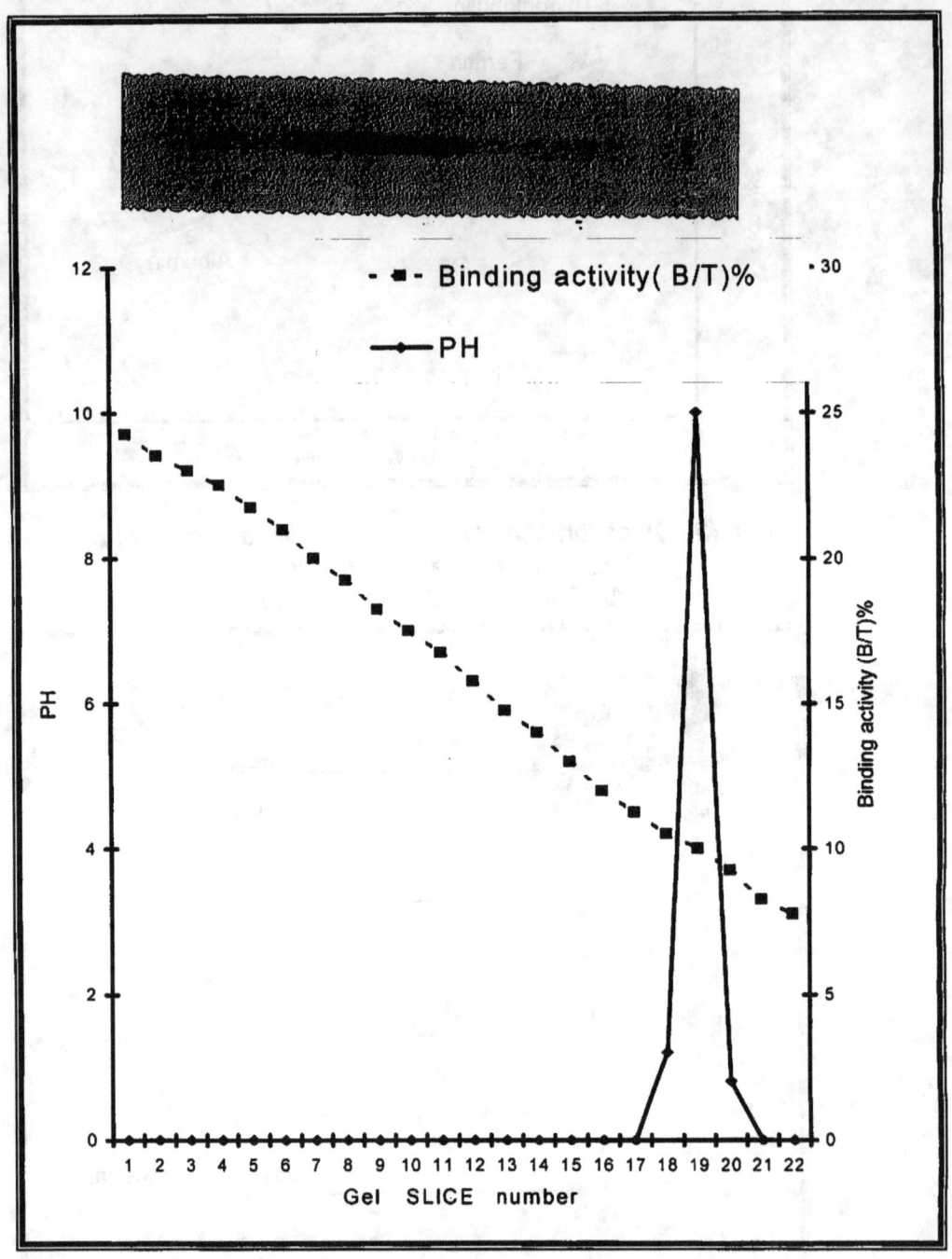

Fig. (3-12): Isoelectric focusing profile of purified CEA
(All details are explained in the text)

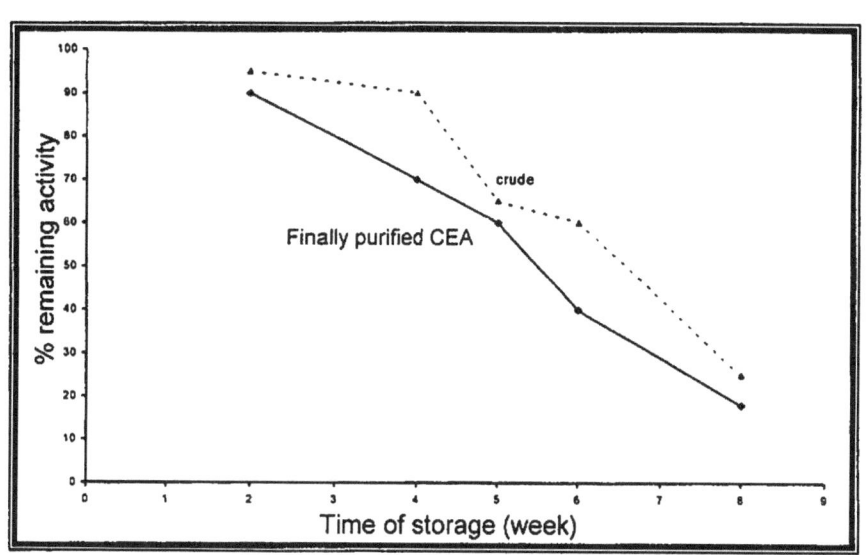

Fig (3-13) : stability of purified CEA and crude CEA storage at -20° C (All details are explained in the text)

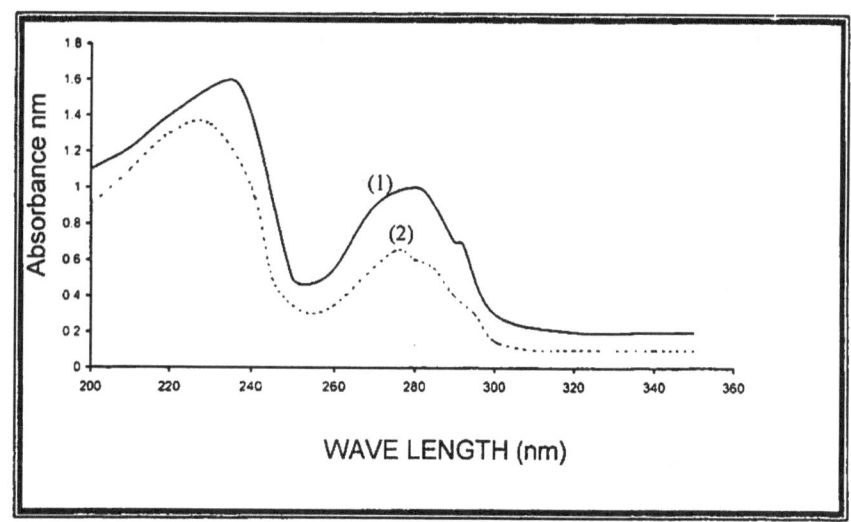

Fig (3-14) : The UV. spectrum of human CEA in Tris buffer at netural pH (7.2) ,(1)highly purified CEA from mammary carcinoma (2) standard CEA (All details are explained in text)

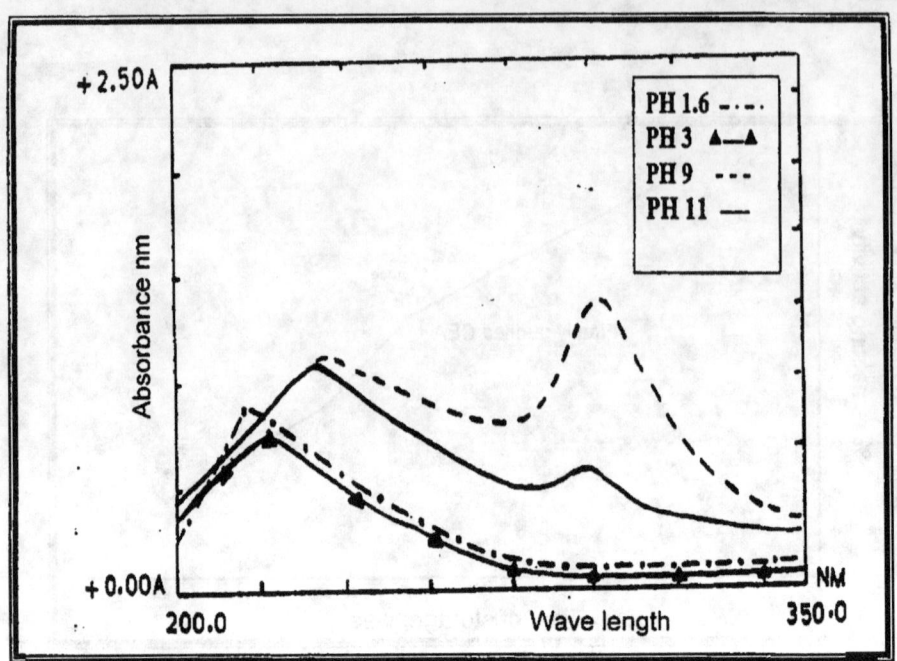

Fig. (3-15): The effect of pH on UV Sepectrum of human mammary Carcinoma
(All details are explained in the text)

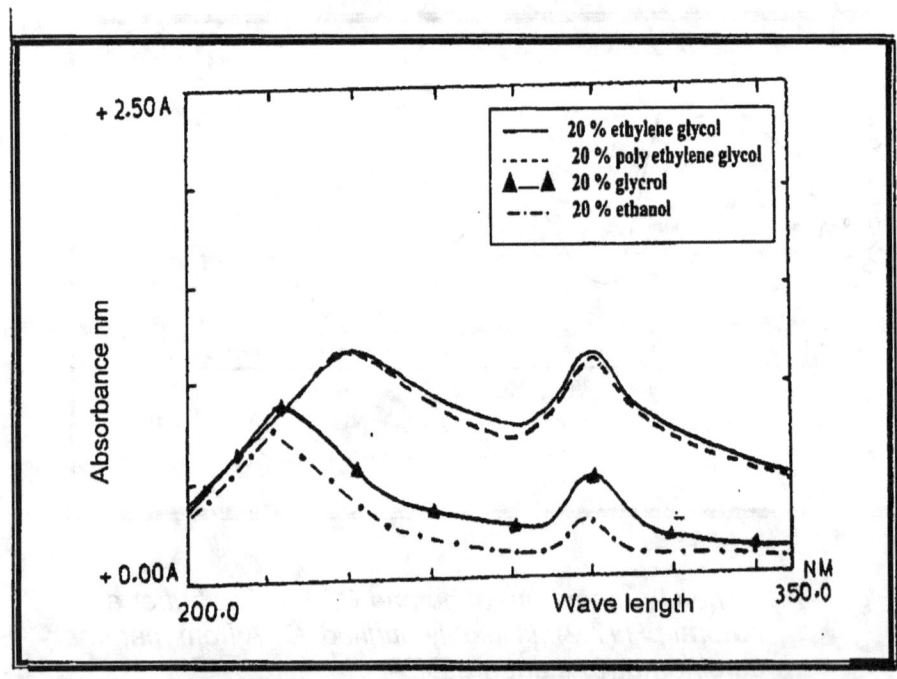

Fig. (3-16): The difference spectra obtained with human CEA from mammary carcinoma at neutral pH (7.2) in presence 20% ethylenglyycol, 20% polyethylenglyycol, 20% glycrol, 20% ethanol.
(all details are explained in the text)

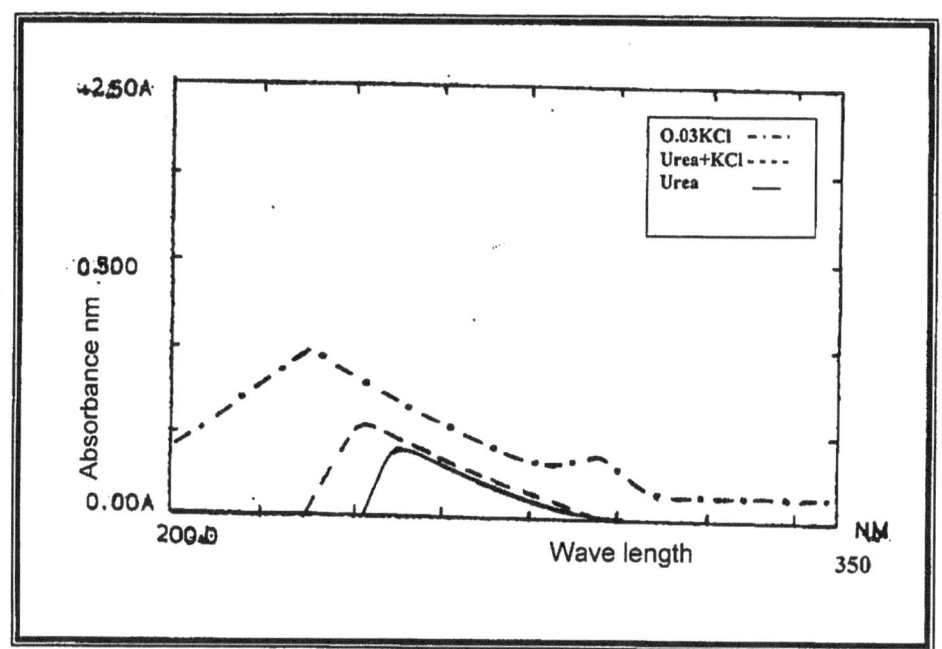

Fig. (3-17): The effect of 8M-Urea, 0.03 MKCl and mix (1:1) of 8M urea+0.03 MKCl on the human CEA UV spectrum at pH 7.2
(All details are explained in the text)

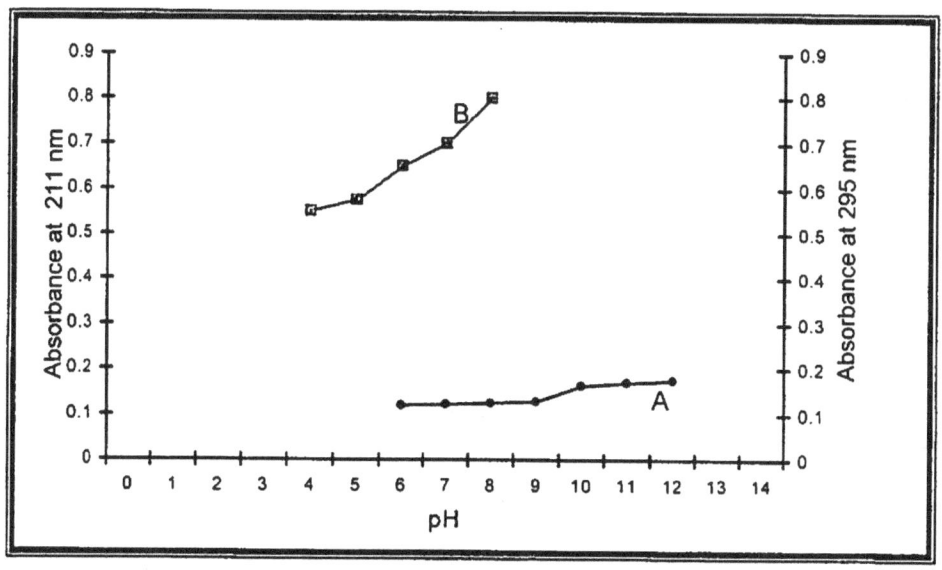

Fig. (3-18): Spectrophotometric titration of human CEA for:
(A) Tyrosine residues
(B) Histidien residues
(All details are explained in the text)

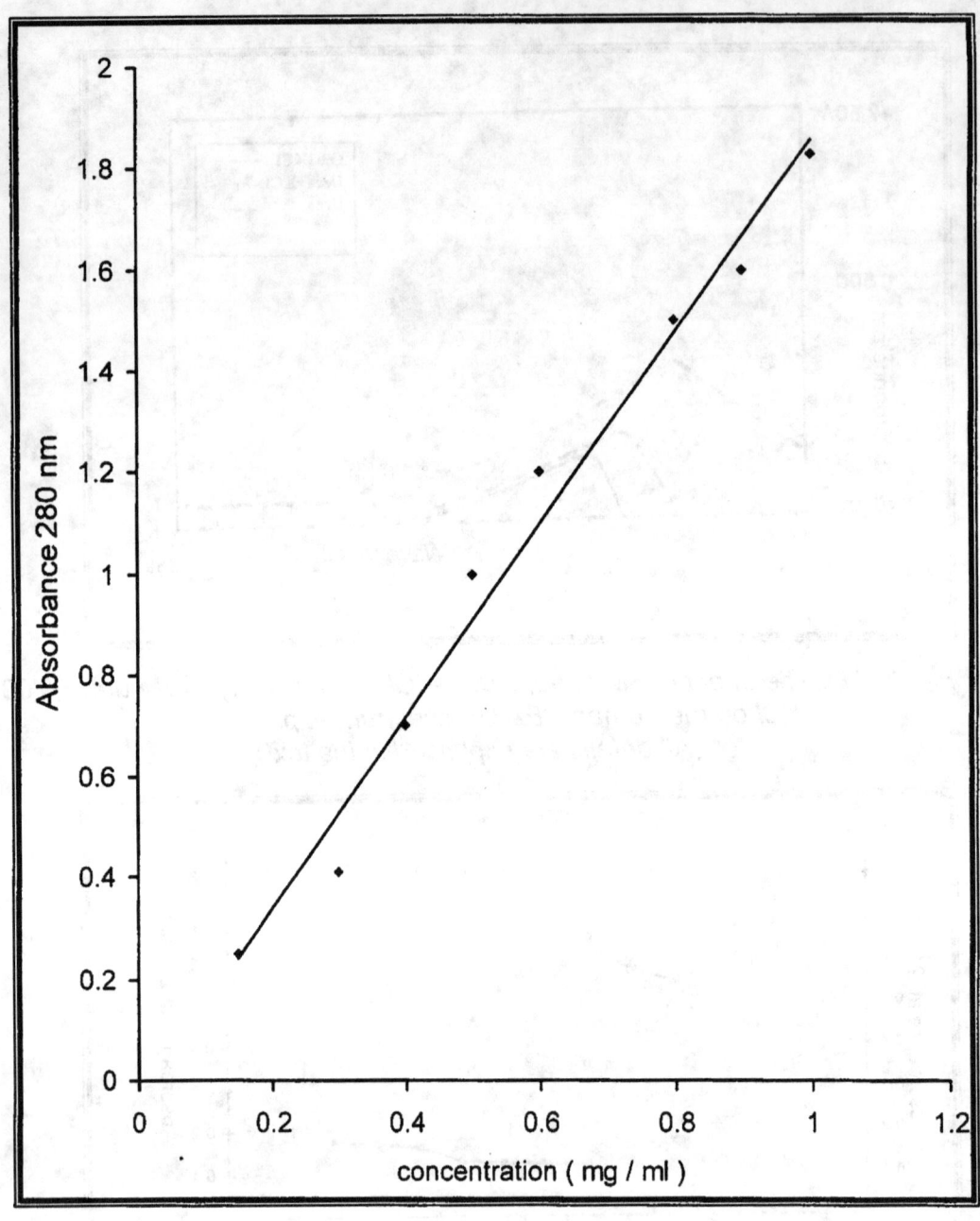

Fig. (3-19): *Calibration curve for estimation of Absorption Coefficient (a_s) (All details are explained in the text)*

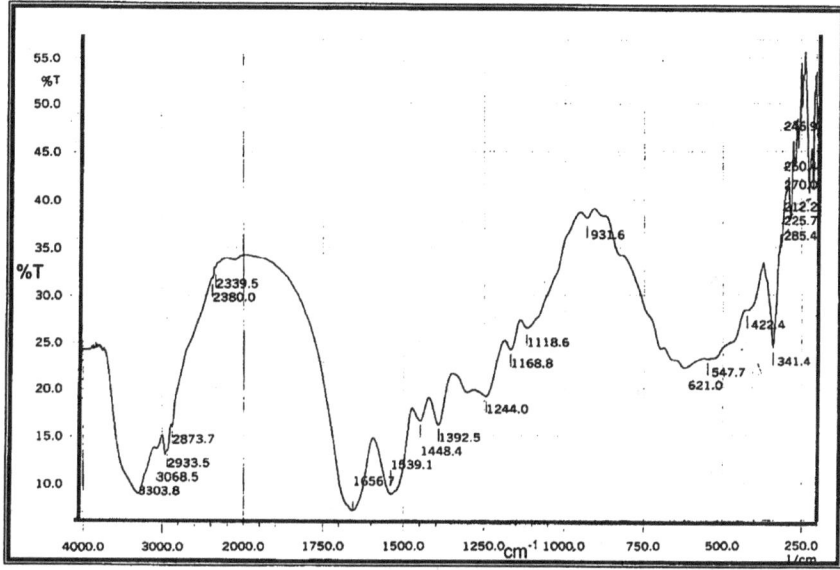

Fig. (3-20): FTIR Spectra of human CEA from mammary carcinoma
(All details are explained in the text)

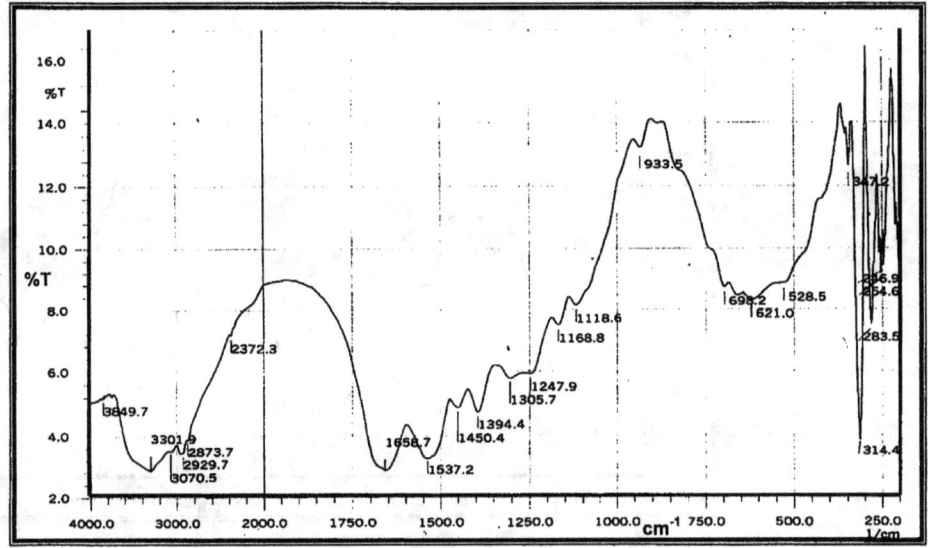

Fig. (3-21): FTIR Spectra of standard CEA
(All details are explained in the text)

CHAPTER FOUR

PREPARATION OF CEA Kit.

Abstract

(1) Highly purified carcinoembryonic antigen (CEA) from Breast carcinoma extracts was labeled with radioiodine according to the chloramine –T– method. The specific radioactivity of radioiodin-ated – CEA was 15.2 µci/µg.

❖ The immunoreactivity of ^{125}I–CEA has been investigated using several immunochemical techniques. The results showed that the ^{125}I–CEA preparation was homogeneous and did not aggregate or losses of antigen reactivity during iodination reaction.

❖ The concentration of the labeled tracer (^{125}I–CEA) preparation, was assessed by self-displacement method. Each milliliter of the radioactive solution was shown to contain 450 nanograms of labelled tracer (^{125}I–CEA).

(2) Antiserum to human CEA was obtained from rabbits by Intravenous inoculation with highly purified CEA.

❖ Monospecific anti-CEA was isolated and purified from other- immunoglobuline subclasses and some serum proteins by ammonium sulfate percipitation at 41% saturation and DEAE-cellulose ion exchange chromatography.

❖ The characterization of purified anti-CEA was carried out through cellulose acetate electrophoresis, ouchterlony double diffusion and by immuno electrophoresis, with these techniques, single precipitin line was observed between the anti-CEA and CEA.

(3) A process is described for the chemical attachment of anti-CEA antibody to the surface of polystyrene tubes. The dizo-polystyrene coupled to rabbit anti-CEA has been used to develop method of solid-phase of radio immuno-assay ((RIA). Incubation is performed in antibody-coated, diazo-polystyrene tubes that are finally washout with water and counted for quantitation of the bound tracer. The solid-phase RIA is simple, rapid, inexpensive, and suitable for automation.

(4) To evaluate the clinical applicability, CEA level was determined in 31 women, including 15 normal (control) and 16 breast cancer patients. Using two immunologic techniques which depended on competition; the techniques used were. Liquid-phase RIA and solid-phase RIA. The results obtained were compared in terms of sensitivity, specificity, simplicity, reproducibility, Accuracy, and convenience for us in routine diagnosis.

Introduction

During the past years various modifications of radioimmunological methods have been applied to the detection, assay and measurement of CEA activity in the biological fluids.

The radioimmunoassay for CEA then becomes important in several respects [128].

(1) It is used, to define the immunological criteria for CEA.

(2) It is used, as method of identification of CEA during isolation, and of demonstration of increase of specific activity with purification.

(3) Chemical manipulations of CEA designed to determine the structure of the tumor site are assessed in terms of their effect on the immunologic activity of molecule as measured by the radioimmunoassay.

(4) The radioimmunoassay, because of its ability to measure small amounts of material in serum, is the method of CEA measurement, which has been applied to the clinical situation.

The radioassay for CEA are most often identified by the procedure used to separate the antibody-bound from free fraction of the antigen.

The original assay procedure [129] referred to as the "Farr" or ammonium sulphate technique, utilizes a perchloric acid extraction step and takes advantage of solubility of CEA in half-saturation of ammonium sulphate.

The z-gel technique [130] also utilizes a perchloric acid extraction step and achieves separation of bound and free antigen by precipitating the anti-CEA-^{125}I-CEA complex with zirconyl phosphate gel. A similar procedure, using zirconyl phosphate gel, but omitting the initial extraction steps has also been developed [131]. An alternative technical approach to the problem of separation of bound and free antigen has been carried out by the precipitation of anti-CEA-^{125}I-CEA by second antibody with specificity toward the anti-CEA antibody [132,133].

Generally, the radioimmunoassay consists of three-steps [134]:

(1) Competitions step in which labeled tracer and either standard antigen competes for limiting specific antiserum.
(2) A separation steps in which antibody-bound label is separated from free label.
(3) The data collection and calculation process.

The RIA for CEA has several advantages over other methods for quantitation of this tumor marker, most importantly, the RIA provides direct measurement of amount of CEA protein and can be performed on the tissue extracts. Further, the RIA is very sensitive, highly reproducible, and simple to perform[135-137].

The goal of this study is to develop successful RIA technique to provide quantitative and sensitive assay that is simple and reliable enough for clinical application.

MATERIALS AND METHODS

4-1 Preparation of Purified CEA Solution (Antigen) for Immunization and Standard

(A) Reagent of the experiment:

1. Physiologic saline solution.
2. Lyophilized CEA.

(B) preparation:

The CEA utilized in this study was prepared as described in chapter 3 – section (3-1). 5mg Dry lyophilized CEA were dissolved in sterile physiologic saline solution. The immunogen solution (CEA) was stored as 0.5-ml aliquots in plastic vials at -20° C, this is a stock CEA solution.

At the time of use, the frozen preparation was thawed and diluted with physiological saline solution. All preparation procedure were carried out under sterile conditions.

4-2 Immunization and Antiserum Generation

(A) Experimental Animals

Twenty-four immature, 3-4 month old, female New-Zealand rabbits were selected at random from the laboratory house of the AL RAZIE center in Baghdad. They were maintained under the same light period and temperature throughout the period of experiment and received food (green fodder) and water.

(B) Experimental Design

The rabbits were randomly assigned to six groups of 4 animals each. Rabbits of each group were placed in a cage 130x70x60 cm. and treated as shown in Table (4-1), each group of rabbits received variable concentration of CEA in marginal ear vein over a period of 21 days. The injection schedule is shown in Table (4-1). Similar volume of the physiological saline solution, instead of CEA solution, was administered in marginal vein to the rabbits of control group. After the last injection the rabbit was left for (7-10) days.

Table (4-1) Injection Schedule for Immunizing Immature Female Rabbits Against CEA
(All details are explained in the text)

Group rabbit	CEA concentration (μg)							Total Does Conc. (μg)
	first day	4th day	8th day	12th day	15th day	18th day	21st day	
1	20	30	45	60	90	120	150	515
2	20	40	55	75	100	150	200	640
3	20	50	65	90	120	180	240	765
4	20	70	85	110	150	200	275	910
5	20	80	100	130	160	220	300	1010
6 (control)	0	0	0	0	0	0	0	0

(C) Isolation of Rabbit Serum Anti-CEA Antibodies:

1. Ten mls of blood were drawn from the heart of immunized rabbit 7th day after last inoculation, then the blood was poured into a sterile centrifuge tube and was left for 30 min, (to let the blood clot).
2. The blood was centrifuged 10 min at 500 xg. Then the serum was aspirated and divided into several 0.5-ml aliquots then stored at −20°C until use.

❖ The detection test of specific antibody (anti-CEA- ABS) was carried out by ouchterlony double diffusion.
❖ The sera obtained from the control group were used as controls in the assay.

4-3 Ouchterlony Double Diffusion in Gel (138,139)

The gel used was 1.1% agarose in barbitone buffer, the pH 8.2, the ionic strength (μ)=0.1 [16 g sodium barbitone, 3g 5,5 diethyl barbituric acid, 0.2g sodium azide, 1000 ml distilled water].

The reagents were dissolved by steaming at 100° C.

Glass plates 10x10 cm were used as a support for the gel. The plates were cleaned with soap and water, rinsed well in water, distilled water and finally dipped in acetone. The clean plates were precoated with molten agarose (0.2% in water) using a small brush, and placed in an incubator at 60° C until they become dry. The precoated plates were then placed on a level surface and 20 ml of 1.1% molten agarose were introduced by means of a prewarmed pipette (60° C) so as to obtain a homogeneous gel of about 2mm thickness. When the gel had settled, wells were prepared using cork borers as cutters to produce wells according to a matrix drawn on paper placed under the gel plate.

The soluble antigen 10µl with concentration (2mg/ml) was placed in the central well (4 mm in diameter) and the concentrated serum samples (10µl) were placed in the six outer wells (12 mm in diameter) at a distance of 7 mm (edge to edge) from the central well. Diffusion was allowed to proceed for 24 hours at 25° C and for a further 24 hours at 4° C in a humid chamber. The plates were subsequently examined directly for presence of precipitation band.

When it was desired to stain the plates, they were washed in phosphate buffer saline (PBS), pH 8.0 (containing 0.1% sodium azide) at 4° C for 2 days; during this time the plates were pressed for 15 minutes twice daily under 1 Kg weight, after being covered with one wet and several dry filter papers, so as to remove as much as possible of the unprecipitated proteins. The plates were then washed in distilled water for 3 hours, pressed, dried completely in stream of hot air stained with ponceau S stain for 10 min, rinsed briefly with distilled water.

Finally destaining was performed in destaining solution (450 ml ethanol, 450 distilled water, 100 ml glacial acetic acid). For 10 min or until a colourless background was obtained in (three washes, 10 min each, were sufficient to obtain a clear background).

4-4 Rabbit Anti-CEA Immunoglobulin Purification (140-142)

Sera with the highest antibody titre, as checked by agar double diffusion, were used for the preparation of mono specific-anti-CEA immunoglobulins. The procedure was as follows:

(A) Salt precipitation:

Dissolve 25 g ammonium sulphate in 100 ml antiserum, the addition was gradual and involved continuous stirring. The mixture was left to stand for at least 3 h at room temperature, centrifuged at 4000 g for 30 min and the supernatant was discarded. The precipitate was washed twice with 41 percent saturated ammonium sulphate.

(B) Dialysis:

The precipitate was transferred to the dialysis bag by adding small amount of distilled water. Dialysis was carried out at 4° C in a 250 ml beaker twice for 12 h against distilled water, once for 24 h against 0.05 M phosphate buffer pH 6, twice for 12 h against water, and once for 24 h against acetate buffer. The precipitate was removed, the supernatant concentrated by dialysis against polyethylene glycol 6000 was conducted. This preparation was then stored at -20° C in 8-ml aliquots and was later used as starting material for isolating anti-CEA by ion-exchange chromatography.

(C) Ion-Exchange Chromatography [143-147] *:*

1. *Preparation of chromatography column:*

    This was conducted on a pre-swollen diethylamino-ethyl cellulose (DEAE), using 40x2.5 cm column. As suggested by the manufacturer and according to the dimensions of the ion–exchanger bed, the required amount of DE52 cellulose was suspended in the required amount of acid component (NaH_2PO_4) of 0.5 M phosphate buffer, pH7. The slurry was then degassed using vacuum pressure, along with continuous stirring using a magnetic stirrer.

The slurry was filtered in a Buchner funnel using a 15cm filter paper (Whatman 54) under reduced pressure provided by a venturi water pump.

The filtrate was discarded and the ion-exchanger then suspended in the basic component (Na_2HPO_4) of the same buffer.

The ion-exchanger was then washed once with a 0.1M phosphate buffer pH7.

Equilibration of ion-exchanger was achieved by repeated buffer washing (using the starting buffer which was always a 5mM phosphate buffer, pH 7) until the filtrate had exactly the same pH of the strating buffer.

Fines were then removed by leaving the slurry to stand for about 30 minutes. After this, some of supernatant buffer containing fines was removed. A fresh starting buffer was then added. This final preparation was then packed into the column.

For re-use, the DE52 column was dismantled and the ion-exchanger was washed with strong salt solution (0.5M NaCl), and then with a 0.1M phosphate buffer, pH 7.6. Equilibration, removal of fines and packing of the column was performed as described before.

2. *Separation Procedure:*

An aliquot (8 ml) of rabbit serum gamma-globulin preparations, which were already dialyzed against the starting buffer, were applied in five ml a liquidate to DE52 columns (with bed dimensions of 30 by 2.5 cm, flow rate 45 ml per hour) This was followed by starting buffer (0.05 M phosphate buffer, pH7).

After elution with 100 ml of 5-mM phosphate buffer, a 5-30 Mm phosphate, pH7, gradient then was begun.

The 3ml fractions were collected until absorbace returns to background.

❖ Follow the absorption at 280 nm for each fraction.

4-5 Methods Used for Identifica-tion of Pure Anti-CEA Immunoglobulins

Both Anti-sera preparations and Anti-CEA immunoglobulin were purified, checked for impurity and specificity by the following techniques.

A- Cellulose acetate electrophoresis [148, 149].

Solutions.

1. Barbital buffer (0·05 M, pH 8. 6)
   The powder of this buffer was dissolved in 1000 ml deionized distilled water to obtain buffer (0.05 M, pH 8.6) This solution was stable for 2 months at (15-30)° C.
2. Ponceau S stain prepared as described in section (3-3 C).
3. Acetic acid (5%).
   Fifty milliliter of acetic acid was completed with deionized distilled water to 1000 ml.
4. Liquid paraffin

Procedure:

1. Cellulose acetate paper was immersed for 5 min. in barbital buffer.
2. Cellulose acetate paper was then dried by filter paper and placed on the Instrument Bridge.
3. Microzone cell was filled with barbital buffer and the bridge was placed in the microzone cell.
4. Fifty microliter serum was withdrawn by applicator and laid continuously above the cellulose acetate paper
5. The cell was connected to power supply and the voltage. Current was raised gradually to reach 200 volts and 1mA respectively. The electrophoresis was continued for (20-25) min.
6. After the 25 min, the paper was immersed in ponceau S stain for 10 min, in order to fix the band in its position.
7. The paper was washed with acetic acid (5%) and the destining solution was changed several times until the stain has been removed.

8. The paper was dried for 30 min, then immeresed in liquid paraffin for 1 min, and the extra paraffin was removed and read in the instrument.
9. Refractometer and the scanned using a densitometer measured total protein concentrations.

B- Immune electrophoresis (IEP)

This was performed as described in chapter 3 section (3-3)

4-6 Preparation of Radiolabeled CEA

A- Radioiodination Reaction [150-152]:

The highly purified CEA (prepared as described in chapter 3) was radioiodinated by chloramin T method [150]. The reaction mixture contain 50 µg of the purified CEA in 50 µl of phosphate buffer (0.05 M. pH 7.3), 50 µg of chloramin – T in 50 µl of same diluent, and 0.5 mci of ^{125}I in 10 µl of dilute NaOH. The final pH of the reaction mixture was 8 to 9. The reaction was permitted to proceed for 60 sec at room temperature (23°) and was then stopped by addition of 100 µg of sodium metabisuifite in 100 µl of the phosphate buffer (prepared immediately before use).

B- Purification of radioiodinated CEA using gel filtration:

1. The gel was prepared by swelling 10 mg of sephadex G-25 in 100 ml of 50 mM phosphate buffer pH 7.4 for 24 hours at room temperature (about 30° C), then stored at 4° C to equilibrate it with the buffer.
2. The suspension was carefully mixed before pouring into vertical column (with diameter of 1.0 cm) containing eluant buffer. After the gel has settled, the column outlet was opened. Packing was continued until the gel reached stable bed high (45 cm), then the column was equilibrated with 50 mM phosphate buffer pH 7.4 with flow rate of 12 ml per hour, then the entire mixture was applied to the surface of the gel carefully to separate bound ^{125}I-CEA from the free ^{125}I.

Elution was carried out using the same buffer of equilibration with flow rate of 12 ml per hour with fraction volume of 1 ml, the radioactivity of each fraction was measured by gamma counter expressed in counts per second (CPS).

C- Calculation:

- The radioactivity of each fraction was plotted vs corresponding fraction number.

- The specific activity (SA) = $\dfrac{\text{Amount of radioactivity } (\mu ci)}{\text{Concentration of CEA } (\mu g)}$

- ^{125}I incorporation% = $\dfrac{\text{Total activity for pooled collection (cps)}}{\text{Total activity for 0.5 mci used in the reaction}} \times 100$

D- Storage of Radioiodinated Tracers:

Radioiodinated tracer could be stored at -20° C, then 10% propylene glycol was added.

4-7 Immunochemical and Physico-chemical Criteria of Iodinated CEA (^{125}I-CEA)

A- Convential disk SDS-PAGE

This was performed as described in chapter three section 3-6

B- Radial-ouchterlony reaction and radioimmunoelect-rophoresis (RIEP)

These were performed as previously described in section (4-3) and in chapter three section (3-3)

CLINICAL APPLICATION

Two radioimmunoassay (RIA) techniques have been established in this work directed toward the investigation of a basic problem in human tumor immunology dealing with breast cancer. These techniques are liquid phase and solid –phase RIA.

The principle of both techniques is based on that the unlabelled antigen competes with ^{125}I-CEA for a limiting amount of antibody. Displacement of ^{125}I-CEA by unlabelled in experimental samples is compared with that of known amount of purified CEA [153].

4-8 Liquid-phase Competition RIA

ASSAY CONDITION

(A) A mount of Anti–CEA

All the following experiments in this section were carried out in three sets, the first set to estimate the total binding, the second sets to determine the non specific binding and the third to measure the total count (CPM) for labeled (CEA) used in each tube (TC)

1. Each binding reaction (total volume 500 µl) was performed in untreated poly styrene tubes and consisted of 100 µl containing different amount of anti–CEA of (0.05, 0.1, 0.2, 0.3, 0.4, 0.5, 0.6, 0.8, 0.9 and 1 mg/ml stock solution) and 50 µl of radioiodinated CEA was added to each tube. The final mixture was completed to 500 µl using phosphate buffer (0.05 M, pH 7.3).
2. The second set of tubes consisted of the same reactants plus 10-fold excess of unlabelled CEA.
3. The third set of tubes (three tubes only) consisted only of 50 µl of radioiodinated CEA (^{125}I-CEA) in order to obtain total count (CPM)
4. All tubes were stopple and incubation was carried out for 24 h at 25°C ±1°C with moderate horizontal shaking.

5. At the end of this period, 500 µl of saturated ammonium sulfate was added to every tube (except the third set) with immediate vortex mixing. The tubes were kept at 4° C for 30 min and then centrifuged at 4000 g for 15 min at 4° C.
6. Aspiration of the contents of all tubes was then carried out carefully, except those for total CPM (third set)
7. Radioactivity was then measured for all tubes, bound count (B) and total CPM (TC); each sample was assayed in triplicate.

Calculations:

1. Correction of the count activity (CPM) of all tubes from background was carried out. (count activity for empty untreated polystyrene tubes)
2. Total binding (TB) represents the amount of radioactivity bound to the particulate fraction (CPM) in the absence of unlablled CEA.
3. The radioactivity of particulate fraction after maximum displacement of the labeled CEA by excess amount of unlabelled CEA is referred to as nonspecific binding (NB).
4. Specific binding (SB) is the difference between radioactivity (CPM) bound to the particulate fraction in the absence of excess unlabelled CEA (TB) and that bound in its presence (NB)

SB (CPM) = TB (CPM) − NB (CPM)

$$SB\% = \frac{SB\ (CPM)}{Total\ count\ (CPM)\ of\ labeled\ CEA\ used\ in\ each\ tube\ (TC)} \times 100$$

5. The value of SB% corresponding to the amount of Anti-CEA was plotted vs concentration (µg) of the anti-CEA.

(B) The amount of radioactive CEA (^{125}I-CEA)

1. In the first set of tubes, 60 µg of anti-CEA was incubated with different volumes of ^{125}I-CEA (10, 20, 30, 40, 50, 60, 70, 80, 90 and 100) µl and the volumes were made up to 500 µl with phosphate buffer (0.05 M, pH 7.3).
2. The second set of tubes consists of the same reactants as in step 1 plus 10-fold excess of unlabelled of CEA.
3. Parallel set of tubes consists of only the same quantity of radioiodinated CEA (^{125}I-CEA) used in step 1. These tubes were used for total count radioactivity (TC).
4. The steps 4, 5, 6, and 7 in section (4-8-A) were followed exactly.

Calculation:

(1) The method of calculation of the experiment (4-8 A) was followed exactly.
(2) The SB% was plotted against the radioactivity CPM corresponding to the concentration ^{125}I-CEA-used.

(C) Effect of Temperature:

Sixty µg of Anti-CEA was incubated with 50 µl of ^{125}I-CEA (0.5 ng, 40000 CPM) and then mixed with or without the addition of 10 fold excess of unlabelled CEA. The volume of the mixture was completed with phosphate buffer 0.05 M, pH 7.3. After incubation for 24 h at 25° C, the bound and free form of CEA were separated as described in the steps of experiment (4-8 A).

This experiment was then repeated at different temperatures (4, 10, 20, 30, 35, 40, 50° C).

The SB% was calculated as mentioned in section (4-8 A) and plotted vs. the temperature of incubation.

(D) Effect of Time

Sixty µg of Anti-CEA were added to 50 µl of ^{125}I-CEA (0.5 ng; 40000 CPM) in final volume of 500 µl (completed with phosphate buffer) with or without the addition of 10 fold excess of unlabelled CEA.

The tubes were then incubated at 25°C±1°C. at certain time intervals (0.25, 0.5, 1, 2, 4, 8, 16, 24, 48, and 72 h). Two tubes of each set were taken and SB% was estimated as mentioned in section (4-8 A) and plotted vs the time of incubation.

(E) Effect of pH:

To demonstrate the effect of pH, 60 µg of Anti-CEA were added to 50 µl (0.5 ng; 40000) of ^{125}I-CEA with or without the addition of 10 fold excess of unlabelled. The volume of the mixture was completed with different buffers at different pH values (2, 3, 4, 5, 6, 7, 8, 8.5, and 9) to 500 µl. The tubes were incubated for 24 hr at 25° C. the SB% was evaluated as revised in section (4-8-A).
The SB was plotted against pH.

(F) Ionic Strength Effect:

In order to investigate the effect of ionic strength on the binding 60 µl of anti-CEA was then added to 50 µl (0.5 ng; 40000 CPM) of ^{125}I-CEA with and without the addition of 10-fold excess of unlabelled CEA. The volume of the mixture was then completed with phosphate buffer pH 7.3 M 0.05 . After incubation for 24 h at 25° C, the SB% was estimated as described in section (4-8 A). The experiment was repeated at different concentration of phosphate buffer range (0.001, 0.01, 0.05, 0.08, 0.1, 0.2, 0.4, 0.6, 0.8, 1M). Also the experiment was repeated by using distilled water. The pH of the buffer solution was fixed at pH 7.3 at all concentration of phosphate buffer.
The SB% was then plotted vs. Molarity.

4-9 The Standard Curve

(A) Solutions:

1. CEA standards; different contentions of CEA were prepared by serial dilutions for stock purified CEA with phosphate buffer.
   The working range of the assay was constructed from 0 to 150 ng/ml. all standard solutions were conserved by sodium azide (< 0.1%) and stored at 4°C.

2. Anti-CEA solution (0.6 mg/ml).
3. ^{125}I-CEA solution (specific activity 15.2 µci per microgram of CEA)
4. Diluent: phosphate buffer pH 7.3, 0.1M
5. Untreated polystyrene tubes (13x50 mm)

(B) Procedure:

1. Number a triplicate series of untreated polystyrene tubes.
2. Sequentially, 100 µl of anti-CEA antibody to the bottom of tubes were added, followed by 100 µl of standard CEA (working range of the assay was from 0 to 150 ng/ml) and then 50 µl (~ 0.5 ng CEA, 40000 CPM) of ^{125}I- CEA was add to each tube The final volume was completed to 500 µl using phosphate buffer pH 7.2, 0.1 M.
3. Incubation of all tubes for 24 hr at 25±1° C with moderat horizontal shaking was carried out.
4. At the end period of incubation 500µl of saturated ammonium sulphate were added to each tube with immediated vortex mixing. The tubes were kept at 4° C for 30 min and then were centrifuged at 4000 g for 15 min at 4° C.
5. The supernatant was then aspirated; and the precipitate was washed once with distilled water.

(C) Calculation:

1. Correction count activity (CPM) for all tubes from background was carried out.
2. The mean of the CPM of standard minus nonspecific binding (assay tubes that contained large enough quantities of unlablled CEA) was divided by the mean of radioactivity bound (Bo) in assay tubes that contained no unlabelled CEA (minus nonspecific binding, and multiplied with the factor 100 in order to obtain the percentage of relative binding (B/Bo)%)

$$(B/B0)\% = \frac{B\ (CPM)_{corr} - NON\ specific\ binding}{B0\ no\ competitor - NON\ specific\ binding} \times 100$$

3. On arithmetic paper, the relative binding of each standard was plotted on y-axis versus the corresponding concentration (ng/ml) on X-axis, as shown in fig (4-14).
4. The concentration of the sample was directly interpolated from the standard curve by the use of their (B/B0)% value.

4-10 Solid-Phase Radioimmunoassay

4-10-1 preparation of Antibody Coated-Tubes [155-160]

A- Activation of Solid Phase Polystyrene Tubes. (50x13mm)

1. **Nitration step:**
   The inner surface of each polystyrene tubes were treated with 3 ml of 47% (v/v) HNO_3 (sp. gr. 1.42)-H_2SO_4 (sp. gr. 1.84). At 0° C, for 45 min, then the nitration reaction stopped by pouring the reaction mixture into a large volume of water, and the tubes was thoroughly washed with large volume of water (ten times with distilled water).
2. **Reduction step:**
   Three ml of 6% (w/v) of $Na_2S_2O_4$-2M KOH were added to each tube left for at least 4 hr, at 70° C, with moderate horizontal shaking.
   The tubes were washed with dil. HCl and then three times with water.

3. **Diazotization step:**

   Prepare solution containing: 1000-ml ice-cold water, 500-ml hydrochloric acid (1M) and 120-ml sodium nitrite (1M). This mixture of solutions was freshly prepared before use these carefully introduced into tubes, up to 3 cm, then left for 20 min, at 0° C. After that the tubes were washed quickly with 0.6 M HCl followed by ice-cold water repeated many time.

   B- Binding of Anti-CEA TO SOLID PHASE

   1. Prepare a stock solution containing 250 µg/ml anti-CEA in PBS, (10 mM, 150 mM NaCl, pH 8.3)
   2. Immediately after diazotization process, the diazo-polystyrene tubes filled with 1 ml of solution containing 250 µg/ml of anti-CEA in PBSpH 8.3. The tubes were capped and allowed to rotate slowly on a horizontal tray shaker for 6 hr at 4° C.
   3. At the end of reaction period (6h), the tube was then centrifuged at 1000 g for 10 min at 4° C. the supernatant was removed and saved. The tubes were washed many times with PBS (10 mM, 150 mM NaCl, pH 8.3) by successive centrifugation until the absorbance of the supernatant was less than 0.01.
   4. The protein content in the first supernatant and the following washing was estimated by Bardford method [161].
   5. Finally, the tubes were washed with distilled water then air drying; storage until use.

   C- Calculation:

   The amount of anti-CEA that bound to the tubes was determined by difference between the initial amount and that found in pooled solutions.

4-10-2 Assay Conditions:

To investigate the optimum conditions of binding ^{125}I-CEA with its diazo-polystyrene coupled to anti-CEA. The same protocol of the experiment in section 4-8 A, 4-8 B, 4-8 C, 4-8 D and 4-8 E were followed exactly except that the bound and free forms of ^{125}I-CEA were separated by aspiration of the contents at the end period of incubation time for each tube, and washing the immuno-complex formed twice with distilled water.

The SB% value was calculated as mentioned in same section (4-8 A, 4-8 B, 4-8 C, 4-8 D, 4-8 E). The condition were investigated included:

1. The quantity of radioactive CEA (tracer).
2. Time of incubation.
3. Temperature.
4. Buffer pH, and ionic strength.

4-11 The Standard Curve for Solid-phase RIA

The standard curve was constructed as described in section 4-9 except that it was performed in diazo-polystyrene coupled to anti-CEA instead of untreated polystyrene tubes.

The percent of binding (B/B0)% value were calculated as mentioned in same section (4-9) and the relative binding of each standard was plotted on Y-axis versus the corresponding concentration (ng/ml) on X-axis, as shown in fig (4-15).

4-12 Evaluation of CEA RIA kit

In this study, normal blood samples were obtained from 15 apparently healthy, (average age 24±5).

Also, blood samples were collected from 16 patients with histological proven breast tumor. (Average age 44.74±1.23)

The level of CEA was determined in duplicate in all sera samples, by both the liquid phase and solid phase RIA assay, using the same procedure mentioned in section 4-9 and section 4-11 were follow exactly.

CEA concentration in sera of samples were directly interpolated from standard curve by the use of their (B/Bo)% values.

4-13 The Assessment of 125I-CEA Concentration [162]

The concentration of the labeled tracer (^{125}I-CEA) was determined according to method of Morris[162] with little modification. The method is outlined in the following steps:

1. In a set of rabbit Anti–CEA coated tubes Marked from 1-12, 100µl of tracer CEA were added.
2. 100µls of each standard of unlablled CEA of concentration ranging from 0-150 ng/ml. were pippeted into each tube and according to the assay protocol described in section (4-11).
3. In another set of the same tubes, different volumes (125,150,175,200,250µl) of tracer CEA were pipetted.
4. All the assay tubes were stopped and incubated for 4 hours (±15 minutes) at 25° C (±1° C), with moderate horizontal shaking (>280 rpm).
5. After incubation time of all tubes, they were decanted carefully, 2 ml of wash solution (distilled water) added and immediately content of the tube aspirated, then the tubes were kept inverted and placed on a pad of cotton. This step lasts at least for 10 minutes in order to allow the complete drainage of any last drops of liquid.
6. The rims of the tubes were blotted with cotton sticks to remove any persistent droplets of the liquid. Care should be

taken not to remove from the precipitate in the bottom of each tube.
7. For all tubes, the radioactivity was counted using gamma counter.
8. To prepare totals (i.e-total count). The same amounts of ^{125}I-CEA prepared in (3) were pippetted into separate set of tubes and the radioactivity was determined using gamma counter.

Calculations:

B is the bound radioactivity (CPM) which represents the precipitate immuno-complex (^{125}I-CEA-antibody complex)

F= is the free radioactivity (CPM) which represents unbound ^{125}I-CEA

F= total count–bound radioactivity

1. The values of the ratio B/F for an ordinary standard curve were calculated.
   This standard curve represents the incubation of different amounts of unlablled CEA standards with constant amounts of ^{125}I-CEA. (Table 4-3)
2. B/F values for the incubation of different amounts of ^{125}I-CEA in presence of zero standard only were also calculated (table 4-4)
3. The data in tables (4-3) and (4-4) were plotted as in (Fig 4-16).
4. Using the two curves I and II in (Fig 4-16), we can get the amount of the radioactivity corresponding to the concentration of unlabelled CEA (table 4-5).
   This was done by drawing a line, which intersects with both two curves at the same increment as shown in fig (4-17).
5. The plot of the data in table (4-5) results in straight line, the increment on the ordinated represents the concentration of the tracer ^{125}I-CEA in nanograms per milliliter fig (4-17).

❖ Concentration of stock radioactive CEA (^{125}I-CEA) preparation = the concentration of tracer used above (ng/ml) x dilution factor.

Results of Liquid –Phase RIA

Assay Conditions:

1- Amount of Antibody (anti –CEA).

In order to demonstrate whether the specific binding is proportional to the concentration of specific antibody in the incubation mixture, increasing amount of specific amount of anti-CEA were incubated with either tracer ^{125}I-CEA or with unlabelled CEA. As shown in Fig (4–12 A) the percentage of ^{125}I–CEA bound specifically to their specific antibody was increased as the later increase in the incubation mixture. The specific binding was increased linearly whereas the non-specific binding was increased somewhat less then that of specific binding.

As noted by others [177,178]. About 10% of ^{125}I –CEA was found in the precipitate when liquid-phase technique was applied to mixture of ^{125}I-CEA and buffer or normal serum, thus explaining why at low concentration of specific antibody (5μg), the specific binding reaches about 25%.

These results indicate that the specific binding is principally dependent on the amount of antibody in the reaction mixture [179,180]. In all subsequent experiments, 60 μg of specific Anti–CEA in the incubation mixture was used. This is minimal quantity of antibody giving the desired level of radioactive antigen binding (generally 30-50% of total radioactive antigen added) as shown in Figure (4-l2 A).

2- The Radioactive CEA:

Most assays are carried out at a level of radioactive CEA of 30 to 50 %. To estimate the suitable concentration of ^{125}I-CEA, the experiment was carried out in the presence of 60 μg of anti-CEA and increasing concentration of radioactive CEA. The results are illustrated in fig (4-12 B). 50 μl of ^{125}I-CEA (~ 0.5 ng) was used in the binding assay at optimum state.

3- Effects of Temperature:

The influence of temperature on the CEA / anti CEA antibody reaction varies with the antiCEA and assay condition. In general, the Ka increases as the temperature is lowered, and CEA binding is maximal at or near 4° C, provided that equilibrium is reached [180]. Fig (4-12 C) shows the results of this analysis, it seemed that specific binding of ^{125}I-CEA to its antibody was maximal at 4° C and at other temperatures lower than 30° C. The binding of CEA by antiCEA antibody is normally improved at low temperature, but only under equilibrium condition. The approach to equilibrium is slowed because of the decreased frequency of collision between CEA and antiCEA. For this reason, many immunoassays utilize a preliminary incubation at ambient temperature. or 37° C, followed by longer period of incubation at low temperature. In immunoassays involving large molecular weight protein antigens, an initial 60 min and incubation at 37° C may shorten the overall time requirement. The use of incubation temperature above 37°C is undesirable because of danger of antibody denaturation [180-182].

4- Time of reaction:

To choose the most appropriate incubation time for binding ^{125}I-CEA with its specific antibody, the experiment was carried out at different incubation time intervals (0.25 to 72 h).

As shown in fig (4-12 D) the optimal binding was achieved at 16 h, then the binding was gradually decreased with increasing incubation time. The loss of the binding percent may be due to irreversible dissociation of the (^{125}I-CEA / Anti-CEA) complexes.

5- Effect of pH:

The analysis of the influence of pH on the binding of ^{125}I-CEA is illustrated in fig (4-12 E). The optimum pH was found to be (6.8) for binding ^{125}I-CEA with anti-CEA, this indicates that the binding was pH dependent. The shift in the pH of the environment may includes the induction of the protonation-deprotonation process occurring within the charge groups on the amino acid residues present in the determinate of antigen. In view of these results, the buffers in all experiments were adjusted at 7.4 [183].

6- Ionic strength:

Fig (4-12 F) shows the effect of ionic strength, on antibody-antigen binding. It is apparent that a significant increase in the binding of anti-CEA to ^{125}I-CEA occurs with increasing ionic strength and it is clear that the binding occurs at morality of 1 or 0.1 better than at 0.01, 0.001 or in distilled water.

The effect of ionic strength could suggest that an electrostatic interaction between the antibody and the antigen is being effected [188].

The Result of Preparation and Properties of Anti-CEA Chemically Attached to Polystyrene Tubes:

All forms of radioimmunoassays used at present include a procedure to separate free and bound tracer antigen when equilibrium is reached in the incubation mixture. This separation may involve precipitation by a second antibody[185,186], electrophoresis[187,188], chromatoelectrophoresi [189], ion exchange[190], solvent fractionation[191], gel filtration [192,193], salt precipitation [194], or adsorption to charcoal [195]. The need to use such formal isolation procedures increases the length and complexity of the assay and introduces a number of possible sources of error.

For these reasons it is introduced in this work system in which both antigen-antibody reaction and the separation of bound and free radioactive antigen could be a chivied in a single step would be a valuable innovation. A polystyrene tube (13x50 mm) is suitable for use in an automatic gamma counter. Specific antibodies can be covalently coupled to internal surface of this, this was performed by activation of solid phase (Polystyrene tube), the activation process include Nitration, reduction and diazotization. These chemical treatments introduce reactive group on the inner surface of polystyrene tubes. The condition described in the section (4-10-1 A) produce an adequate degree of substitution without solubilization of polystyrene.

The mechanism of antibody coupling to the polystyrene tubes is illustrated in fig (4-2).

(A) Activation Process

1. Nitration:

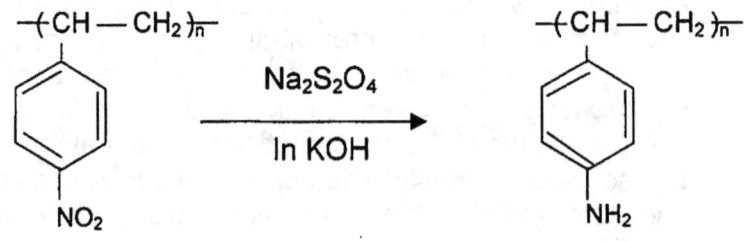

Polystyrene → polynitrostyrene

2. Reduction:

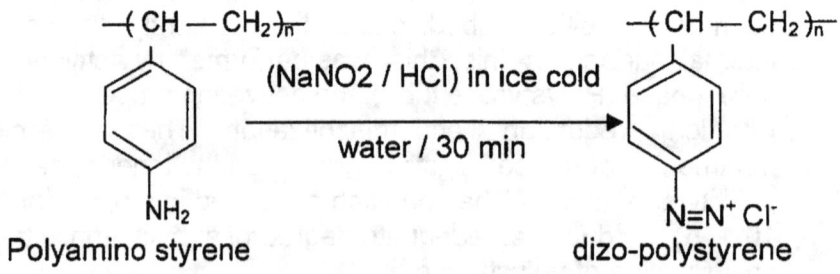

Polynitrostyrene → polyaminostyrene

3. Diazotization:

Polyamino styrene → dizo-polystyrene

(with (NaNO2 / HCl) in ice cold water / 30 min)

(B) Binding of Antibodies to Activated polystyrene tube

Fig (4-2)
steps in coupling specific-anti-CEA to polystyrene tubes

Under the conditions described in section (4-10 A) about 50 µg of anti-CEA remain bound to the tubes (50 µg / tube). The specific antibody to CEA is believed to be covantely attached to the Diaz-polystyrene tube, since then prolonged subjection of the tubes to washing procedures described in section (4-10 B) and solid-phase RIA in section (4-11) does not reduce the antibody activity (amount of radioactivity bound to the antibody coated tubes).

Preparation of specific- antibody chemically attached to polystyrene tubes has been used over a period of several weeks without any significant loss in activity, the tubes stored at 4° C.

RIA Solid Phase- Assay Conditions

The followings are the optimal conditions for the binding of ^{125}I-CEA to anti-CEA coated tubes:
(a) Amount of radioactive CEA: 0.3 ng about 32×10^3 CPM fig (13-A).
(b) Incubation: 3 h or more (fig 13-B).
(c) Temperature of reaction: 15° C (fig 13-C).
(d) pH 7.2 (fig 13-D).
(e) Molarity: 0.1 M. phosphate buffer (fig 13-E).

The finding show that anti-CEA is strongly attached to the tube surface by forces that are unaffected by conditions far more rigorous than those occurring during the assay. The coupled specific anti-CEA provides the site for competitive binding of labelled and unlabelled forms of CEA to the inner surface of the tube. In contrast to the substantial binding of radioactive-CEA to the tube coated with specific antibody, only negligible binding (about 1 percent of added counts) occurred when tubes were untreated, coated with nonimmune rabbit serums.

The optimal condition for the assay of solid phase RIA is useful not only for the clinical application but also to elucidate the structure – function relationship, mechanism of anti-CEA / CEA binding and for engineered CEA molecule or engineered monoclonal antibodies against CEA with specific binding activity. These changes in the optimal conditions are due to variation in the structure of antiCEA itself, modification of amino acid residues in the active binding site, conformational change, change in the charge, formation of diffusion layer around anti-CEA, steric hindrances effect and electrostatic interaction between two molecules of anti-CEA and CEA. The observed changes of binding properties on solid phase are resulted from complicated interaction of these factors and it is difficult to determine the exact effect of a given factor in term of change of binding properties.

The following changes in optimal assay condition were observed when compared with those of Liquid assay. These changes include the followings:
1) The time of incubation (3h).
2) Temperature of reaction (15-25° C).
3) Molarity of buffer (0.1 M).
4) Amount of radioactive CEA (0.3 ng).

The standard curve

Standard curve was constructed, using a broad range of antigen concentration (0 to 150 ng/ml) in the two assays (fig 4-14) and (fig 4-15).

Inhibition experiments using the two assays showed that ^{125}I-antigen/antibody reaction in solid phase was sharply reduced by the addition of as little as 0.1-0.5ng/ml. These suggest that the coated tubes give standard curves of a more sensitive comparable to that obtain by Liquid phase.

The specificity of binding of ^{125}I-CEA in the both assays were indicated by inhibition of the binding produced by increasing amounts of unlabeled CEA added to ^{125}I-CEA for antigen-binding phase (fig 4-14, 4-15) curve, while other proteins in excess (rabbit serum albumin, normal serum), failed to inhibit ^{125}I-CEA binding.

In general, when large enough quantities of unlabeled CEA are added (150ng/ml) radioactive antigen binding is reduced to the nonspecific antigen binding.

Result of Evaluation of CEA by the Prepared Kit

Aliquots from 31 blood samples (15 normal, and 16 from breast cancer) were tested in duplicate by both liquid and solid-RIA.

Table (4-2) summarizes the comparative analysis of the sensitivity, specific, accuracy and efficiency. The solid phase assay was most useful in separating cancer from non-cancer patients.

The notable features of solid phase RIA procedure are the simplicity and economy resulting from the use of antibody-coated plastic tubes.

The use of antibody-coated tubes provides the simplicity inherent in all solid-phase forms of radioimmunoassay, because the isolation of bound radioactive CEA is readily affected by washing-out of the tube on completion of the immune reaction.

All separation methods fail to discriminate fully between the two fractions and some misclassification occurs. Erros in discriminating between the two fractions are detailed as follows:

1. Supernatant in the interstices of the precipitate.
2. Tracer adsorbed non-specifically to tube.
3. Tracer adsorbed to non-specific proteins in precipitate.
4. Tracer impurities behaving differently to tracer, e.g. higher adsorption to tube and non-specific binding.

Solid-phase do not require precipitation at all because of the ease of separation using solid-phase antibodies, extensive washing of the antibody bound fraction becomes a practical proposition. This can lead to removal of erroneous counts in the precipitate and the precise identification of the bound fraction.

Expense is minimized by the use of the same tube for all phases of the assay procedure; thus incubation, separation of bound and free tracer, and counting of the bound tracer are all performed in a tube coasting low, also large numbers of tubes can be coated with anti-CEA and stored prior to distribution without loss of antigen-binding capacity for many months, thus reducing the influence of batch variability of antibody on the assay and reducing the time necessary to perform the assay. The assay can be easily done on a large number of patient samples with a minimum of equipment.

The solid phase assay appears to be as good a diagnostic aid for cancer than liquid phase.

Determination of ^{125}I-CEA Concentration

The concentration of ^{125}I-CEA preparation was determined according to self-displacement method suggested by B.J. morris (1976) for the assessment of the concentration of any radioactive tracer.

This method uses increasing amounts of labeled antigen for the incubation with constant amount of antibody under conditions similar to those employed in normal radioimmuno assay for which the tracer is used. Specific radioactivity and concentration of the tracer (ng/ml) is then determined by comparing the ratio of bound to free (B/F) at each increment of the tracer with B/F for the normal RIA standard curve.

Self-displacement method necessitates the presence of standard solution of the labelled CEA with concentration higher than that used in the normal RIA. The final volume of all solutions used in both paralleled experiments must be equal.

The method was modified by adding different but comparable volumes of the labelled CEA (125, 150, 175, 200, 250 µl). Different volumes of the labelled CEA added cause a little difference in the final volume incubated in RIA tubes. These little differences result in an approximate estimation of the concentration of ^{125}I-CEA (i.e. 450 ng/ml). This method can be used to determine the approximate concentration and specific activity of any labelled antigen.

Table (4-2): Compression of Sensitivity and Specificity of Lquid-Phase and Solid-Phase RIA Assay for Detection of CEA on Same Blood-Sample (All details are explained in the text)

Variable	Liquid-phase assay RIA	Solid-phase assay RIA
Normal blood sample	15	15
Breast cancer blood sample	16	16
TP	10	12
TN	3	7
FP	12	8
FN	6	4
Sensitivity (TP/(TP+FN))x100	62%	75%
Specificity (TN/(TN+FP))x100	20	46.6
Accuracy ((TP+TN)/(TP+TN+FN+FP))x100	41.9	61.3
Efficiency: PV(-ve)%=(TN/(FN+TN))x100	33.3	63.6
PV(+ve)%=(TP/(TP+FP))x100	60	60

CEA level considered positive (+) when above 3 ng/ml
CEA level considered negative (-) when equal to or below 3 ng/ml
Abbreviation:
- TP true positive are those with the disease who are positive.
- TN true negative are those without the disease who are negative.
- False positive are those without the disease who are positive.
- False negative are those with the disease who are negative.

PV = predictive value

Table (4-3): B/F Value Corresponding to Different Concentration of Purified CEA Standard Used in Standard Curve
(All details are explained in the text)

The concentration of standard ng/ml	Bound / free B/F
0	0.75
1	0.66
5	0.5
10	0.26
20	0.16
50	0.1
100	0.09
150	0.08

Table (4-4)
B/F Value Corresponding to Different Amounts of (^{125}I-CEA) Used Incubation
(All details are explained in the text)

Amount of tracer ^{125}I-CEA in CPM (T)	Bound radioactivity in CPM (B)	B/F
141659	60600	0.74
158654	62500	0.65
192192	65500	0.517
233800	66800	0.4
260157	67500	0.35

Table (4-5)
The Mass of the Standard in Nanogram Per Milliliter Corresponding to a Given Amount of the Tracer (^{125}I-CEA)
(All details are explained in the text)

Bound radioactivity in CPM	Amount of the standard CEA ng/ml
63500	1
64000	2.5
64750	3.5
65750	5
66000	6
67230	7.5

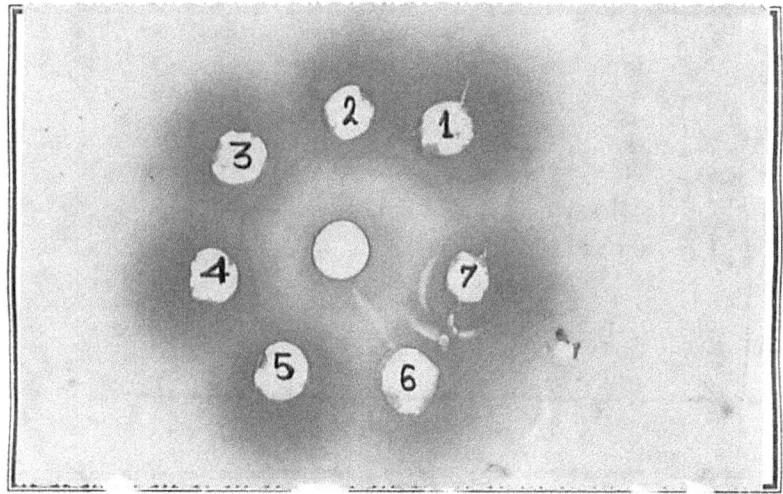

Fig (4-3):
Photograph of Ouchterlony Gel Diffusion Plate Central Well Contains Purified CEA, periphera well contain serum rabbit as fallow:
(1) Serum rabbit group No. 1
(2) Serum rabbit group No. 2
(3) Serum rabbit group No. 3
(4) Serum rabbit group No. 4
(5) Serum rabbit group No. 5
(6) Serum rabbit of control group (unimmunization)
(7) Dose not contain serum
(All details are explained in the text)

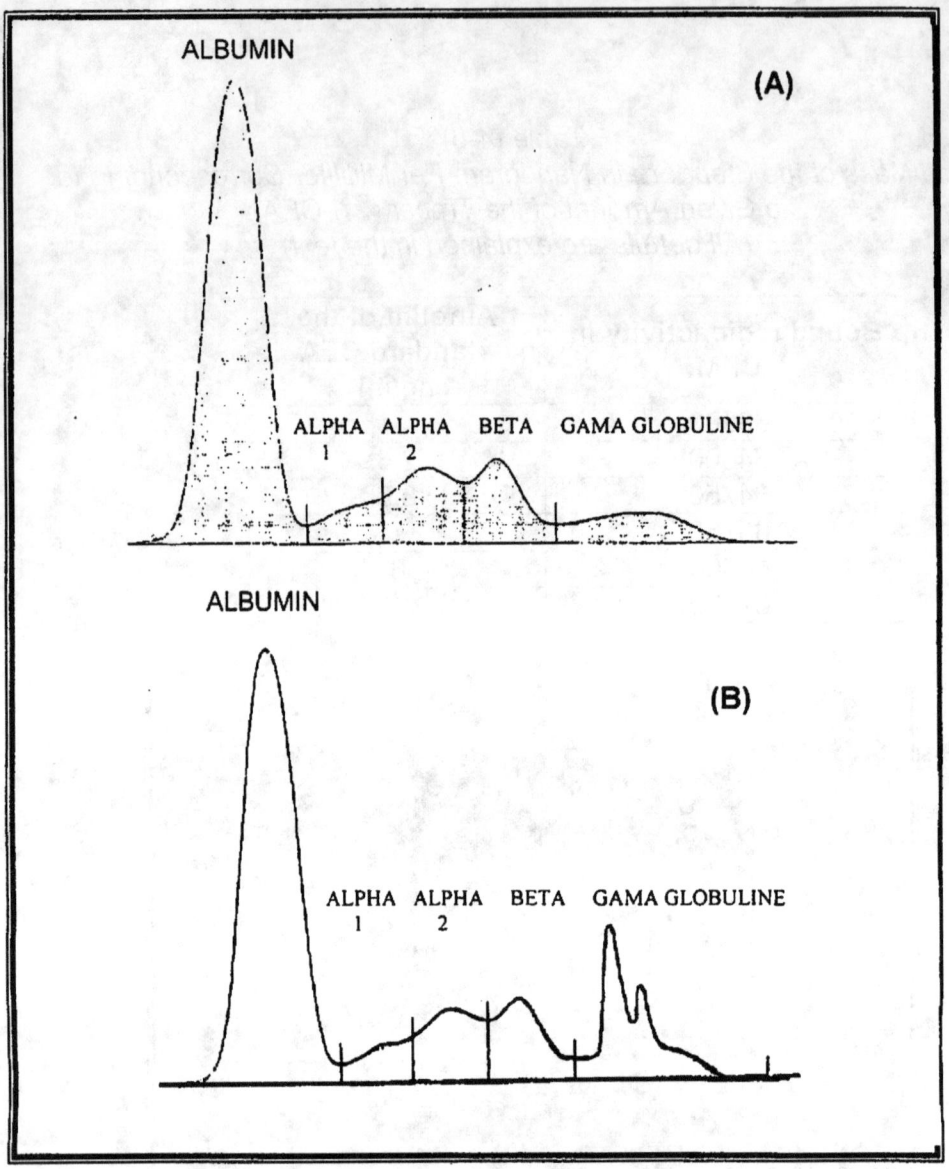

Fig. (4-4):

Rabbit serum protein electrophoresis (Zone electrophoresis) on cellulose acetate
(A) control rabbit serum (unimmunized)
(B) immunized rabbit serum
(All details are explained in the text)

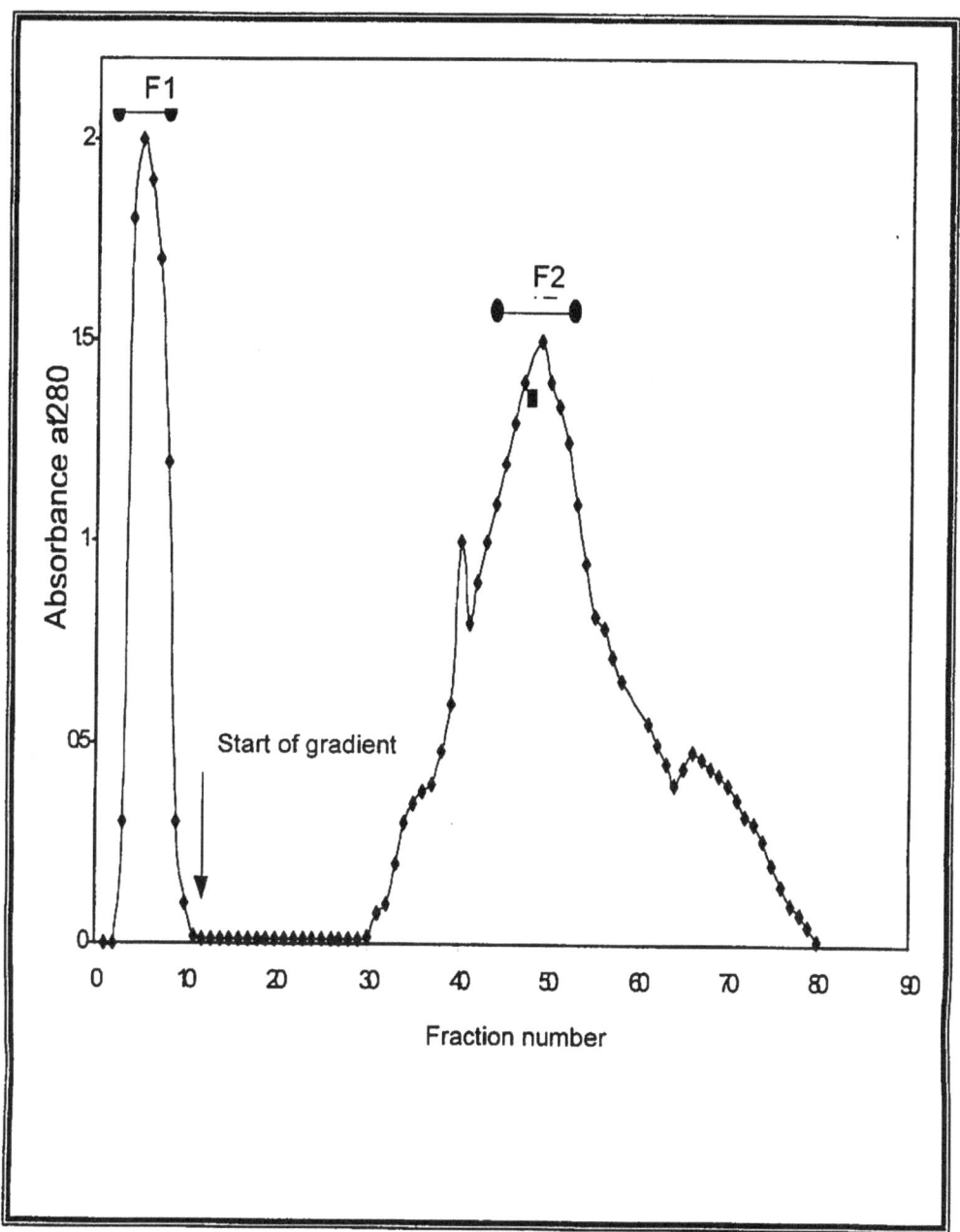

Fig. (4-5): Fractionation of immune rabbit serum on DEAE-cellulose. Two distinct immunoglobuline peaks were obtained and pooled, to give fraction 1 and 2 as follows:
F1: Indicates wash fraction pooled without any binding activity against CEA
F2: Indicates elution fraction pooled with binding activity against CEA
  (All details are explained in the text)

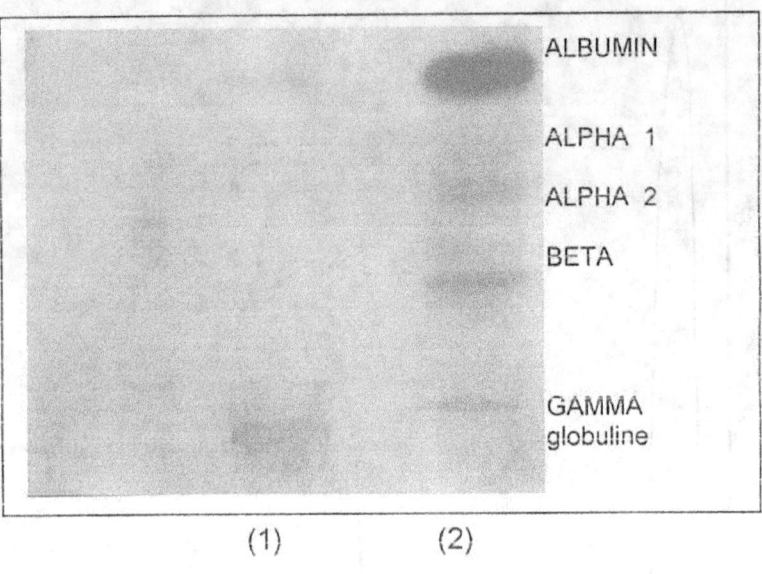

Fig. (4-6): Cellulose acetate electrophoresis of rabbit anti-CEA immunoglobulin purification fraction
- Line 1 finally purified anti-CEA
- Line 2 immunized rabbit serum
    (All details are explained in the text)

Fig. (4-7): immunoelectrophoretic of purified CEA against purified anti-CEA
(All details are explained in the text)

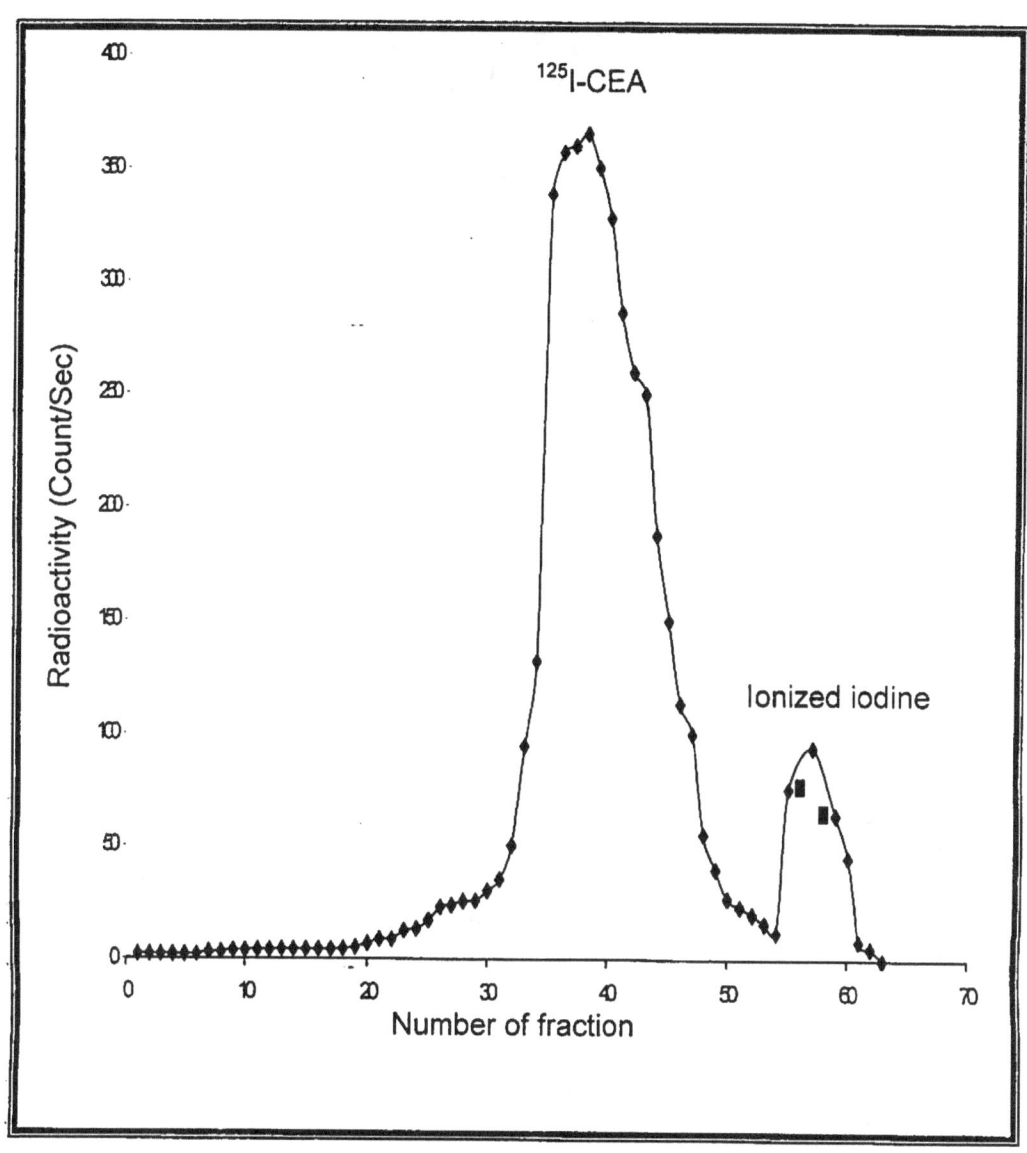

*Fig. (4-8): Separation of ^{125}I-CEA lablled CEA from (^{125}I- iodine on Sephadex G-25 columns
(All details are explained in the text)*

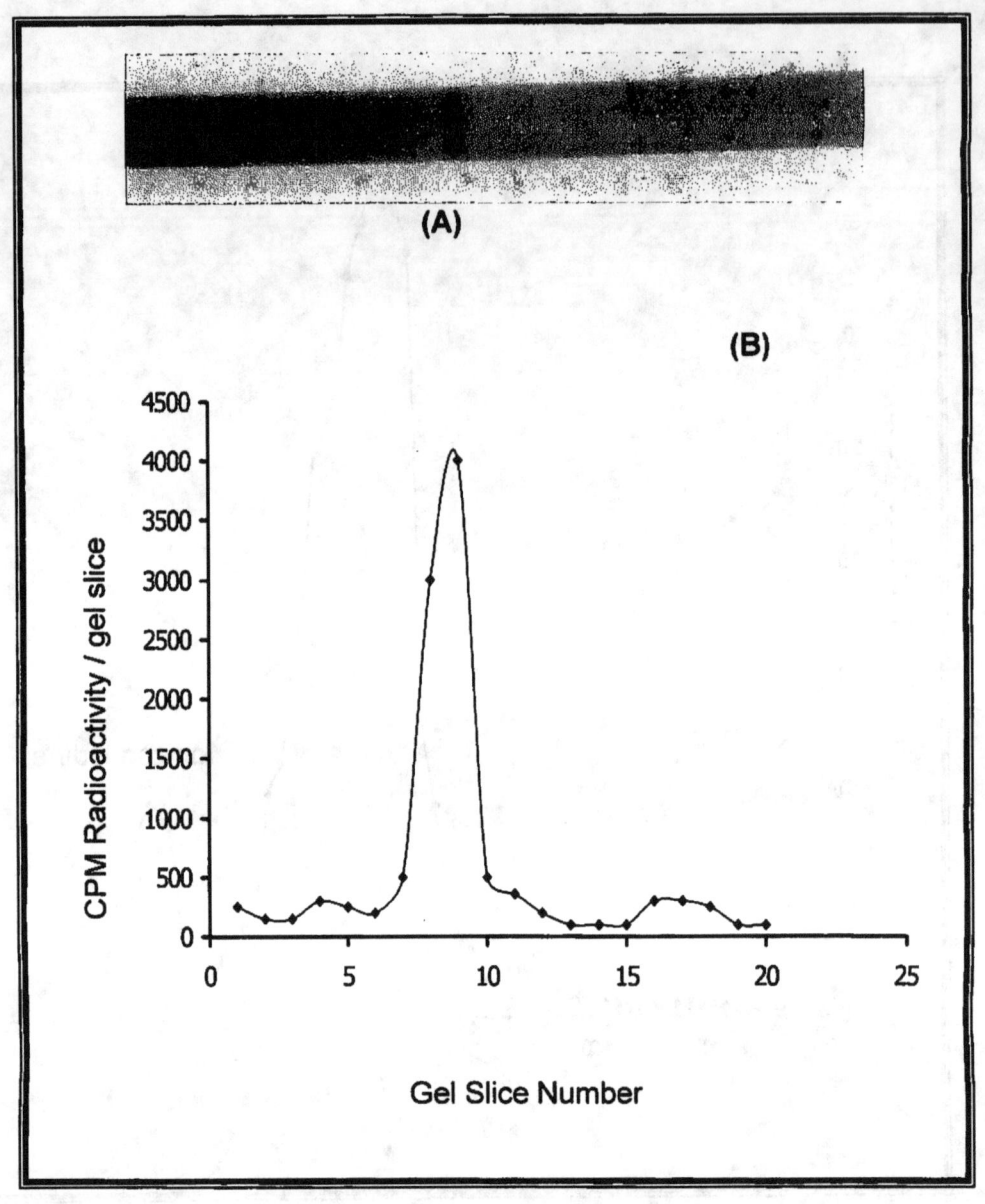

Fig. (4-9): Conventional disc polyacryamid gel electrophoresis of ^{125}I-CEA (A) and the radioactivity in each 5mm gel slice (All details are explained in the text)

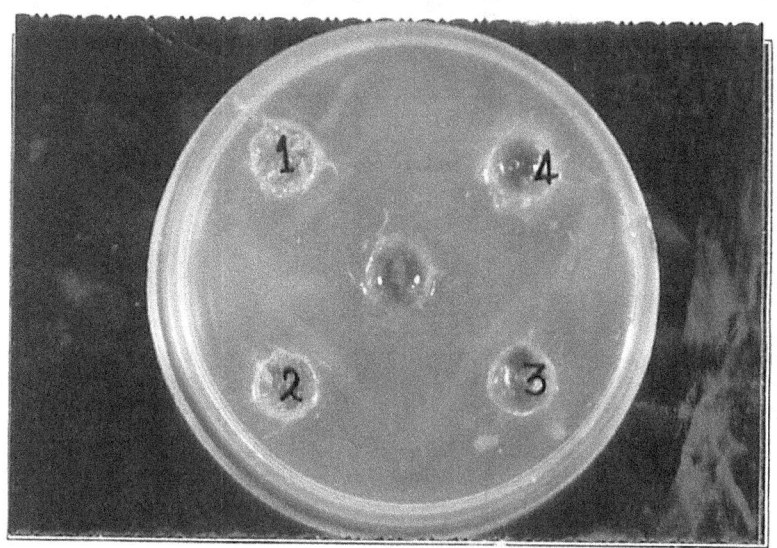

Fig. (4-10)
Photograph of Radio-Ouchterlony Gel Diffusion Plate. Central well Contains Rabbit anti-CEA. The Peripheral Wells Contain (1) unlabelled CEA (2,3) ^{125}I-CEA (4) rabbit serum albumin (standard)
(All details are explained in the text)

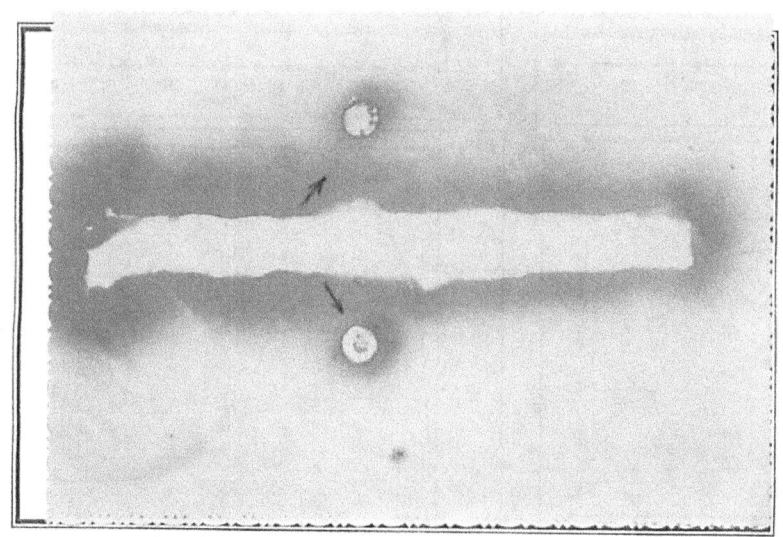

Fig. (4-11)
Immunoelectrophoresis of labelled and unlabelled CEA
(All details are explained in the text)

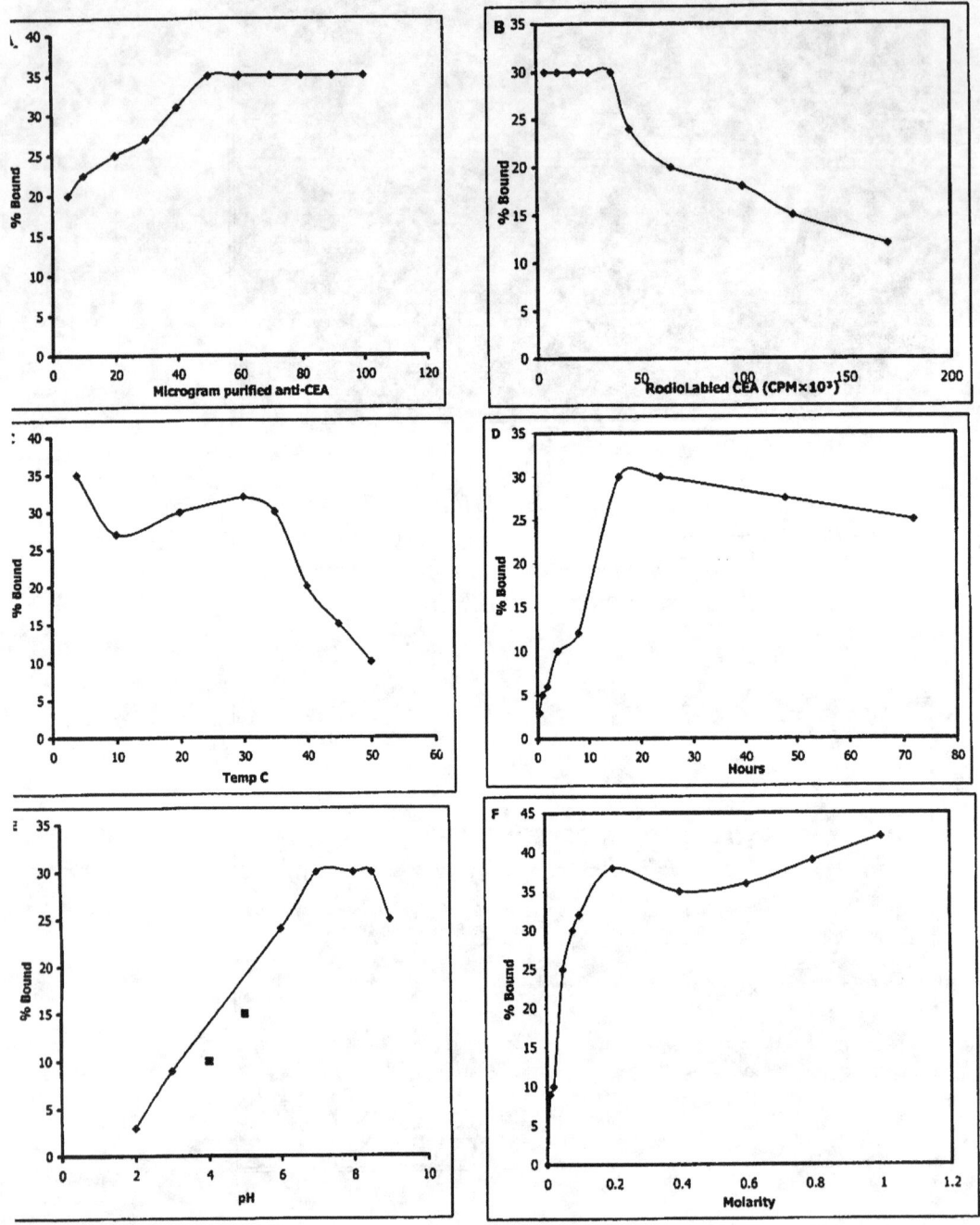

Figure (4 - 12) A - F
Assay condition of liquid-phase Radioimmumoassay binding of anti-CEA to ^{125}I-CEA.
Antibody concentration effect (the optimal concentration 60 mg) B:Concentration of rdioactive CEA (about 50000 CPM). C:Temperature effect (lower than 30 C).
D:Time effect (about 16 h). E:pH effect (pH 7). F:Molarity of the buffer(0.1 or more)
(All details are explaind in the text)

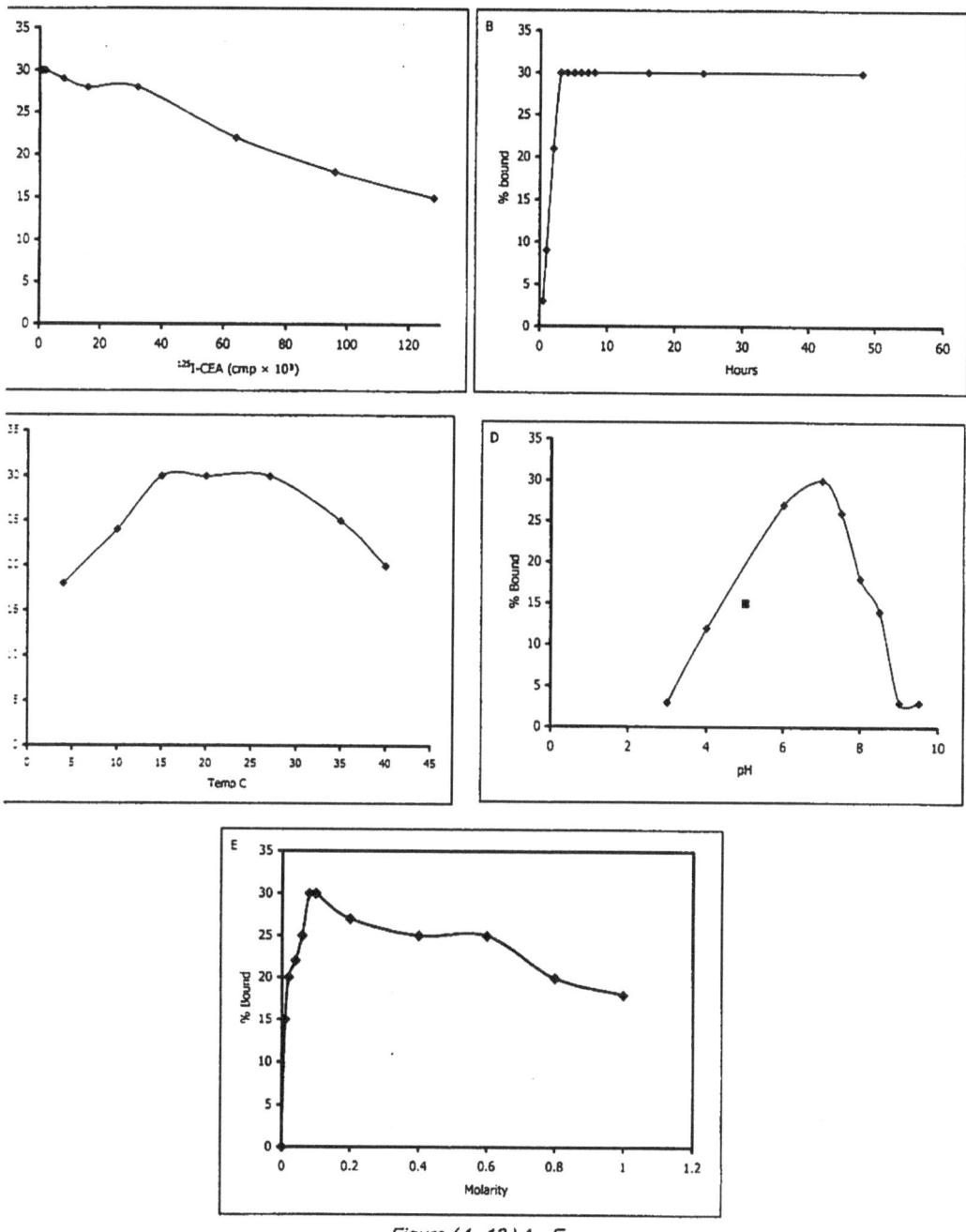

Figure (4 - 13) A - E

Assay condition of Solid-phase Radioimmunoassay binding of anti-CEA to coated polystyrene tube to ^{125}I-CEA
A: Amount of tracer (about 30000 CPM). B: Incubation time (aboyt 3 h). C:Temperature of reaction (15 - 25).
D: pH effect (pH 7). E:Ionic strength (0.1 or more)
(All details are explaind in the text)

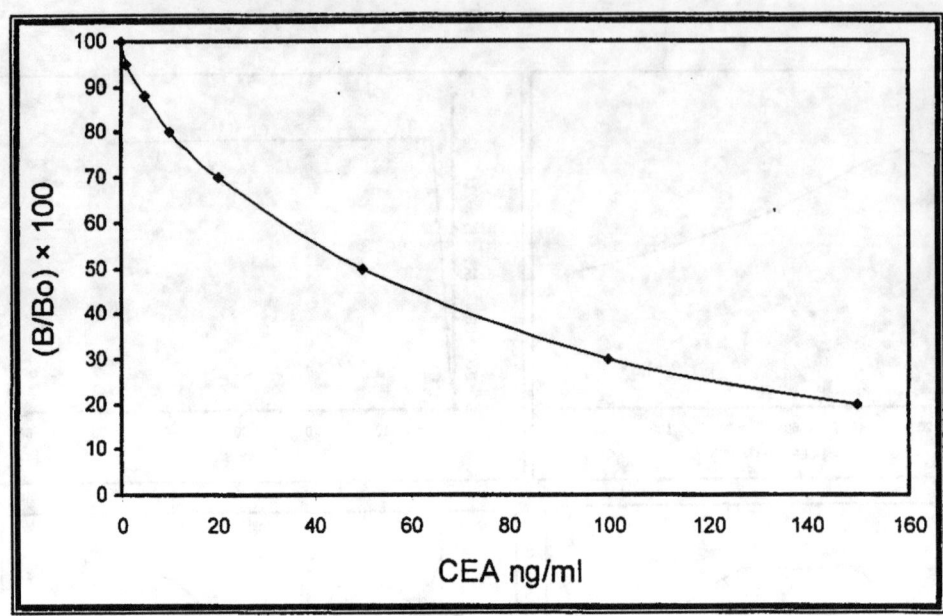

Fig. (4-14): Standard curve for radioimmunoassay of CEA in liquid-phase (arithmetic plot). Each point represent the mean of triplicate determination (All details are explained in the text)

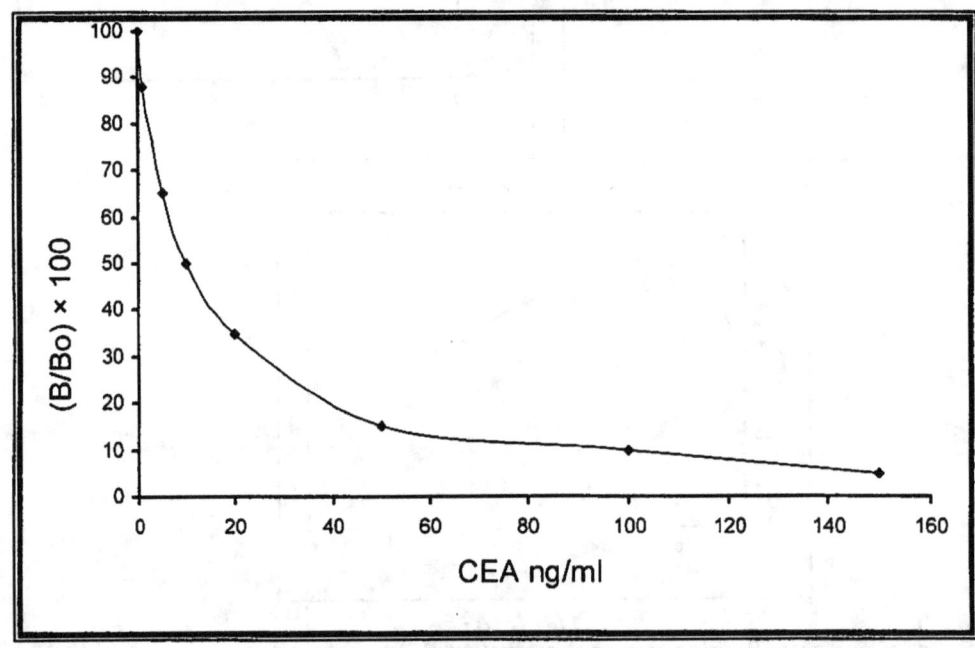

Fig. (4-15): Standard curve for radioimmunoassay of CEA in solid-phase (arithmetic plot). Each point represents the mean of triplicate determination (All details are explained in the text)

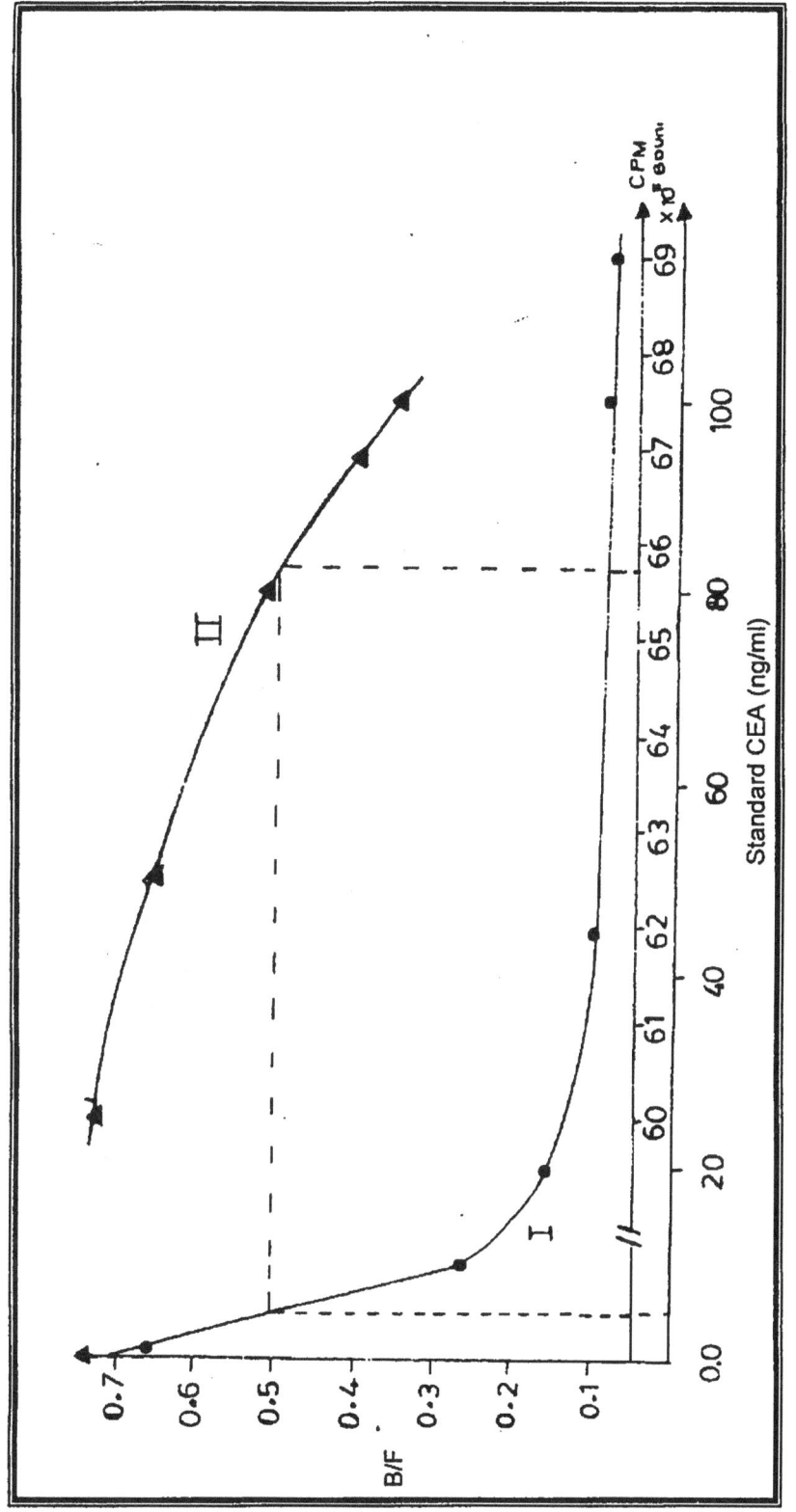

Fig. (4-16) Ratio of bound radioactivity to free radioactivity (B/F) for ordinary standard curve, were different amounts of human CEA incubated with constant amount of ^{125}I-CEA in the absence of unlabelled CEA
(All details are explained in the text)

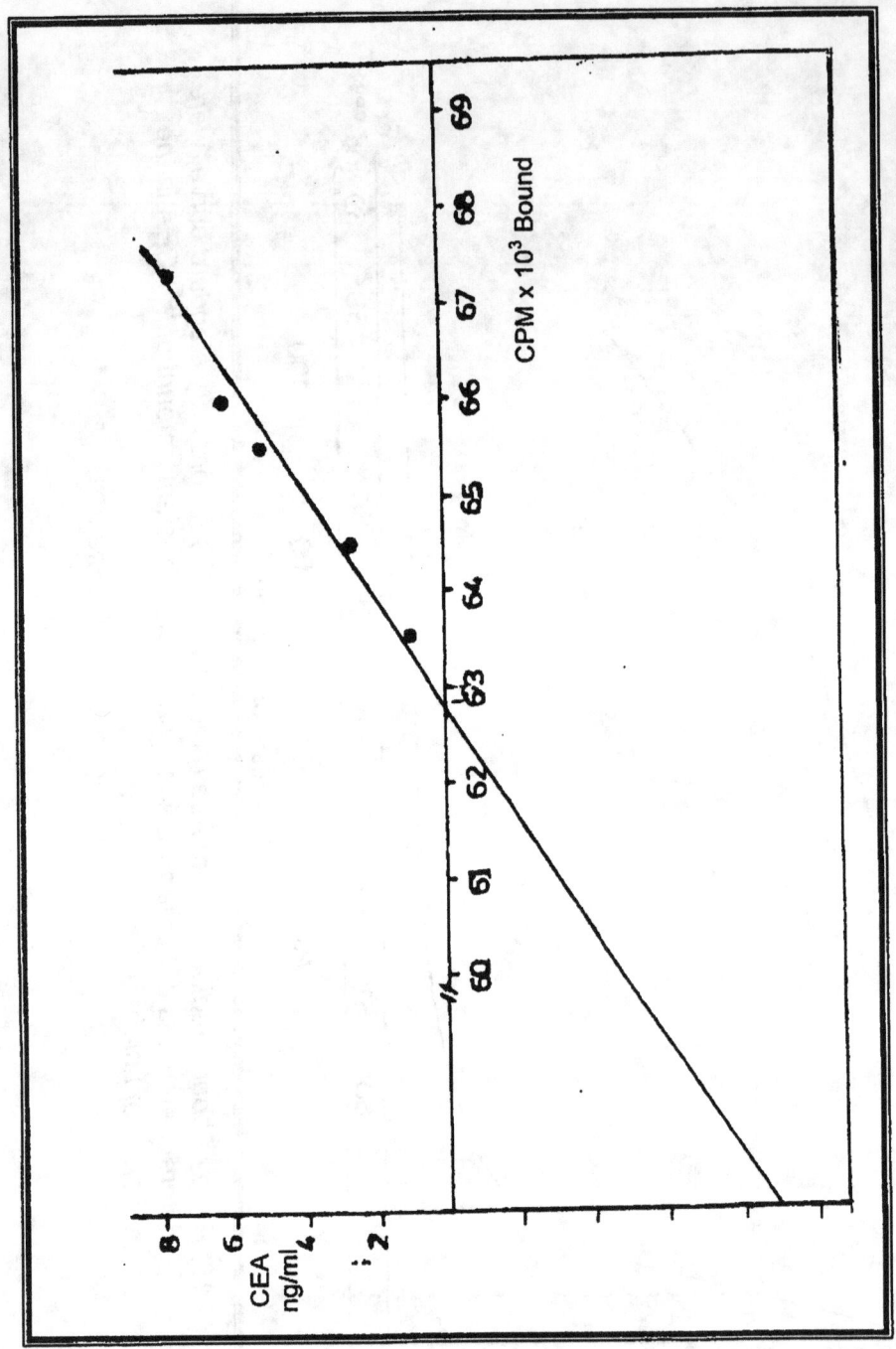

Fig.(4-17): A plot of the mass of CEA standard against the CPM of ^{125}I-CEA having the same B/F from fig (4-16) result in a stratigh line, the intercept on the ordinate corresponds to the concentration of ^{125}I-CEA in (ng/ml)
(All details are explained in the text)

Chapter five

Thermodynamic and Kinetic Studies of CEA Receptor-Binding

Abstract

1. Two groups of breast cancer patients were used to investigate the presence of cytosolic and nuclear CEA receptor. Radioreceptor assay procedure has been developed for the determination of cytosolic and nuclear CEA receptors. The optimum conditions obtained for estimation of cytosolic CEA receptors as follows; receptor concentration 200 µg protein, ^{125}I-CEA concentration 0.5 ng (50,000 CPM), temperature 4° C, time 8h and pH 7.4 . the typical conditions observed for quantitation of nuclear receptors were receptor concentration: 150 µg DNA, ^{125}I-CEA (0.7 ng) temperature 4° C, pH 7.4, time: 8h, also, the CEA binding to their receptor seemed to be affected by mono and divalent chloride salts.
2. Kinetic and thermodynamic parameters associated with the binding of ^{125}I-CEA in both cytosolic and nuclear homogenate were investigated. It was shown that the reaction in all cases studied follow pseudo-first order reaction kinetics.
3. The value of kinetic parameter K_a, K_d, K_{obs}, K_{+1}, K_{-1}, $(t_{1/2})_{ass}$, $(t_{1/2})_{diss}$ and maximal binding (B_{max}) at 4°C for the binding of ^{125}I-CEA with its cytosolic receptor in mammary of adenocarcinoma from postmenopausal patient tissue were found to be: 94.73×10^2 µg^{-1}.ml, 10.5×10^{-5} µg^{-1}.ml, 13.6×10^{-3} (min^{-1}), 135 (µg.ml.min^{-1}), 12.7×10^{-3} (min^{-1}), 30 min, 54 min and 85×10^{-5} µg.ml^{-1} protein respectively, while 77.77×10^2(µg^{-2}.ml), 10.5×10^{-5} (µg.ml^{-1}), 11×10^{-3} (min^{-1}), 150 (µg.ml.min^{-1}), 17×10^{-3} (min^{-1}), 60 min, 47 min, and 78×10^{-5} µg.ml^{-1} protein respectively for the binding of ^{125}I-CEA with its cytosolic receptor in mammary adenocarcinoma from premenopausal patient tissue.
4. The van't Hoff plot demonstrated a linear relationship between ln K_a and 1/T, using the homogenate as the receptor source. Arrheniuns plot indicates that there was a linear relationship between log K_{+1} and 1/T. the transtion state thermodynamic parameters for the formation of (^{125}I-CEA-R) complex represented by E_a, ΔG^*, ΔS^* were determined.
5. Thermodynamic data show that the binding reaction is as an entropically driven reaction and suggest an involvement of

hydrophobic forces in the stabilization of ^{125}I-CEA-receptor complex.

Introduction

Tissue-receptor-binding proteins that have been used in competitive binding assays fall into two categories, arbitrarily designated in this discussion as type A and type B receptors. Type A receptors are derived from the external cell membrane. Most are receptors for hormones that act at the cell surface to modulate adenylate cyclase activity, including ACTH, glucagon and growth hormone. The type B receptors are cytoplasmic or nuclear proteins with an affinity for agents that act inside the cell, including cyclic Amp and estrogen.

The procedure used in competitive binding assays tends to be similar regardless of wether an antibody or plasma or a tissue-binding protein is involved. A radiolabelled ligand is used, and competitive binding is measured by diminished binding of radiolabelled to receptor protein. In receptor binding assay systems, optimal condition for binding varies with the particular protein. Some time the assay can be applied directly to crude tissue extracts, but frequently the sample must be partially purified first. When the binding receptor is on the cell surface, the assay may be attempted with intact cells.

CEA receptors deserves special attention, these receptors are known to be found on the surface of embryonic, and all types of tumor cells, while they are absent on the surface of normal mammalian cell [198-205].

Some of the previous studies reported that CEA may bind to specific receptor on monocytes, macrophage, activated human T-lymphocytes with malignant [198-205].

Analysis of temperature dependence of kinetic and equilibrium constants allows determination of energetic of binding and methods are presented for calculation of the changes in Gibes free energy, enthalpy and entropy that are associated with the binding of antibody to its antigen [210].

In other word, thermodynamic measurement of reactions interactions under equilibrium conditions provide information about differences between the initial, final states of each reactant, while kinetic studies supply that information for the differences between those states and an intermediate activated complex, (i.e. the pathway taken by the reactants reach the final product) [211].

There were no references to evaluate CEA receptor, there for, this chapter develops Radioreceptor assay to carry out determination of cytosolic and nuclear CEA receptor in mammary adenocarcinoma tissues, and the basic mathematical analyses that could be used to explain the mechanism of binding of CEA to their receptor to form (^{125}I-CEA~R) complex in human breast tissue.

Materials and Methods

5.1 Chemicals:
All laboratory chemicals and reagents were of analor grade. Tris (hydroxymethy/amino methane), dithiothreitol, glycerol, EDTA, KCl, NaCl, $CaCl_2$, $MgCl_2$.

5.2 Apparatus:
The apparatus during this study were, LKB gamma counter type 1270 Rack, Beckman model -25 spectrophotometer, cooling centrifuge type Hettich, cooling centrifuge type MLW k_{24}, pye-unicam pH meter, Memmert water bath, Memmert incubator.

5.3 Buffer and Reagents:
All buffer solutions were prepared by dissolving the appropriate amount of salts in distilled water and the required pH was adjusted.

Other reagents were prepared as described previously
1. TED buffer (pH 7.4): Tris (0.01 M) buffer containing 0.15 mM EDTA, 1.2 mM diethiothreitol and 10% glycerol pH 7.4 .
2. Standard unlabelled CEA solution: stock solution were prepared by dissolving the appropriate amounts of highly purified CEA in fewest buffer then the volume was complete with distilled water (as described in chapter 4 section)
3. Radioactive CEA ^{125}I-CEA were used, the specific radioactivity of ^{125}I-CEA approximately 15.2 µci/µg as described in chapter 4.

5.4 Collection of Specimens and Preparation of Tissue Homogenate:

The tumor tissues were surgically removed from breast tumor patients by either mastectomy or lumpectomy. The specimens were cut off and stored immediately at -20° C. prior to the study the frozen tissue was pulverized on ice bath then homogenized at 4° C in Tris buffer (TED buffer, pH 7.4) with a ratio of 1:3 (weight: volume) using a manual homogenizer. The homogenate was filtered through a nylon mesh sieve in order to eliminate fibres of connective tissues then centrifuged at 200 xg for 10 min at 4° C. the pellet was neglected and the supernatant was centrifugation at 2000 xg for 10 min at 4° C. the pellet was neglected and the supernatant was centrifuged at 2000 xg for 10 min at 4°C. The sediment was used to obtain the nuclear fraction and the supernatant was used to isolate the cytosolic fraction. Nuclear fraction was obtained by rehomog-enization of the sediment in 3ml TED buffer in a manual homogenizer, then centrifuge at 2000 xg for 10 min at 4° C. the supernatant was discarded and the sediment was rehomogenized again in 3 ml TED buffer. The mixture was filtered through a nylon mesh sieve. Crude cytosol fraction was isolated by centrifugation of the supernatant of the cytosolic fraction at 1500 xg for 20 min at 4° C. the sediment was discarded and the supernatant was used in the experiments involved cytosolic fraction. The cytosolic and nuclear, fractions were used as sources of CEA receptor through out this study.

Two groups of breast cancer patient's were included in this study. Group 1-permenopausal patients with breast cancer. Group 2 postmenopausal patient with breast cancer.

5.4 Estimation of Protein and DNA Contents:

Protein was measured by the method of Lowry et.al.[93] Using bovine serum albumin as standard. DNA was determined according to Burton method[212] with thymus DNA as standard.

5.6 Binding studies of ^{125}I-CEA with their receptors located in Malignant Mammary tissues:

5.6.1 Preliminary Tests of ^{125}I-CEA binding with its cytosolic and nuclear receptors in malignant mammary tissues.

The binding of ^{125}I-CEA to their receptors in the homogenate was primary checked according to the following:

A. Cytosolic CEA receptor

1. 100 µl of homogenate (protein concentration 200 µg) was incubated with 100 µl ^{125}I-CEA (1 ng ^{125}I-CEA) at 4° C for 24 h. the final volume was completed up to 1 ml with TED buffer pH 7.4 .
2. After incubation, the bound CEA was estimated, for this purpose 0.8 milliliter of saturated ammonium sulphate solution were added with moderate horizontal shaking (>280 rpm) for 10 min.

    The tubes were kept at 4° C for 30 min and then centrifuged at 4000 xg for 15 min. each supernatant was decanted in another tubes, the rims of the tubes were blotted with cotton sticks to remove any persistent droplets of supernatant. Care should be taken to remove the precipitate in the bottom of each tube.
3. Radioactivity, of bound (CPM) in each tube was counted using gamma counter (the amount of bound and free radioactivity were determined)
4. The steps from 1-3 were repeated with the addition 50-fold excess of unlabelled CEA.

5. Two additional tubes containing 100 μl of ^{125}I-CEA only (for total radioactivity) were counted.

B. Nuclear CEA receptor

It was primary checked as follows:
1. One hundred microliter of nuclear fraction (150μg DNA) was incubated with 100μl of ^{125}I-CEA and the volume of the mixture was completed to 1ml with TED buffer (pH 7.4).
2. Steps 2,3,4 and 5 of experiment A were repeated.

Calculation:

1) Total binding (TB) represent the amount of radioactivity bound to the particulate fraction (expressed in counts per minute CPM) in the absence of unlabelled CEA.
2) The radioactivity of the particulate fraction after the maximum displacement of labelled CEA by excess amount of unlabelled CEA is referred to as nonspecific binding (NB).
3) Specific binding (SB) is the difference between radioactivity (CPM) bound to the particulate fraction in the absence of excess unlabelled CEA and that bound in its presence.

SB(CPM)=TB(CMP)-NB(CPM)

4) %SB can be got from the following formal:

$$\%SB = \frac{SB(CPM)}{Total\ count\ (CPM)\ of\ labelled\ CEA\ used\ in\ each\ tube\ (T)} \times 100$$

5.6.2 Influence of ^{125}I-CEA on the binding

All the following experiments were carried out with two sets, The first one was used to estimate the total binding and the second to determine the nonspecific binding.

A. Cytosolic receptor:

Increasing concentrations (0.1-1ng) of labelled CEA were added to 100μl (200mg protein) of crude cytosol in the first set of tubes with final volume of 1 ml (completed with TED buffer).

The second set of tubes consisted of the same reactants plus 50-fold excess of unlabelled CEA. After incubation for 24 h at 4°C the bound CEA was determined as described in section (5-6-1).

B. Nuclear CEA receptor:

The same experiment A was repeated using 100 μl (150 μg DNA) of nuclear fraction, and increasing concentration (0.1-1 ng) of labelled CEA with or without the addation of 50 fold excess of unlabelled CEA. The final volume (1 ml) of the incubation mixture was made up with TED buffer. After incubation for 24 h at 4°C the bound CEA was determined as described in section (5-6-1). The precentage of specific binding (SB%) was calculated according to the following formula

$$SB\% = \frac{\text{Specific binding (CPM)}}{\text{Total radioactivity of }^{125}\text{I-CEA}} \times 100$$

The SB% was plotted against the concentration ^{125}I-CEA.

5.6.3 Influence of receptor concentration on the binding with ^{125}I-CEA

A) Cytosolic CEA receptor:

50 μl of labeled CEA (0.5 ng=50000 CPM) were added to 100 μl of increasing amount (25,50,75,100,150,200,250 μg protein) of crude cytosol in final volume of 1 ml (complete with TED buffer) with or without the addition of a 50

fold excess of unlabelled CEA. After incubation for 24 h at 4° C the bound-CEA were determined as mentioned in section (5-6-1).

B) Nuclear CEA receptors:

The same experiment A was repeated using 100 µl of increasing amount (25, 50, 75, 100, 150, 200, 250 µg DNA) of nuclear fraction added to set of tubes contained 75 µl (0.75 ng) of labelled CEA. The volume of the mixture was completed to 1 ml with TED buffer. After incubation time the bound CEA to nuclear receptor was estimated.

The SB% was calculated as mentioned in section (5-6-1) and plotted vs, the amount of receptor included in each tube.

5.6.4 Temperature dependency of the binding

A) Cytosolic CEA receptor:

50 µl (0.5 ng=50000 CPM) of radioactive CEA and 100 µl (200 µg protein) of crude cytosol were mixed with or without the addition of 50 fold excess of unlabelled CEA. The volume of mixture was completed with TED buffer to 1 ml. After incubation for 24 h at 4° C the bound CEA to cytosolic receptor was estimated as described in section (5.6.1). The experiment was repeated at different temperature (10,20,25,35,45° C).

B) Nuclear CEA receptors:

To evaluate the temperature dependency of nuclear receptor binding, 100 µl (150 µg DNA) of this fraction were added to 75 µl of radioactive CEA (0.75 ng ^{125}I-CEA $\cong$ 75000 CPM) with or without the addition of 50 fold excess of unlabelled CEA.

The volume of mixture was completed to 1 ml with TED buffer pH 7.4 . After incubation for 24 h at 4°C, the bound CEA to nuclear receptor was determined as described in section (5-6-1).

The experiment was repeated at different temperatures (10,20,25,37,45). The SB% was calculated as mentioned in sections (5.6.1) and plotted vs the temperature.

5.6.5 *Time course of receptor binding*:

Crude Cytosolic fraction (200 µg protein in 100 µl) was added to 50 µl (0.5 ng) of radioactive CEA in a final volume of 1 ml (complete with TED buffer) with or without the addition of 50 fold excess of unlabelled CEA. The tubes were incubated at 4° C. at certain time intervals (30, 60, 120, 150, 180, 240, 480, 600, 660, and 720) min, two tubes from each set were taken and the bound CEA was estimated as mentioned in section (5.6.1).

The experiment was repeated at 10,20,35,45° C. the same protocol was repeated for the nuclear fraction using 100 µl (150 µg DNA) of this fraction add to 75 µl (0.75 ng ^{125}I-CEA) of radioactive CEA with or without the addition of unlabelled CEA. The final volume was completed to 1 ml with TED buffer and the bound CEA was estimated as described in section (5.6.1). the SB% was calculated and plotted vs the time of incubation.

5.6.6 *Effect of pH on the receptor binding:*

To demonstrate the effect of pH, 100 µl (200 µg protein) of crude cytosol were added to 50 µl (0.5 ng≈50000 CPM) of radioactive CEA with or without the addition of 50-fold excess of unlabelled CEA. The volumes were completed with TED buffer of differ pH (7,7.2,7.4,7.6,7.8,8) to 1 ml. The tubes were incubated for 8 h at 4° C. the bound CEA and SB% was evaluated as revised in section (5.6.1).

The experiment was repeated using 100 µl (150 µg DNA) of nuclear fraction added to 75 (0.75 ng) of tracer CEA with or without the addation of a 50 fold excess of unlabelled CEA. The volumes of the mixtures were completed in the same manner.

After incubation for 8 h at 4° C. the bound CEA and SB% were estimated as mentioned in section (5.6.1). the SB% was plotted against the pH.

5.6.7 Effect of monovalant and divalent salt on Binding ^{125}I-CEA to its receptor

(A) Cytosolic CEA Receptor:

(1) Stock solution containing 25mM, 50mM, 75mM, 100mM, 125mM, 150mM, 175mM, 200mM, 225mM and 250mM of each of the following salts were prepared respectively in TED buffer pH 7.4
   a. NaCl   b. KCl   c. $MgCl_2$ d. $CaCl_2$

(2) 100 µl crude cytosol (200 µg protein) were added to 50 µl of radioactive CEA (0.5 ng ^{125}I-CEA) with or without the addition of unlabelled CEA in a final volume of 1 ml, completed with TED buffer (pH 7.4) containing different concentration (25-250mM) of each following salts (NaCl, KCl, $CaCl_2$, $MgCl_2$), in addition a sample of Cytosolic fraction without the addition of any salt was used as a control, then the tubes were incubated for 8 h at 4° C.

All other steps of experiment (5.6.1) were performed as outlined, to get the pellet of CEA-receptor complex.

(B) Nuclear CEA Receptor:

(1) The same experiment mentioned in A was repeated using 100 µl (150 µg DNA) nuclear fraction added to 75 µl of radioactive CEA (0.75 ng ^{125}I-CEA) with or without the addition of unlabelled CEA in a final volume of 1 ml, completed with TED buffer (pH 7.4) containing different concentration (25-250mM) of each of the following salts (NaCl, KCl, $CaCl_2$, $MgCl_2$), also the sample without addation any salt was used as a control.

(2) All other steps of experiment (5.6.1) were repeated.

5.6.8 Stability of CEA-Receptor Complex:

In order to investigate the effect of temperature on receptor properties, the stabilities of CEA receptor complex have been measured. The experiment was performed on Cytosolic and nuclear fraction of mammary malignant tissues as described in section (5.6.4), except that was performed at optimum condition. After the evaluation of the bound CEA, the ^{125}I-CEA-receptor complex was reincubated at two temperatures 4, 30 ° C. between 0 and 10 h the remaining bound CEA in each tube was measured and SB% was calculated and plotted against the time of incubation.

5.7 Determination of affinity constant (Ka) and the maximal binding capacity (Bmax) of ^{125}I-CEA association with their Cytosolic and nuclear receptor.

(A) Cytosolic CEA receptor:

(1) Cytosolic receptor was measured by addition of 100 μl (200 μg protein) of crude cytosol to 20, 40, 50, 75, 100, 125 μl) of ^{125}I-CEA (concentration 9 ng/ml).
(2) TED buffer (pH 7.4) was added to each assay tube to give final volume of 1 ml.
(3) The experiment was carried out in duplicate. A parallel set of assay tubes was used to determine nonspecific binding as outlined in the previous experiments.
(4) All tubes were incubated for 8 h in order to attain an equilibrium state.
(5) The steps 2,3,5 in experiment (5.6.1) were preformed as outlined.
(6) All the previous steps of the experiment were performed at different temperatures.
   (10,20,35,45°C)The times of incubation needed to get the Equilibrium State at each temperature was obtained from the related time course pattern.

(B) Nuclear CEA Receptor:

(1) Nuclear receptor were determined using 100 µl (150 µg DNA) of nuclear fraction added to (20, 40, 50, 75, 100, 125 µl) of ^{125}I-CEA (concentration 9 ng/ml).

(2) All other steps (2-6) of experiment A were repeated.

Calculations

1. Values of TB, T, F were determined, where

   TB: is the bound radioactivity means (C.P.M), which represent (^{125}I-CEA/receptor) complex

   F: is the free radioactivity mean counts (CPM, which represent the non bound ^{125}I-CEA

   T: is total radioactivity mean counts (CPM)

   $$F = T(CPM) - TB(CPM)$$

2. The values of ^{125}I-CEA which is bound specifically (µg/ml) were calculated using the following formula:

   $$B_{specific} = \frac{\text{Total binding (TB)} - \text{non specific binding}}{\text{Total count (T)}} \times \text{Conc. Of } ^{125}\text{I-CEA}$$

3. The affinity constant and the maximal binding capacity were determined according to scattered equation [213].

   $$\frac{B}{F} = \frac{1}{K_d}(B_{max} - B)$$

   $$K_a = \frac{1}{K_d}$$

   Where:
   K_a = Affinity constant
   K_d = Dissociation constant
   B_{max} = Maxmal binding capacity

4. The values of the ratio B/F were plotted against the value of B in µg/ml, gives a linear relationship.

The values of the affinity constant of the binding (Ka) at each temperature can be calculated from the slope of the straight line, while the value of the total concentration of CEA (B_{max}) in mammary carcinoma tissues was calculated from the intercept with the X-axis.

5.8 Kinetic Studies of Receptor Binding:

Kinetic parameters were evaluated from the data of the time course of association of CEA protein with their receptors. The experiment was followed as described in section (5-7) except that the mixtures were incubated at 4° C for several time intervals. After each time interval, the assay tubes were withdrawn and the bound CEA was estimated as mentioned in section (5.6.1). To evaluate the data of association at further temperatures, this experiment was carried out at 4 temperatures (10,20,35,45° C). The specific binding was estimated as described in section (5.6.1) and plotted against the time of incubation. Using the data obtained from the time course, the following equation was used to calculate the rate constant of receptor association with CEA protein [214].

$$Ln \left[\frac{(^{125}I\text{-}CEA/R)_e}{(^{125}I\text{-}CEA/R)_e - (^{125}I\text{-}CEA/R)_t} \right] = t\, K_{obs}$$

$$K_{obs} = K_{+1} \left[\frac{(^{125}I\text{-}CEA)_T \times (R)_T}{(^{125}I\text{-}CEA/R)_e} \right]$$

Where:

$(^{125}I\text{-}CEA/R)_e$: concentration of (^{125}I-CEA / receptor) complex at equilibrium.

$(^{125}I\text{-}CEA/R)_t$: concentration of (^{125}I-CEA/ receptor) complex after time t, t: the time.

K_{obs}: the observed value of first order rates constant.

K_{+1}: the first order rates constant.

$(^{125}I\text{-}CEA)_T$: the total ^{125}I-CEA concentration.

$(R)_T$: the total receptor concentration.

$$\ln \frac{[^{125}I\text{-}CEA/R]_e}{(^{125}I\text{-}CEA/R)_e - (I\text{-}CEA/R)_t}$$ Was plotted against the time t, and the K_{obs} was determined from the slope of the stright line obtained. Subsequently K_{+1} was calculated at the five temperatures studied. On the other hand the dissociation constants (K_{-1}) were calculated from the values of Ka estimated at the five temperature, since:

$$Ka = \frac{K_{+1}}{K_{-1}}$$

5.9 Estimation of Hill coefficient (n) of Receptors:

To assess the cooperatively of the binding, the experiment was performed as described in section (5-7) - using 100 µl crude cytosol and nuclear fraction (200 µg protein, 150 µg DNA) respectively.

The bound CEA was measured as mentioned in section (5.6.1). The equation of Hill was used for the determination of Hill coefficient (n) [102,215].

$$\text{Log}\left[\frac{B}{B_{max} - B}\right] = n \text{ Log L} - \text{Log K}`B_{max}\text{-}B$$

L: ^{125}I-CEA concentration in the incubation medium.
n: Hill coefficient.
K`: Constant comprising the interaction factors and the intrinsic dissociation constant.

* $\log\left[\dfrac{B}{B_{max}\text{-}B}\right]$ Was plotted against the log L. The slope of the straight line gave the Hill coefficient (n) value.

5.10 Thermodynamic Studies of CEA Binding to Its Receptor.

(1) One hundred microliter of cytosolic and nuclear fractions (200 µg protein, 150µg DNA) respectively were mixed with ^{125}I-CEA (50 µl, 75µl) for cytosol and nuclear fractions respectively .the volumes were made up to 1ml with TED buffer (pH7-4).

(2) All other steps of experiment in section (5-8)were carried out.

Calculation

1. The thermodynamic parameter of standard state ($\Delta H°$, $\Delta G°$, $\Delta S°$) were obtained from Van't Hoff plot, the value of the nature logarithm of equilibrium constant (affinity constant Ka) obtained at different temperatures were plotted against the reciprocal values of absolute temperature in Kelvin (1/T) & was calculated according to the following equation

$$\text{Ln Ka} = \frac{\Delta S°}{R} - \frac{\Delta H°}{Rt}$$

Where:
$\Delta H°$ = The enthalpy change of standard.
$\Delta S°$ = the entropy change of the standard state.
R: The gas constant (8.31414 J.K^{-1}.mol^{-1})
$\Delta H°$ value obtained from the slope of the linear relationship of the plot.
The change in Gibbs free energy of the standard state ($\Delta G°$) was obtained from the following equation:

$$\Delta G° = -R\, T\, \text{Ln Ka}$$

Where Ka is the affinity constant, while the standard state entropy change was obtained from Gibbs equation:

$$\text{Ln Ka} = \frac{\Delta S°}{R} - \frac{\Delta H°}{RT}$$

(154)

2. The thermodynamic parameters of the transition state were obtained from Arrhenius plot of Ln K_{+1} values against $1/T$ values, that gives a linear relationship according to the following equation:

$$Ln\ K_{+1} = Ln\ A - \left[\frac{E_a}{RT}\right]$$

Where:
A: Arrhenius constant.
Ea: Apparent energy of activation.
T: Absolute temperature in kelvin

The value of Ea of the binding reaction can be determined from the slope of the straight line.

The enthalpy of transition state (ΔH^*) was obtained from:

$$\Delta H^* = E_a - RT$$

The free energy change of transition state (ΔG^*) was calculated using the following equation:

$$\Delta G^* = -RT\ Ln\ K_{+1} + RT\ Ln\ (KT/h)$$

Where:
K: Boltzmann constant = 1.38×10^{-23} J. deg^{-1}
h: Plank constant = 0.662×10^{-33} J. Sec^{-1}

The change in entropy of the transition state (ΔS^*) was calculated from following equation:

$$\Delta S^* = \frac{\Delta H^* - \Delta G^*}{T}$$

Results and Discussion

Tissue homogenization was carried out in 10% glycerol because glycerol is a hypotonic solution, which enhances the rupture of plasma cell membrane and preserves other cell organelle [217].

Homogenization was carried out in a cold medium (i.e 2-4° C) so that protein denaturation due to the pressure of the pestm of the homogenizer is nearly prevented, on the other hand the proteolytic enzyme activity decrease with the lowering of the temperature [218].

The filtration of the tissue homogenate through layer of the nylon gauze facilitated the removal of any suspended pieces of unhomogenized tissue and blood vessels, while homogenate centrifugation at 2000 xg removed the unruptured cells and intact nuclei of the ruptured cells, leaving mitochondrial / Golgi fraction and cell microsomes in the supernatant [217].

The study of the binding of any antigen (e.g. hormon, drug, virus etc) to its receptor necessitates the choice of the most appropriate conditions that lead to the maximum specific binding. Hence, the study of each of the following effects on the extent of the binding of CEA to its receptor is quite necessary:

1. The quantity of the receptor source and the labelled antigen.
2. Effect of pH.
3. Effect of time and temperature on the extent of the binding.
4. Effect of ionic strength.

◁ **Preliminary tests of ^{125}I-CEA binding with its receptors in mammary carcinoma.**

Cytosolic and nuclear fractions in mammary carcinoma were used as sources of CEA receptors in this study. The tumors were considered to have CEA receptors if they contained whatever amounts of specific binding (SB%). The preliminary conditions used in this experiment result are presented in table (5-1). The measurement of CEA receptor concentration would be carried out after the development of radioreceptor assay. However, there were no published data to evaluate these findings.

The receptor source and the labelled CEA were incubated at 4°C for 24 h. the choice of this long time period is attributed to the hypothesis that the interaction of tissue-proteins with its receptor is a diffusion-controlled process [219,220].

The separation of the bound CEA from unbound is carried out by the addition of saturated ammonium sulphate to the incubation mixture, takes the advantage of solubility of CEA in half-saturated ammonium sulphate.

The specifity of the binding was further investigated by introducing different concentrations of unlabelled CEA in to the incubation medium. The concentration of the unlabelled CEA (in ng/ml) necessary to cause amaxium displacement of the labelled CEA was about 50 time that of ^{125}I-CEA. About 85% of the bound ^{125}I-CEA was displaced from its receptor and the amount of nonspecifity remained constant whatever higher concentration of unlabelled CEA used.

◄ Influence of ^{125}I-CEA Concentration:

One of the most important criteria of the true receptors is the saturability. To fulfil of this criterion and to estimate the suitable concentration of ^{125}I-CEA, the experiment was carried out as mentioned previously in section (5.6.2). The results are illustrated in fig (5-1) A, B, it is shown that the specific binding of radioactive CEA with receptor proteins is a saturable process but complete saturation however is theoretically never reached unless the amount of tracer used reaches infinity[219]. As shown in the same fig., the cytosolic receptor protein used in the incubation mixture under the conditions of the experiments were saturated with tracer (^{125}I-CEA) when the amount of the latter in the incubation mixture was equivalent to 50 μl (approximately equal to 0.5 ng). On the other hand, nuclear fraction appeared to be saturated with ^{125}I-CEA at concentration that equivalent to 75 μl (≈ 0.7 ng). According to the results of this experiment, 50 and 75 μl of ^{125}I-CEA were used in the binding studies of cytosolic and nuclear receptors respectively.

◄ Effect of receptor concentration on the binding:

In order to demonstrate whether the specific binding is proportional to the concentration of CEA receptor actually present in the incubation mixture, increasing amount of cytosolic or nuclear homogenate were incubated with either tracer CEA or with unlabelled CEA. As shown in fig (5-2) the percentage of tracer CEA bound specifically to their receptors was increased as the latter increase in the incubation mixture. The specific binding was increased linearly whereas the nonspecific binding was increased somewhat less than that of the specific binding. These results indicate that CEA-receptor binding are principally dependent on the amount of receptor protein in the reaction mixture[221]. In all the subsequent experiment, 200 µg of receptor protein or 150 µg of nuclear DNA in the incubation mixture were used.

◄ Effect of Temperature

The temperature dependency of the association of tracer CEA with their cytosolic and nuclear receptor isolated from malignant breast tumors was investigated. Fig (5-3) shows the results of this analysis. It seemed that specific binding of tracer CEA to their receptor was maximal at 4°C and low at other temperatures used for incubations particularly at 45°C. The loss of binding activity may due to degradation of the receptor and or the irreversible dissociation of CEA-receptor complex. As a result of the temperature sensitivity of CEA-receptor complexes, it is decided to study the time course of the association of CEA with their receptor at different temperature.

◄ Time Course of Receptors Binding:

To examine the characteristics of the association of tracer CEA with their receptor, the experiment was carried out at five temperatures (4,10,20,30,45). As seen in fig (5-4 A ► D) the time course of the binding reaction after incubation of tracer CEA with or without unlabelled CEA. The specific binding of tracer to its receptors was maximal at 5 h and 4°C, and remained unchanged for 5 additional hours of incubation. At 30°C and 45°C the apparent equilibrium was reached in 4 h and was maintained for additional 1 h before a gradual loss of binding activity was observed. Fig (5-4 B). The specific binding of postmenopausal cytosolic fraction was more stable and less sensitive to elevated temperature than that of cytosolic receptor form permenopasual patient. These results revealed the low stability of CEA-receptor at elevated temperature. The loss of the binding activity may be due to either the degradation of the receptors or the irreversible dissociation of CEA-receptor-complexes.

According to the results of this experiment the binding studies of the subsequent investigations were carried out with 8 h at 4° C for cytosolic and nuclear receptor.

≺ Effect of pH on the Binding

Fig (5-5 A, B) show the effect of increasing pH from 7 to 8 on the binding of ^{125}I-CEA to its binding receptor in the homogenate. Maximum value of specific binding occurred at pH 7.4 (exhibits a narrow pH-optimum). The results indicate that in general, binding was pH-dependent and the shift in the pH of environment may affect the properties of particulate involved in the binding.

The pH dependence of the binding indicates that protonation deprotonation reactions are important to the energetic of ^{125}I-CEA-receptor, the destabilization of the complex at low pH may be due to increase in the dissociation rate of the complex.

In view of these results, the buffers in all experiment were adjusted at 7.4 pH.

≺ Effect of Monovalent and Divalent Salts on the Binding:

When monovalent salts (NaCl and KCl) and divalent salts ($CaCl_2$ and $MgCl_2$) were added with different concentrations (50-250 mM) to the reaction mixture, the results obtained indicated significant effect on the ^{125}I-CEA binding with their receptor. As in (fig (5-6),(5-7)). these results indicate that a small amount of salt causes a high specific binding of ^{125}I- CEA to their receptor, any further increase in salt concentration more than 50 mM causes instability of the ^{125}I-CEA-R complex, the reason may be due to the electrostatic interactions. Indeed if hydrophobic interactions were the force which stabilize ^{125}I-CEA-R, then increasing ionic strength would be expected to facilitate ^{125}I-CEA-R interactions.

In general, the mechanism by which these salts dissociate protein-protein interaction is not completely clear, one hypothesis assumes that salt may alter the nature of the hydrophobic forces controlling the stabilization of protein-protein complex formed [223]. The high concentration of salt ten to destabilize the complexes as a result of their interaction with water molecules leading to diminution of protein-protein interaction and reversible denaturation of the protein [223,224].

≺ Stability of CEA Receptors Complex

The influence of temperature on the stability of CEA-receptor complex as a function of time was studied. The complex was reincubated at two different temperatures (4 and 30°C) and at an certain time intervals the remaining bound CEA was estimated. As seen in fig (5-8 A, B), the rate of dissociation of CEA-cytosolic receptor complex was increased as the temperature increase leading to almost complete elimination of specific binding at 30° C after 4 h.

However after 4 h, about 75% of the specific binding of nuclear receptors at time zero was still tightly bound. The dissociation at 4°C of CEA–receptor complexes is very weak. The results of this experiment stated clearly the temperature sensitivity of CEA-receptor complex at elevated temperature (more than 4°C)

Scatchard Scattered Analysis and Kinetics of CEA Binding to their Receptor:

The simplest proposed model representing the interaction of ^{125}I-CEA with their receptor is expressed by the following equation:

$$\underbrace{^{125}\text{I-CEA}}_{L} + \underbrace{R}_{\text{receptor}} \underset{K_{-1}}{\overset{K_{+1}}{\rightleftharpoons}} \underbrace{^{125}\text{I-CEA} - R}_{\text{product}} \quad \ldots(1)$$

K_{+1} is the rate of association of ^{125}I-CEA with their receptor and K_{-1} represents the rate of the reverse reaction i.e., the dissociation of the complex formed under the same condition:

$$\text{At equilibrium; } Ka = \frac{[L-R]}{[L][R]} \quad \ldots(2)$$

$$Kd = \frac{[L][R]}{[L-R]} \quad \ldots(3)$$

$$\text{Thus; } Ka = \frac{1}{Kd} = \frac{K_{+1}}{K_{-1}} \quad \ldots(4)$$

Where:

Ka is the equilibrium constant of the association (i.e., affinity constant).

kd is the equilibrium constant of the dissociation of ^{125}I-CEA-R complex.

The values of Ka and total receptor concentration (B_{max}) were calculated from scatchard plot at five different temperatures in fig (5-9 A,B,C-D).

It is clear from table (5-2), that the affinity constant (Ka) is dependent on the type of tumor (postmenopausal or permenopasal), the receptor source (cytosolic or nuclear) and on temperature. Generally Ka decrease with increased temperature for the same type and source of tumor (e.g., in cytosolic fraction from menopausal patient, Ka decreased from 94.73µg^{-1}.ml at 4° C to 12.85 µg^{-1}.ml at 45° C. where the values of dissociation constant (Kd) were calculated using equation (4), and show that the lowest Kd value of ^{125}I-CEA-R complex occurs at 4° C at the time of incubation.

On the other hand, determination of maximal binding capacity (B_{max}) of CEA in each type of tissue source homogenate revealed similar result for Ka value, it is temperature dependent, B_{max} decreased with increasing temperature.

However, Scatchard plot analysis always gave straight line fig (5-9A → D) indicating that probably only one species of receptor site is present, or more but with the same affinity and number of binding sites. All parameters obtained from Scatchard plot are shown in table (5-2).

The time-course data shown in fig 5-4 (A → D) could be used to determinate the reaction order of CEA binding to their receptor using the following equation [211].

$$Ln[L-R]_e \left[\frac{[L]_T - [LR]_t [LR]_e / [R]_T}{[L]_T[LR]_e - [LR]_t} \right] = K_{+1} t \left[\frac{[L]_T[R]_T - [LR]_e}{[LR]_e} \right] \ldots\ldots(5)$$

The equation (5) could be simplified to equ (6) in order to fit the data of the first order kinetics:

$$Ln \frac{[LR]_e}{[LR]_e - [LR]_t} = K_{+1} t [L]_T [R]_T / [LR]_e \ldots\ldots(6)$$

Where:

K_{+1}: is the kinetic association constant in µg.ml.min^{-1}.
$[L]_T$: is the total concentration of ^{125}I-CEA in µg.ml^{-1}.
$[R]_T$: the total concentration of CEA-receptor in µg.ml^{-1}.
$[LR]_e$: the concentration ^{125}I-CEA-receptor complex formed at equilibrium.
$[LR]_t$: the concentrations of the complex formed after time (t).

The simplification of equation (5), which corresponds to second order reaction kinetics to equation (6), was carried out for one important consideration:

Most of the labeled CEA (i.e., ^{125}I-CEA) remained free and only a small fraction of $(L)_T$ is bound even at equilibrium (pseudo-first order condition). Weiland & Molinoff [214] reported that equation (6) could be used when 10% or less of ligand is specifically bound to its receptor.

On the other hand fig 5-10 (A → D) shows the plot of $\ln \dfrac{[LR]_e}{[LR]_e - [LR]_t}$ against time (t) gives a straight line with a slop equal to the observed value of first rate constant (K_{obs}) in min^{-1}.

The rate constant (K_{+1}) in µg^{-1}.ml^{-1}.min^{-1} was calculated at five different temperatures using the following equation [102].

$$K_{obs} = K_{+1} \frac{[L]_T [R]_T}{[LR]_e} \quad \quad \quad (7)$$

Also, the value of K_{-1} at five temperatures was calculated using equation (4). Whereas, the half life time of association $(t_{1/2})_{ass.}$, which represente the time needed for formation of half amount of the complex at equilibrium was determined from the concentration of the complex at equilibrium and the time-course curve.

The half-life time of dissociation $(t_{1/2})_{diss.}$, was calculated from the following relation:

$$(t_{1/2})_{diss} = \frac{\ln 2}{K_{-1}} = \frac{0.693}{K_{-1}} \quad [119]$$

The values of K_{obs}, K_{+1}, K_{-1}, $(t_{1/2})_{ass.}$, and $(t_{1/2})_{diss}$ at five different temperatures are summarized in table (5-3). Data analysis of this table show that the highest rate for association reaction K_{+1}, in malignant tumor homogenate occurs at 4° C while the lowest rate occurs at 45° C. when the reaction temperature was elevated from 4°C to 45° C, the value of association rate constant K_{+1} decreased by approximately 4 fold. These phenomena may be due to the change in the suitable conformation of the protein and affect the suitable binding sites.

Many investigators working on kinetic of association of CEA with specific monoclonal antibody reported the complete dependency of the reaction rate on temperature change [112,119]. AL-Kazzaz [119] observed that the rate of binding of ^{125}I-antiCEA to carcinombryonic antigen in crude colorectal tumor at 4°C is about 2.5 folds that at 45° C.

Table (5-3) also shows the value of rate constant for the reveres reaction K_{-1} calculated from equation (4). Results show that the rate of dissociation of ^{125}I-CEA from their receptor is temperature dependent.

In this study the kinetic finding with tissue homogenate from pre and postmenopausal breast cancer patient are in agreement with that obtained by previous studies on antibody-CEA system which reported that the binding reaction was time and temperature-dependent process [112,119].

Estimation of Hill Coefficients (n) of Nuclear and Cytosolic Receptor in Human Malignant Breast Tumors:

The Hill equation is an appropriate tool for binding analysis only when cooperative is very strong or non-existent [225,226]. Fig. (5-11 A, B) represents the Hill plots of ^{125}I-CEA binding to their nuclear and cytosolic receptor in (pre-post menopausal) malignant breast tumors at optimum condition.

The results shows that Hill coefficient for this binding is approximately 1.7, this value indicates that the reaction between ^{125}I-CEA and their receptors is characterized by high affinity and cooperation.

Many authors reported that when the Hill coefficient was ranged between (1-2), this indicates that the reaction has a high affinity and cooperatively [224,227,228].

Many investigators showed that the mechanism of cooperative attachment of steroid to its receptor is in dispute but two basic models have been proposed; the symmetrical, allosteric effector hypothesis of Monod and the induced fit, sequential hypothesis of koshland [225]. Although Walent and Gorski (1990) presented a cooperative receptor model. According to this model, steriod (S) binds to a receptor and forms a non-activated monomeric (SR) complex. The monomeric complex forms an activated (SR) dimer only after undergoing a cooperative dimerization reaction that is dependent on the concentration of (SR) monomerric complex. Cooperatively dimerization is therefor required for activation of (SR) complex in this model [226].

The Thermodynamic of Receptor Binding Result

(1) Thermodynamic Parameters of Standard State:

The dependence of the equilibrium constant (affinity constant) for binding of ^{125}I-CEA to cytosolic and nuclear fraction of mammary adenocarcinoma tissue on the temperature can be observed from Van't Hoff plot, as showing in fig (5-12 A, B). The result obtained from Van't Hoff plot revealed that $\Delta H°$ in the general has small negative value table (5-4).

The negative value of $\Delta G°$ reflect the stability of complex hence, the high affinity of the reactions. The high negative values of $\Delta G°$ for the binding reaction are controlled by high positively $\Delta S°$ as shown in table (5-4). So, the present system is characterized by the sole contribution of $\Delta S°$ to the stability of the complex formed, while $\Delta H°$ has little or no effect [229].

The high values of positive $\Delta S°$ suggest that the reaction was entropically driven and indicate that the hydrophobic interactions are essentially important in stabilizing the complex [230].

(2) Thermodynamic Parameters of Transition State:

The transition state theory proposes that the association of two substances to form the final product proceed through the formation of an active complex (Transition State). Consequently, the interaction of ^{125}I-CEA with cytosolic or nuclear receptor can be represented as follows:

$$CEA + R \longrightarrow [CEA \ldots R]^* \longrightarrow CEA\text{-}R$$

State A — An activated complex (Transition state) State B — Final Product State C

The thermodynamic parameters of the transition state (Ea, ΔH^*, ΔS^*, and ΔG^*) could be determined from Arrhenius equation and the kinetic constants. Fig (5-13 A and B) shows the Arrhenius plots of Ln K_{+1} against 1/T values. The slope of the straight line represents the activation energy (Ea).

Table (5-5) show the values of thermodynamic parameters of the transition state (Ea, ΔH^*, ΔS^*, and ΔG^*). The high values of activation energy 9.972 KJ.mol^{-1} and 6.23 KJ.mol^{-1} of cytosolic and nuclear fractions respectively; represent the required energy to overcome the energy barrier of the transition state for the formation of (^{125}I-CEA-R) complex. Also the value of activation is in accordance with the high positive values of ΔG^*, which indicates that the formation of the activated complex is a non-spontaneous process and required a lot of energy (equal to Ea) to overcome the transition state energy barrier and giving the final product, whereas the high negative ΔS^* revealed that the activated complex had a more order structure than reactions.

From the results obtained for the thermodynamic parameters in the Transition State. It can be concluded that the positive values of ΔH^* and high positive values of ΔG^* are favorable to overcome the energy barrier of the transition state, the high negative values of ΔS^* mean more arranged structure for the activated complex. The positive values of ΔG^* is mainly attributed to the decrease in entropy of the transition state ($\Delta S^* < 0$). In addition the positive values of ΔH^* shows that the heat content of the activated complex is more than that of isolated species [214,231].

The values of thermodynamic parameters of the binding reaction gave an overall idea about the nature of forces that regulate the formation of complex. The thermodynamic model describe the formation of the complex was suggested using the thermodynamic parameters of both the standard and the transition states. The model is illustrated in figure (5-14). This model proposes that the formation of the (^{125}I-CEA-receptor) complex undergo three thermodynamic states [232]. The thermodynamic state A represents the initial energy level of ^{125}I-CEA and cytosolic or nuclear receptors. In the thermodynamic state B, the tow species bind to form the activated complex (^{125}I-CEA-receptor) the last thermodynamic state C, represents the fully interacting (^{125}I-CEA-receptor) complex.

In step 1 of the reaction, the binding of ^{125}I-CEA to cytosolic or nuclear receptor was associated with positive ΔG^* values. This indicates that the initial step of the reaction requires input of energy for the system. The negative entropy change ΔS^* for this step of the reaction reflects the change of (^{125}I-CEA/receptor) transition complex to a more arranged structure.

In - step 2 the activated complex contributes in further interactions, giving fully interacting complex (^{125}I-CEA/ receptor). It is proposed that the formations of a protein-ligand complex occur in these two steps. The first is the stabilization of the complex by hydrophobic interactions and the second is the stabilization by short-range interactions, such as electrostatic interaction, hydrogen bonding and Van der Waals interaction [233].

Hydrophobic interactions contribute to the complex stability via high positive entropy change ($\Delta S^* > 0$), while electrostatic interactions, hydrogen bonding and Van der Waals interactions contribute to the stability of the complex via negative entropy change ($\Delta S^* < 0$) [233,234].

The thermodynamic data indicate that the binding of ^{125}I-CEA to cytosolic or nuclear receptor are entropy driven in agreement with the concept that hydrophobic interactions play an important role in (^{125}I-CEA-receptor) interactions.

Table (5-1)
Preliminary Tast of ^{125}I-CEA Specific Binding to Their Receptors in Breast Adenocarcinoma and benign Tissue
(All details are explained in the text)

Tissue source	Type of Mammary tumor	Type of fraction	Number of cases	SB%
Pre-menopausal patient	malignant	Cytosolic	14	7%
		Nuclear	14	5%
Post-menopausal patient	malignant	Cytosolic	19	10%
		Nuclear	19	7%
	benign	Cytosolic	5	2%
		Nuclear	5	1%

Table (5-2) The Kinetic Parameters of ^{125}I-CEA Binding with Cytosolic & Nuclear receptor in mammary adenocarcinoma tissues (All details are explained in the text)

Temp (°C)	Ka x 10^2 (µg^{-1}.ml)				Kd x 10^{-5} (µg.ml^{-1})				B$_{max}$ 10^{-5} (µg.ml^{-1})			
	Postmenopausal patient		Premenopausal patient		Postmenopausal patient		Premenopausal		Postmenopausal		Premenopausal	
	cytosolic	Nuclear	cytosolic	Nuclear	cytosolic	Nuclear	cytosolic	Nuclear	cytosolic	Nuclear	cytosolic	Nuclear
4	94.73	87.5	77.77	87.5	10.5	11	12.85	11.42	85	70	73	78
10	88.88	77	70	81.25	13.3	12.9	14.2	12.3	57.5	48	50	42
20	88.23	78.4	65	75	15	12.7	13	13.3	40	40	35	39
35	55	57	45	40	17.2	17.5	22.4	25	32	30	22.5	28
45	12.85	16.66	11.25	17.5	80	60	88.88	57	12	11	9.5	9.5

Table (5-3) The effect of temperature on the kinetic parameters of ^{125}I-CEA binding with cytosolic & Nuclear receptor in mammary adenocarcinoma tissue. (All details are explained in the text)

Temp	$K_{obs} \times 10^{-3}$ (min^{-1})				K_{+1} (µg^{-1}.ml.min^{-1})				$K_{-1} \times 10^{-3}$ (min^{-1})				$(t_{1/2})_{ass}$ (min)				$(t_{1/2})_{diss}$ (min)			
	Postmenopausal		Permenopausal		Postmenopausal		Permenopausal		Postmenopausal		Permenopausal		Postmenopausal		Permenopausal		Postmenopausal		Permenopausal	
	cytosolic	Nuclear	cytosolic	Nuclear	cytosolic	Nuclear	cytosolic	Nuclear	cytosolic	Nuclear	cytosolic	Nuclear	cytosolic	Nuclear	cytosolic	Nuclear	cytosolic	Nuclear	cytosolic	Nuclear
4	13.6	14	11	16	135	150	115	145	12.7	17	14.76	16	30	30	60	45	54	41	47	43.3
10	10	9	8.5	9	131.7	140	108	143	14.8	17.5	15	17	60	30	30	30	37	38	46	39.4
20	8	8.8	7	8	128	141	110	135	14.5	18	17	18	30	60	60	60	48	38	41	39
35	6	8	6.6	7	84	128	99	83	15	19	22	20	10	60	30	60	46	36.5	31.5	35
45	5	6.6	5	6	30	39	39	40	23.3	23	24	23	150	90	60	60	24	24	29	30

Table (5-4) Thermodynamic parameters of standard state of ^{125}I-CEA binding with cytosolic & Nuclear receptor in mammary adenocarcinoma tissue (All details are explained in the text)

| Temp (°C) | Tumors of postmenopausal patients ||||||| Tumors of Premenopausal patients |||||||
| | Cytosolic Fraction ||| Nuclear Fraction ||| Cytosolic Fraction ||| Nuclear Fraction |||
	ΔH° KJ.mol^{-1}	ΔG° KJ.mol^{-1}	ΔS° J.mol^{-1}.K^{-1}	ΔH° KJ.mol^{-1}	ΔG° KJ.mol^{-1}	ΔS° J.mol^{-1}.K^{-1}	ΔH° KJ.mol^{-1}	ΔG° KJ.mol^{-1}	ΔS° J.mol^{-1}.K^{-1}	ΔH° KJ.mol^{-1}	ΔG° KJ.mol^{-1}	ΔS° J.mol^{-1}.K^{-1}
4	-11.62	-21.03	34.06	-19.4	-20.87	5.3	11.08	-20.6	34.36	18.99	-20.7	6.17
10	-11.62	-21.35	34.385	19.4	-21.04	5.7	11.08	-20.81	34.38	18.99	-21.16	7.68
20	-11.62	-22.08	35.70	19.4	-21.81	8.2	11.08	-21.35	35.05	18.99	-21.71	9.28
30	-11.62	-22.01	33.73	19.4	-22.11	8.5	11.08	-21.17	33.3	18.99	-20.87	6.20
45	-11.62	-18.87	22.79	19.4	-19.6	0.62	11.08	-18.5	23.3	18.99	-19.55	1.76

Table (5-5) Thermodynamic parameters at Transition state of ^{125}I-CEA binding with cytosolic & Nuclear receptor in mammary adenocarcinoma tissue (All details are explained in the text)

Temp (°C)	Tumors of postmenopausal patients									Tumors of Premenopausal patients								
	Cytosolic Fraction				Nuclear Fraction				Cytosolic Fraction				Nuclear Fraction			
	Ea*	ΔH*	ΔG*	ΔS*	Ea*	ΔH*	ΔG*	ΔS*	Ea*	ΔH*	ΔG*	ΔS*	Ea*	ΔH*	ΔG*	ΔS*
	KJ.mol^{-1}	KJ.mol^{-1}	KJ.mol^{-1}	J.mol^{-1}K^{-1}	KJ.mol^{-1}	KJ.mol^{-1}	KJ.mol^{-1}	J.mol^{-1}K^{-1}	KJ.mol^{-1}	KJ.mol^{-1}	KJ.mol^{-1}	J.mol^{-1}K^{-1}	KJ.mol^{-1}	KJ.mol^{-1}	KJ.mol^{-1}	J.mol^{-1}K^{-1}
4	9.972	7.67	56.34	-175.70	5.193	2.84	56.09	-192.07	9.418	7.118	56.71	-179.06	6.23	3.93	56.188	-188.65
10	9.972	7.63	57.66	-176.78	5.193	2.85	57.52	-193	9.418	7.07	58.11	-180.68	6.23	3.89	57.711	-190.180
20	9.972	7.54	59.87	-178.6	5.193	2.76	59.65	-194.17	9.418	6.98	60.23	-181.76	6.23	3.8	59.44	-191.788
30	9.972	7.42	64.14	-184.144	5.193	2.64	63.19	-196.6	9.418	6.86	64.77	-191.14	6.23	3.68	63.67	-194.80
45	9.972	7.3	69.02	-194.1	5.193	2.55	68.33	-206.8	9.418	6.77	69.20	-196.29	6.23	3.6	68.28	-203.40

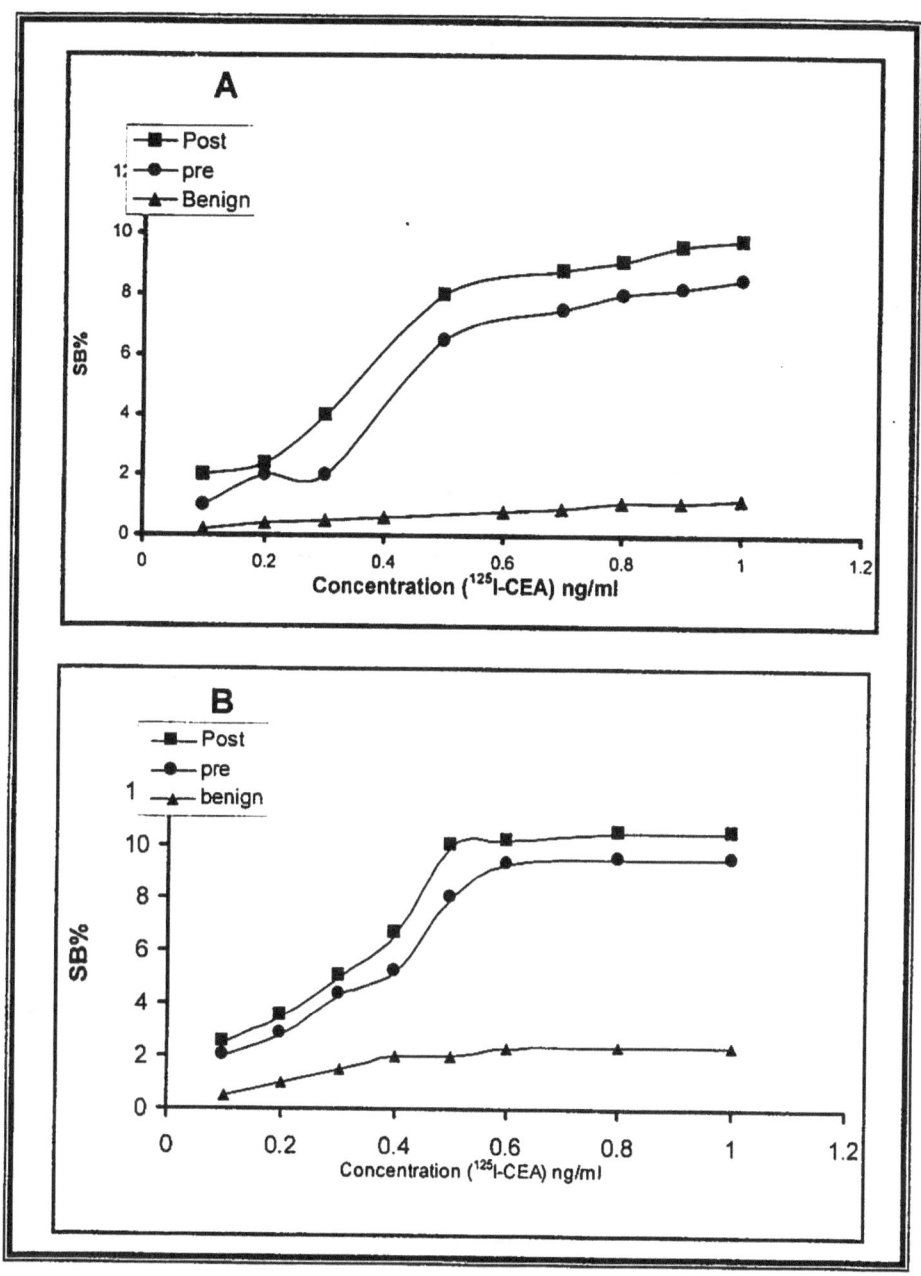

Fig. (5-1): Effect of the concentration of radioactive CEA on the binding with cytosolic (A) and nuclear (B) receptors.
(All details are explained in the text)

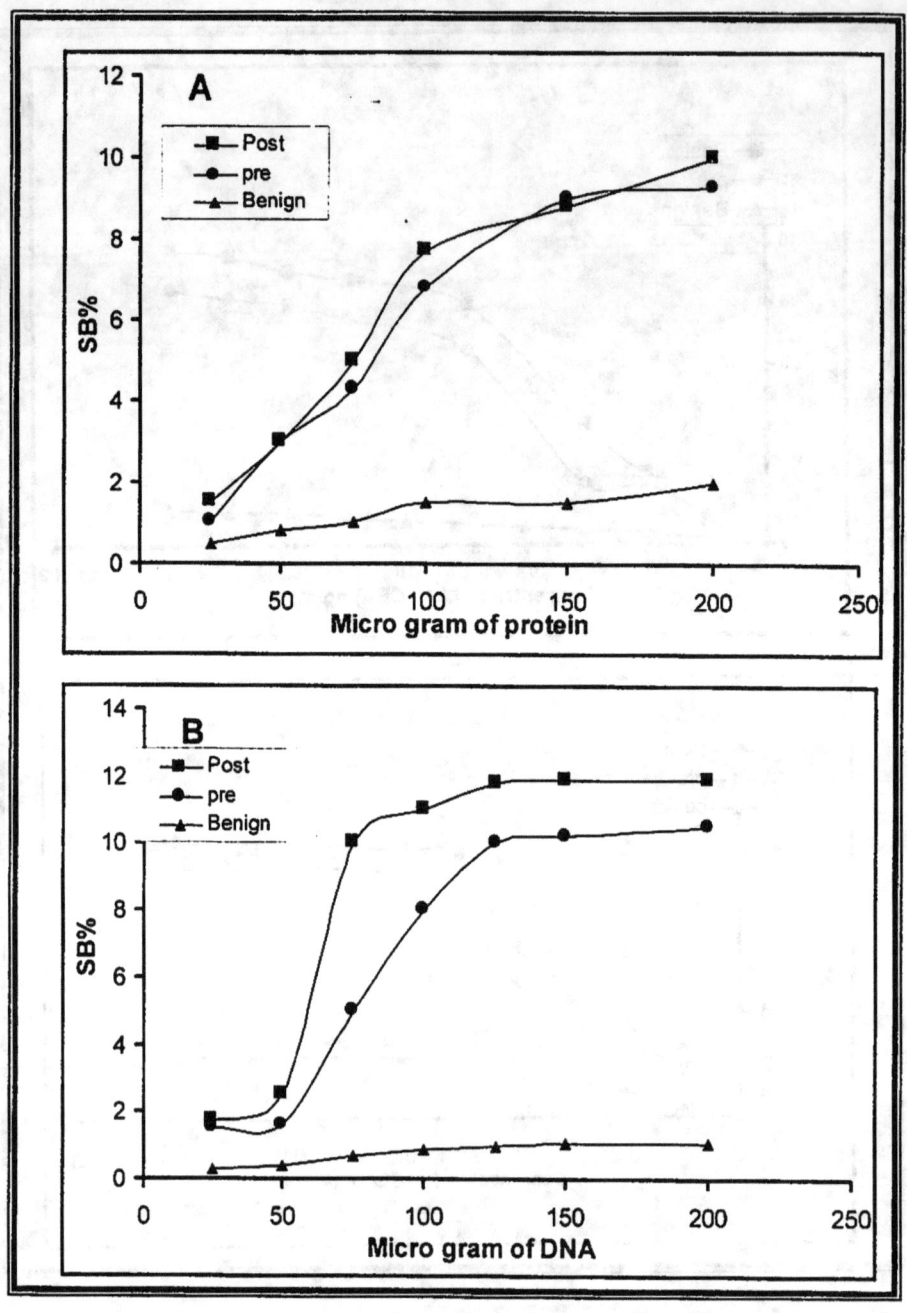

Fig. (5-2) Influence of cytosolic (A) and nuclear (B) receptor concentration of the binding with radioactive (CEA). (All details are described in text).

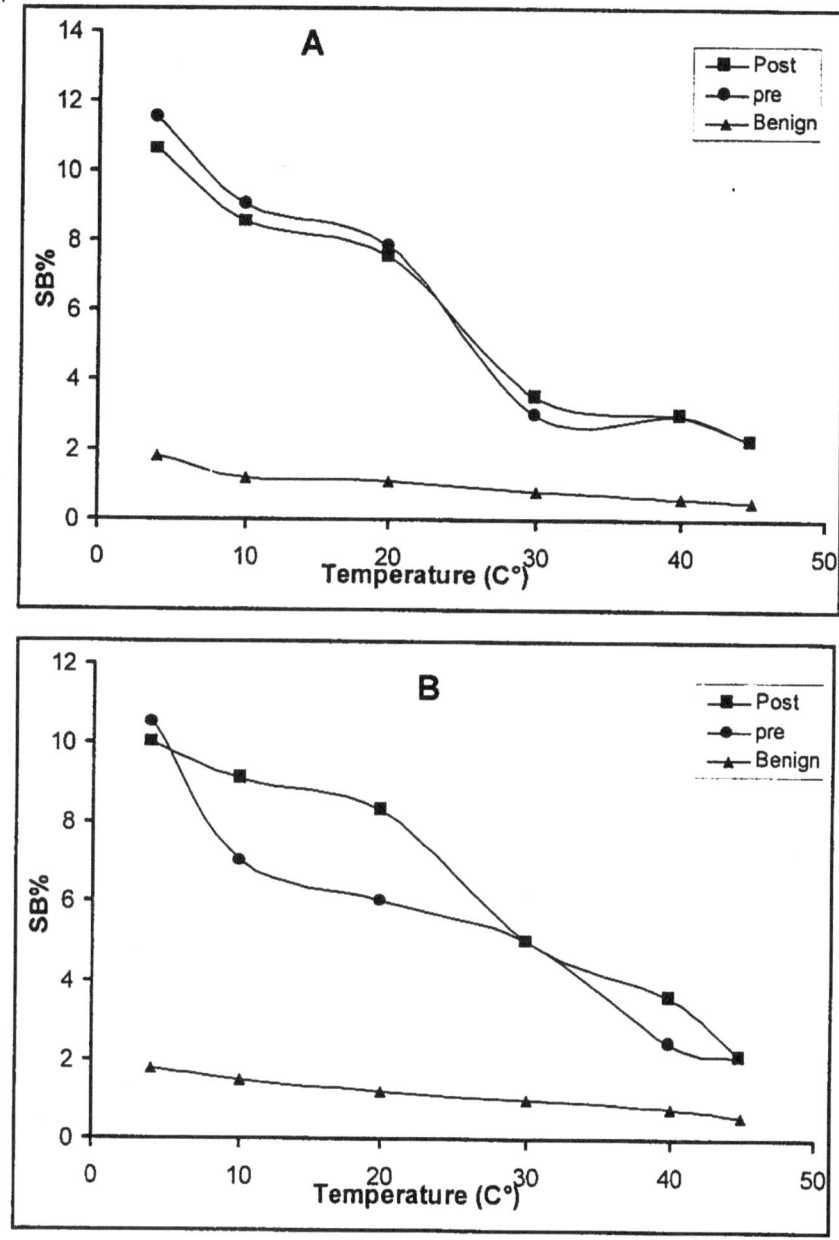

*Fig. 5-3 Effect of temperatures on ^{125}I-CEA binding with their cytosolic (A) and nuclear (B) receptors.
(All details are explained in the text)*

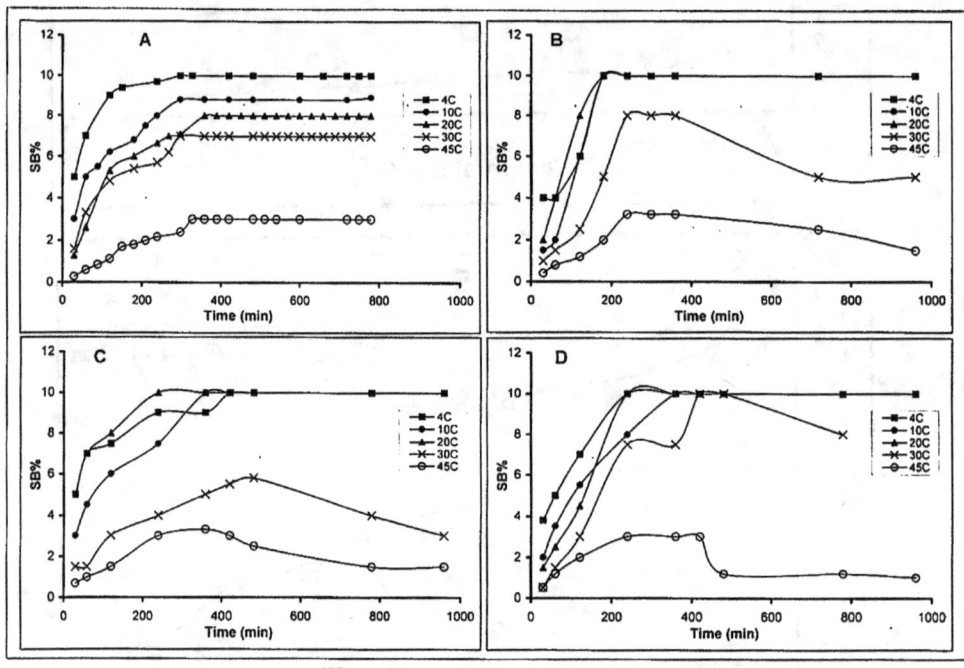

Fig. 5-4 Time course of ^{125}I-CEA binding with their cytosolic and nuclear receptors
A: Cytosolic fraction / postmenopasual patient., B: Cytosolic fraction / premenopasual patient., C: Nuclear fraction / premenopasual patient., D: Nuclear fraction / postmenopasual patient
. All details are described in text.

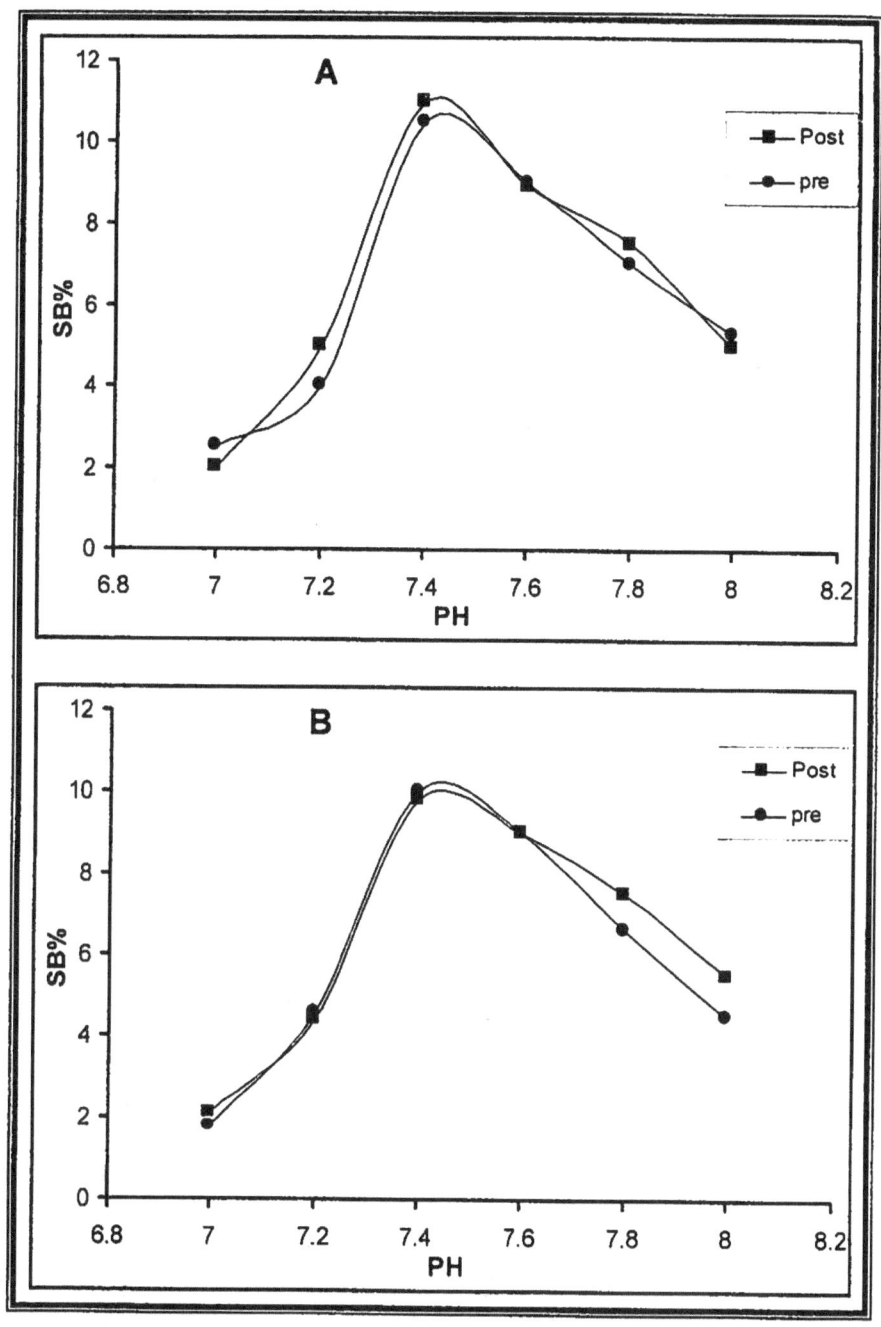

Fig. 5-5 pH dependency of ^{125}I-CEA binding with their cytosolic (A) and nuclear (B) receptors.
(All details are described in the text).

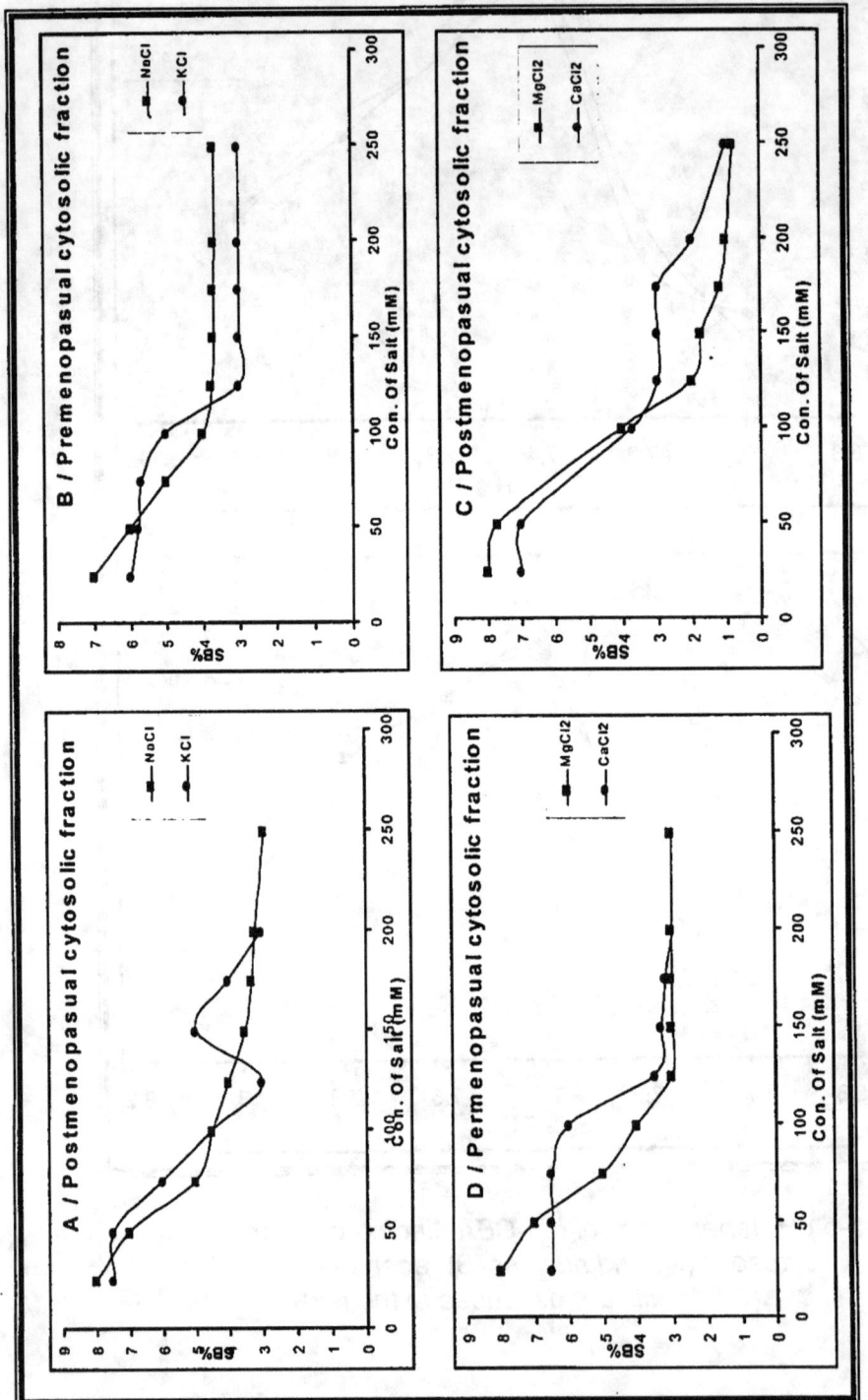

Fig. 5-6: The effect of salt concentration on the ^{125}I-CEA binding to their cyyosolic (A,B,C,D) receptor
(All details are explained in the text)

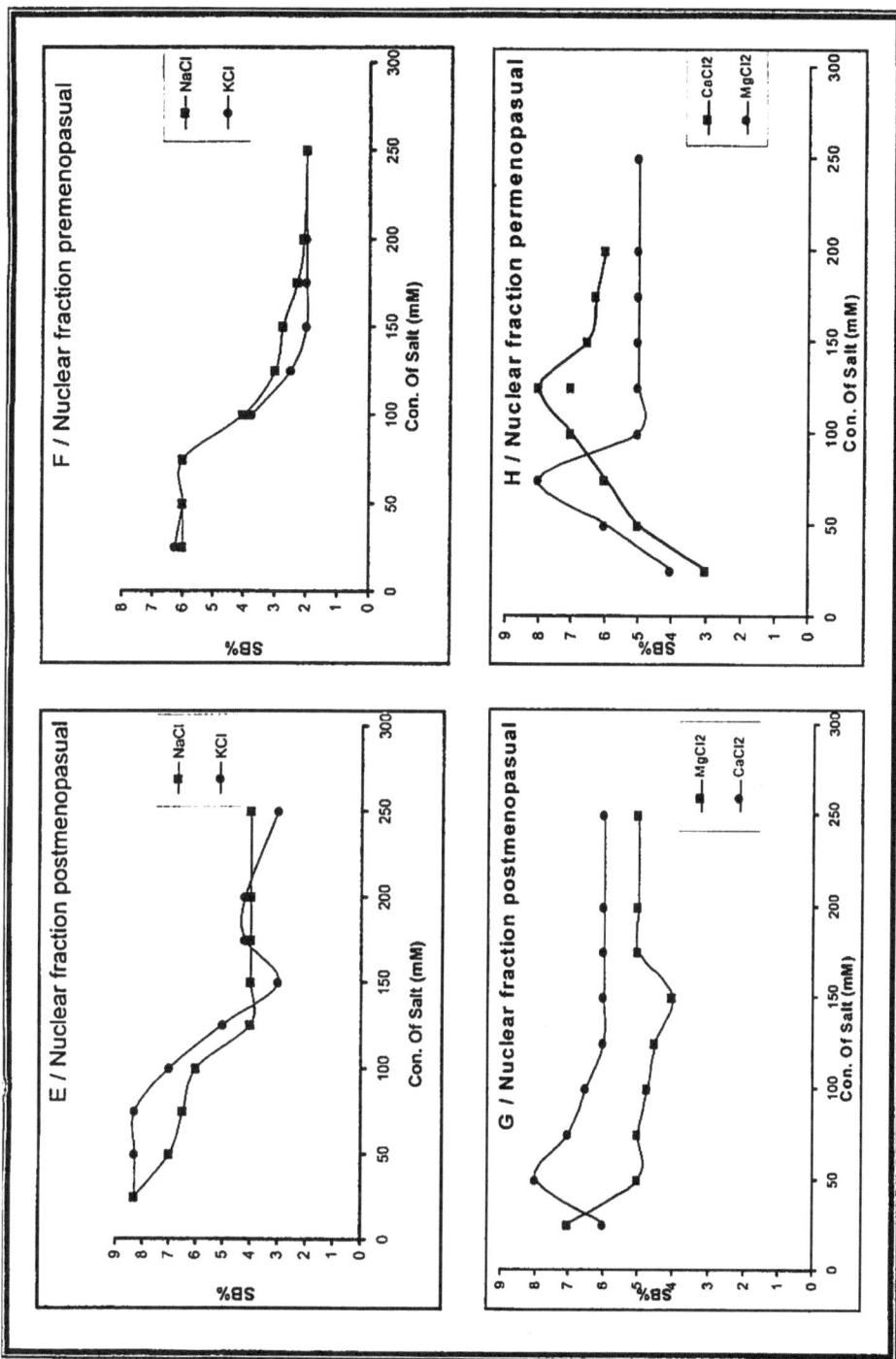

Fig. 5-7 The effect of salt concentration on the ^{125}I-CEA binding to their nuclear (E,F,G,H) receptor (All details are explained in the text)

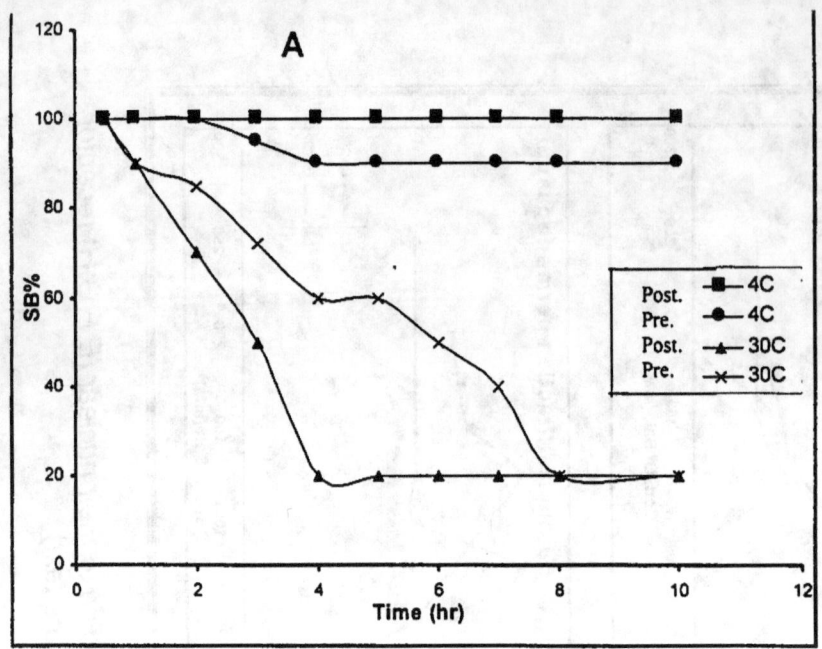

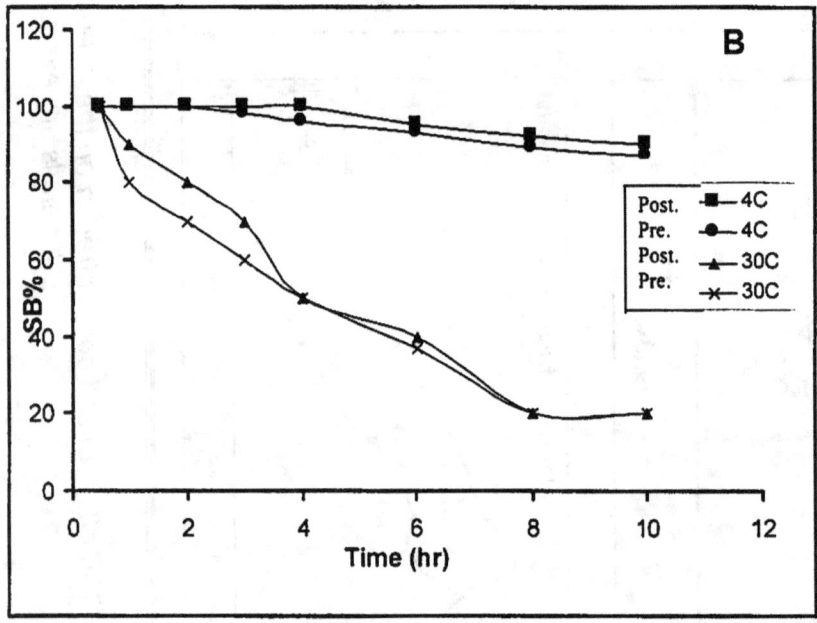

Fig. (5-8) Stability of ^{125}I-CEA receptors complex, (A) Cytosolic fraction from pre-post,menopasual. (B) nuclear fraction from pre-post,menopasual at two different temperatures. All details are explained in the text

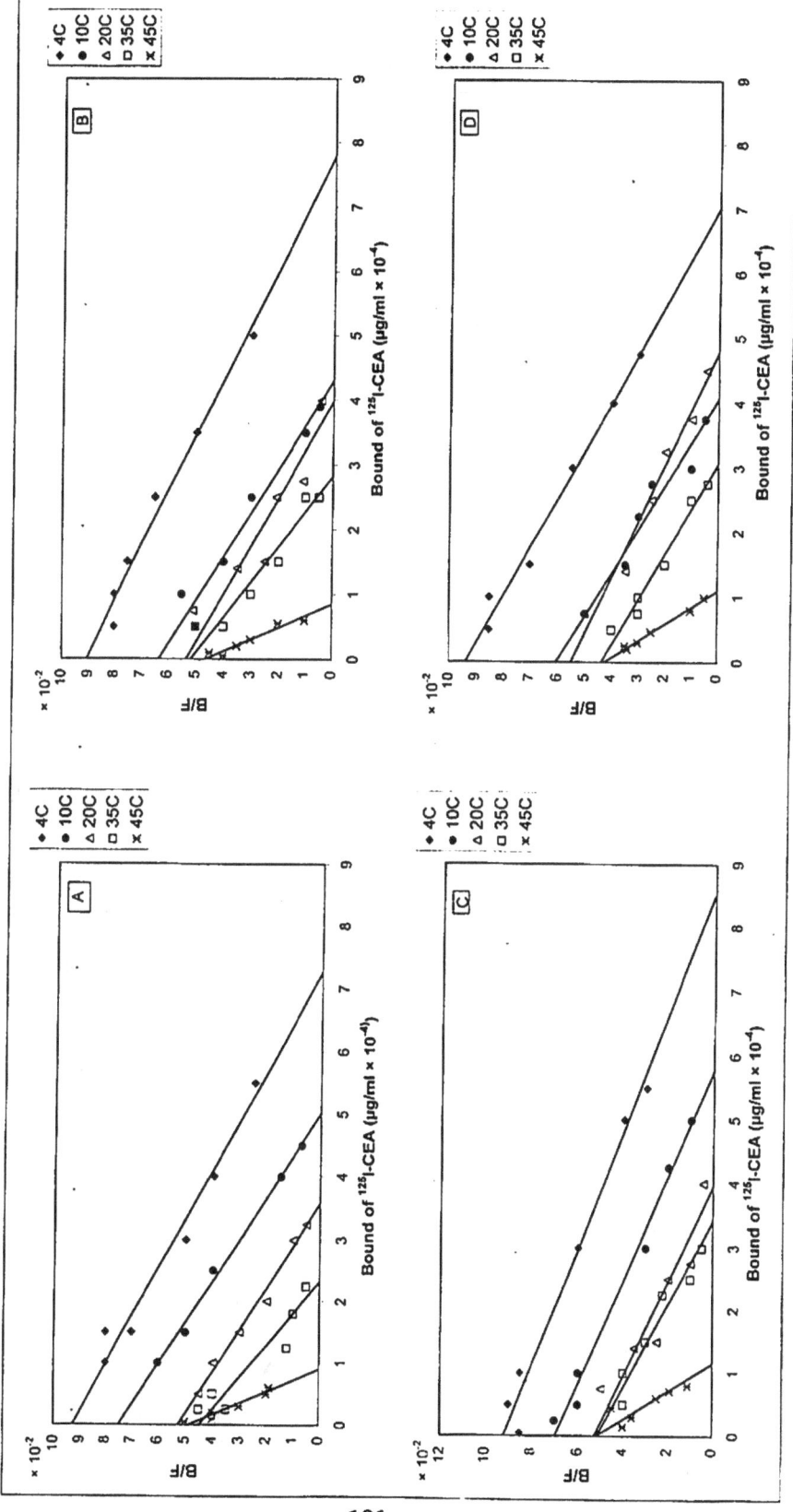

Fig. (5-9): Scatchard plots of ^{125}I-CEA binding with their receptors in:
A: Cytosolic fraction from premenopasual adeno-carcinoma tissues. B: Nuclear fractions from premenopasual adeno-carcinoma tissues.
C: Cytosolic fraction from postmenopasual adeno-carcinoma tissues. C: Nuclear fraction from postmenopasual adeno-carcinoma tissues.
All details are discribed in text.

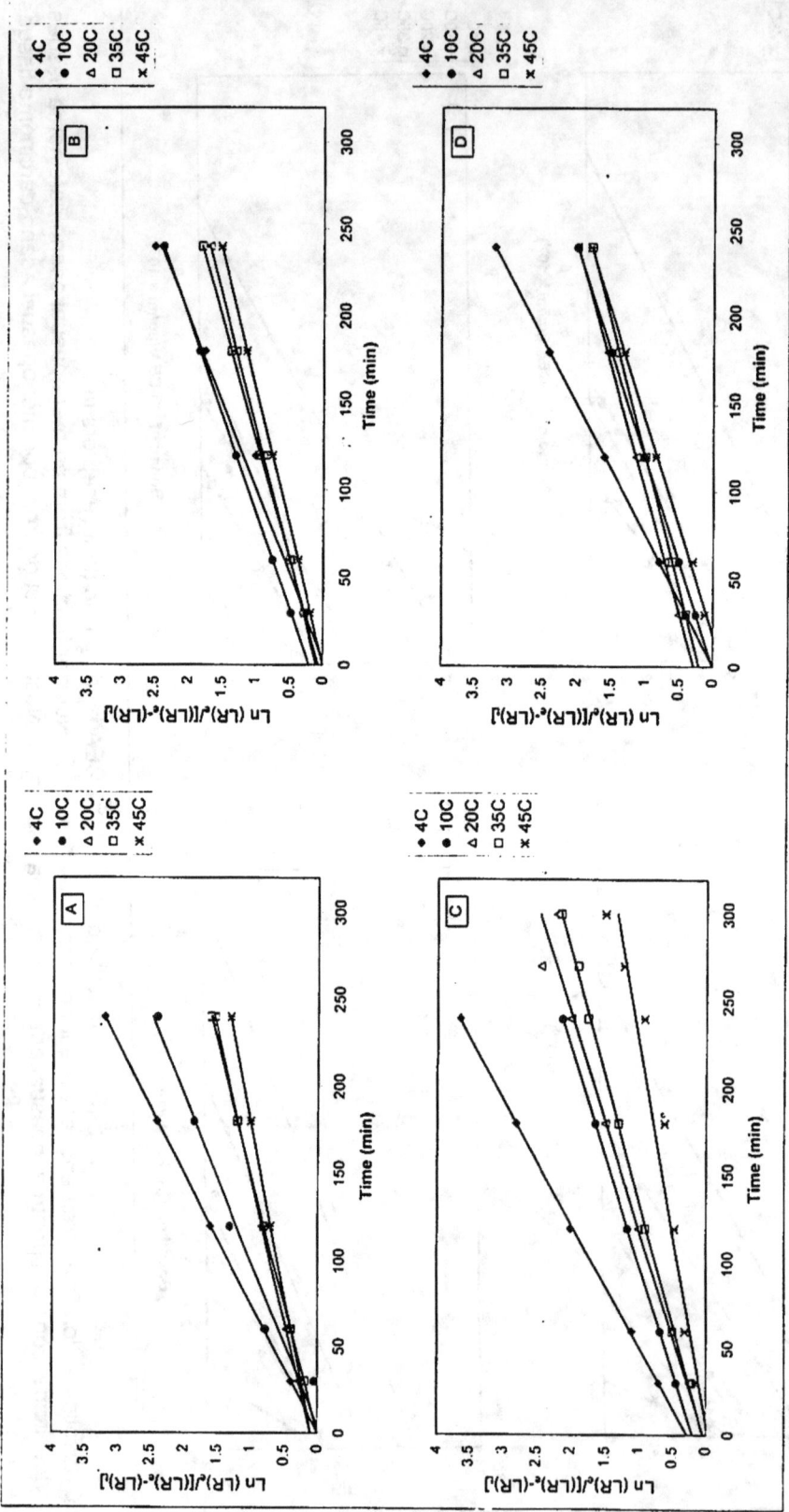

Fig. (5-10) : Kinetic of ^{125}I-CEA binding with their receptors in :
A: Cytosolic mammary adeno-carcinoma tissues from premenopasual patient.
B: Nuclear mammary adeno-carcinoma tissues from premenopasual patient
C: Cytosolic mammary adeno-carcinoma tissues from postmenopasual patient.
D: Nuclear mammary adeno-carcinoma tissues from postmenopasual patient.
All details are discribed in text.

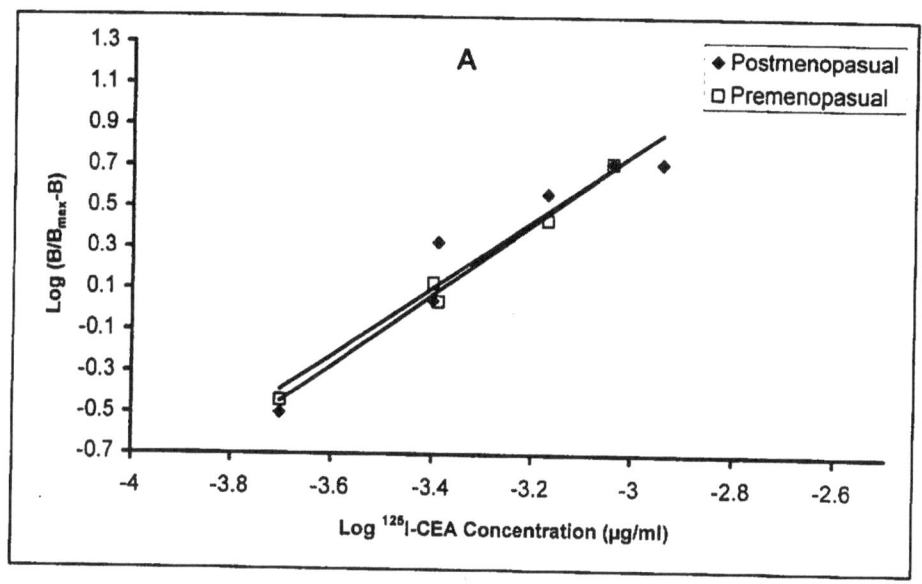
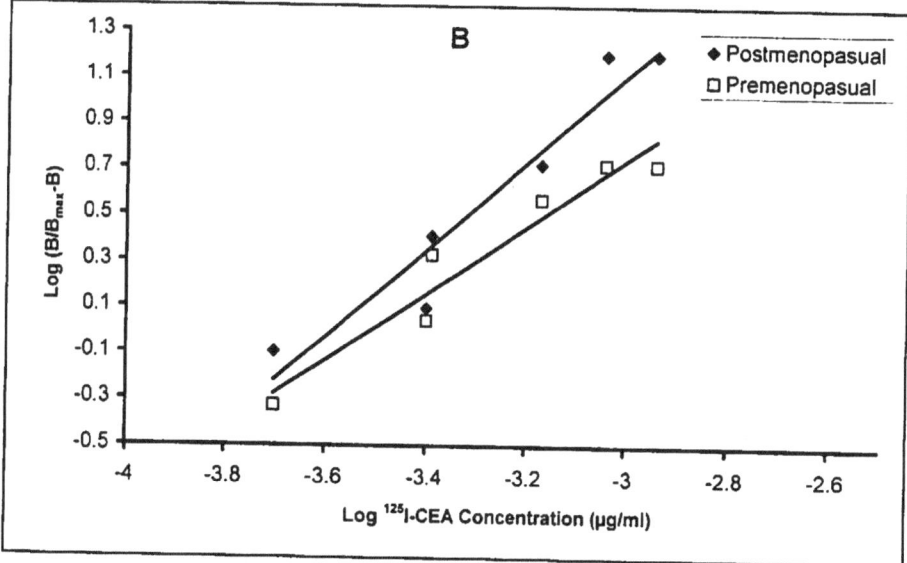

Fig (5-11): Hill plot of ^{125}I-CEA binding to their receptors
A: Cytosolic (pre-post menopasual) malignant breast tumors
B: Nuclear (pre-post menopasual) malignant breast tumors
(All details are described in text)

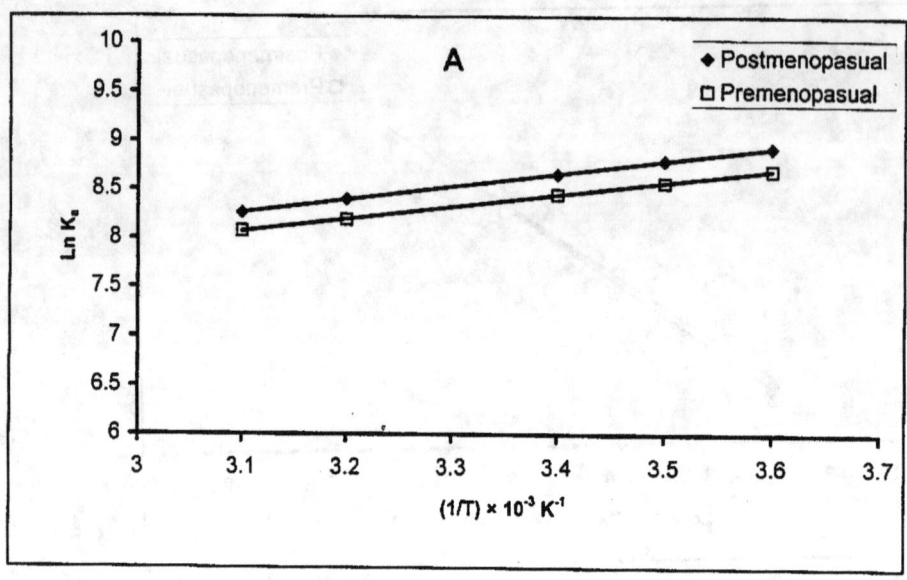
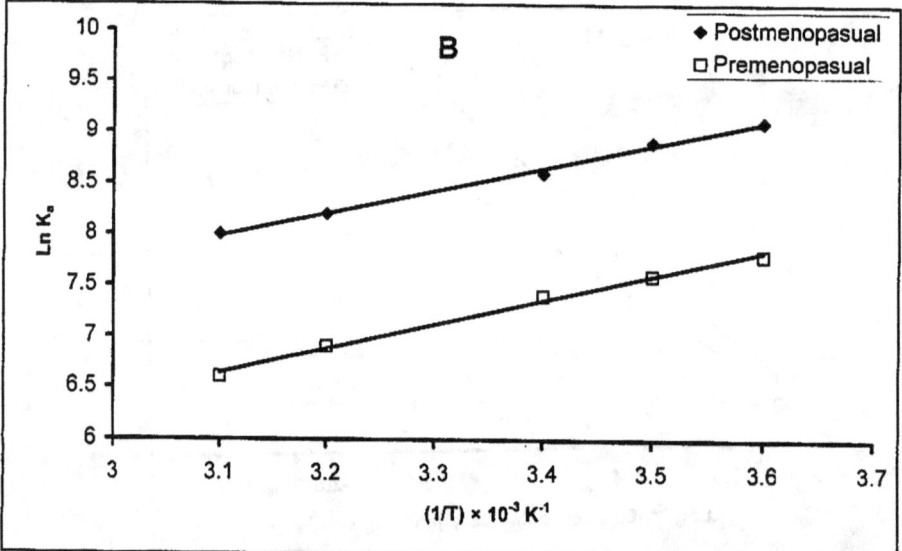

Fig (5-12): Van't Hoff plot for the ^{125}I-CEA binding to their receptors
A: Cytosolic (pre-post menopasual) malignant breast tumors
B: Nuclear (pre-post menopasual) malignant breast tumors
(All details are described in text)

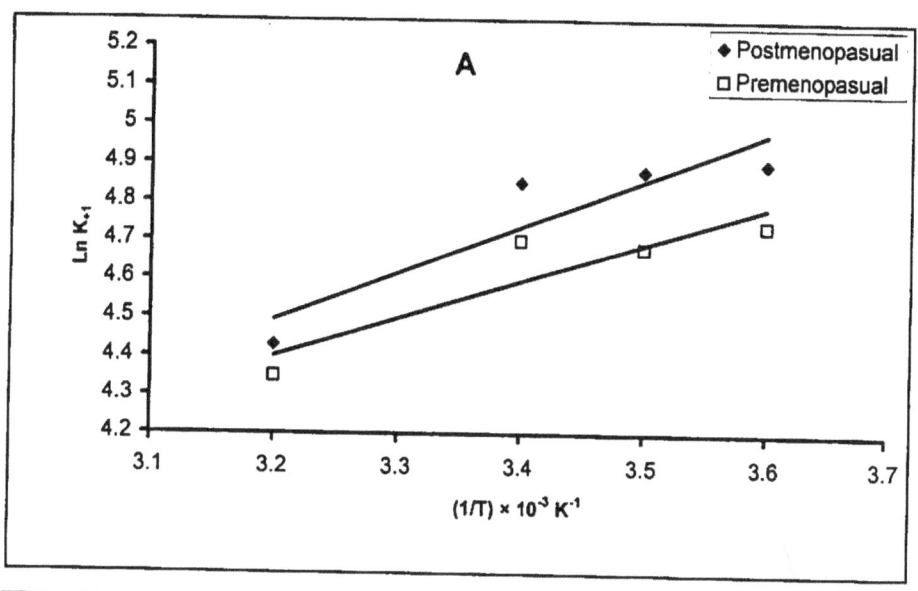
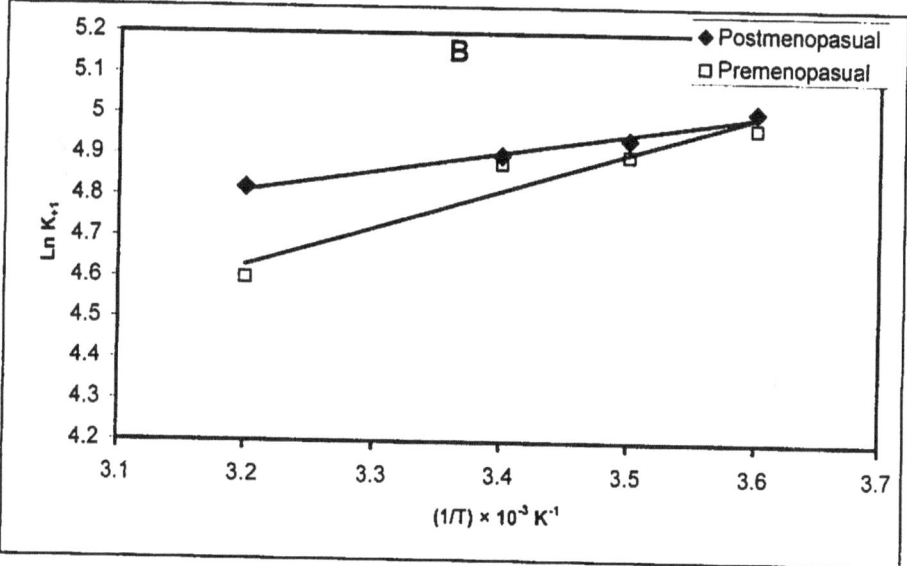

Fig (5-13) : Arrhenius plot for the ^{125}I-CEA binding to their receptors
A: Cytosolic (pre-post menopasual) malignant breast tumors
B: Nuclear (pre-post menopasual) malignant breast tumors
(All details are described in text)

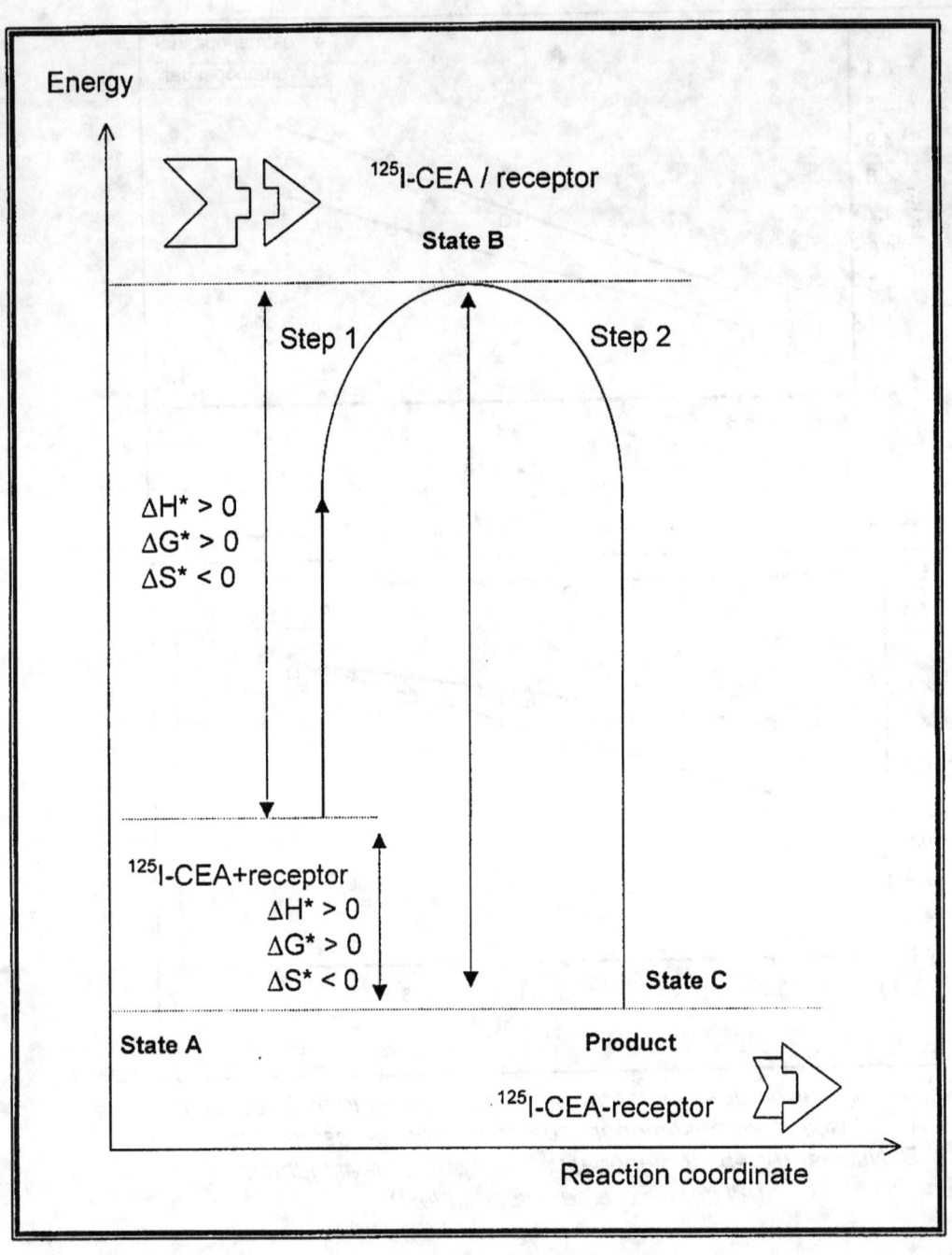

Fig (5-14): General energy diagram and thermodynamic model applied to the complex formation between ^{125}I-CEA and receptor

CHAPTER SIX

Isolation and Characterization of CEA Receptors in Mammary Tissues

Abstract

This is the first trial to isolate purified and characterize CEA receptor from mammary adenocarcinoma tissues. The purification procedure included Fractionation with ammonium sulfate, ion exchange chromatography (DEAE and CM-cellulose) and gel-filtration in sepharose 6B. The results revealed the presence of two types of receptors mainly .The first type Acidic cytosolic receptor, while the second type designated as cationic cytosolic receptors.

Characterization experiments show that cationic receptor has molecular weight 83000 dalton, stock radius 37° A and it contains 15.8% Carbohydrate .In isoelectric focusing one band was observed with isoelectric points (pI) 6.8

UV spectral studies showed that ^{125}I–CEA–receptor complex absorption maximum occurs at 241 nm while the absorption of the receptor was at 280 nm.

Introduction

The behavior of malignant tumor cells in vivo differs from that of normal cell in that they continue to proliferate and showing altered strength and specificity of adhesion to other cells and differs in migratory property [233]. Thus, Malignant cells are not constrained by the normal controls which regulate growth and keep cells of a give tissue in place; they cross basement membranes (invasion) and move around the body and implant in appropriate place (metastasis). Cell–type specific sorting involves surface molecules, as does adhesion in general; both migration and invasion involve interaction of the cell surface with environment, and stimulation and inhibition of cell division may also involve cell surface contacts, either with hormones, or with neighboring cells [236-240].

A major and interesting facet in the biologic spectrum of neoplastic phenomena is the production by malignant cells of products generally recognized only during the early oncogenic stages of development (i.e embryo antigens). The etiology leading to the occurrence of such embryo antigens remains unknown and intriguing. For example, it has been postulated that tumor with fetal receptor characteristics represent embryonal rests which have undergone expansion and re-expression. Alternatively, it has been suggested that the reappearance of embryo antigen is due to an antigenic (perhaps mutagenic) shift with progressive dedifferentiation (i.e antigenic reversion) [238]. Nonetheless, although this theoretical basis is poorly understood, embryo antigen can often be identified in sera and tissues of several human and murine tumors. The qualitative and quantitative nature of this expression may be critical to the cell biology of cancer. Furthermore, a continued and dramatic emphasis is being placed upon the identification of embryo antigen profiles in human sera as a diagnostic tool for cancer identification.

In particular, the influence of embryonic antigen on both general host immunocompetence and on specific tumor immune responsiveness is an intriguing issue [241-242].

Little is known about the physiological roles of CEA and very little attention on CEA receptors. These receptors to be found on the surface of embryonic and tumor cells while they are absent on the surface of normal mammalian cells [198-202].

In this chapter we will concentrate on the techniques used to purify and characterize CEA receptor. The potential application of these finding to cancer diagnosis and treatment. There were no references to evaluate CEA receptor in cancer tissue.

Materials and Method

6-1 Buffer and Reagents

1- All buffer solution were prepared by dissolving the appropriate amount of salt in distilled water and the required pH was adjusted[243].
2- Most of buffers and reagents are mentioned in chapter 3 and chapter 4. Other solutions used are indicated in each experiment.

6-2 Patients and Specimens

The tumor tissues were surgically removed from breast tumor patient (postmenopausal patients with breast cancer). Breast specimens were immediately immersed in ice-cold isotonic saline solution.

They were collected individually in plastic receptacle and stored at −20° C until homogenization.

6-3 Preparation of Cytosol

All operations were carried out at 0-4° C, tissues were thawed at 4° C, minced, and weighed. Two milliliter of ice-cold TED buffer pH 7.2 were added for each gram of tissue.

The tissue is then homogenized using a manual homogenizer. The temperature must be continuously monitored and kept at 0 °C. the homogenate was filtered through four layers of nylon gauze in order to eliminate fibers of connective tissues, then centrifugation at 4000 xg for 15 min at 4° C was carried out in order to precipitate the remaining intact cells and the intact nuclei. The supernatant was used throughout this study for the purification and characterization of cytosolic receptor of CEA.

6-4 Purification of CEA Receptors:

6-4-1 Ammonium sulphate fractionation of crude cytosolic receptors:

Successive fractions were made by addition, at 0 c° with stirring of increments of solid ammonium sulphate .The amount of ammonium sulphate to be added can be obtained from table 1 in refrance (137). The pH should be monitored and sufficient 1N NH_4OH was added to keep the pH 7.4 . When all the ammonium sulphate was dissolved, the mixture was allowed to stand for 15 min and then centrifuged at 4° C at 6000 xg for 30 min. The supernatant fluid was decanted and used as the starting material for the next fraction.

Fractions can be successively precipitated at saturation of 20,30,40,50,60,70.80 and 90%. The individual precipitate fraction should be drained, and the side of the vessel wiped free of adhering solution. The material should be dissolved in small amount of TED buffer.

Removal of ammonium sulphate can be accomplished by dialysis. For dialysis, the material should be transferred quantitatively and dialyzed at 0-4° C against several changes of the same buffer, stirring the dialyzing medium constantly. At the end of the dialyzing period, the sack should be emptied and the protein content, specific bindings for each fraction were measured.

Calculation:

1- Assay performed for protein content by lowry method [93].
2- The amount of radioactivity bound to the pellet was expressed as specific binding (SB) and was calculated by the following formula.

a- Specific Binding = $\dfrac{\text{Total binding} - \text{nonspecific binding}}{\text{Total count (T.C)}}$ x con. of Tracer(ng)

b- specific binding activity = $\dfrac{\text{Specific Binding (ng)}}{\text{Total protein in assay sample (mg)}}$
(ng/mg protein)

3- Total activity (ng)= Specific Binding activity (ng/mg) x total protein in pellet

4- purification fold = $\dfrac{\text{Specific binding of purified receptor ng/mg protein}}{\text{Specific binding of homogenate ng/mg protein}}$

5- Yield % = $\dfrac{\text{Total activity of purified receptor (ng)}}{\text{Total activity of crude (ng)}}$ X 100

6-4-2 Ion exchange chromatography of cytosolic receptor:

6-4-2-1 Anion-exchange

(A) preparation of DEAE-sephadex A-50 ion exchange column :
A column of 1.8 x 20 cm was used and packed as described in chapter three section (3-1-B).

(B) Separation procedure:
The concentrated protein (2-ml) obtained by ammonium sulphate fractionation (50-90% saturation) was loaded on the column. After an initial pre wash with 120 ml Tris-HCl buffer pH 7.4 at flow rate 40 ml/h. protein, was eluted using linear gradient of sodium chloride 0.0 M to 1 M in Tris buffer.

Fractions of 4 ml were collected. The elute was constantly monitored for its spectrophotometeric absorption at 280 nm, and specific binding using ^{125}I-CEA as described in chapter five (5-6). The specific binding of each fraction was calculated and plotted against the fraction number. Selected fractions containing high concentration of receptor were poold, dialyzed at 4° C against several change of the same buffer and then concentrated to 5 ml with dialysis against sucrose. The protein content of this pooled fraction was determined using lowry. et. al method [93]. Also specific binding activity, total activity and the purification fold were calculated as mentioned in section (6-4-1).

6-4-2-2 Cation exchange

(A) Preparation of carboxymethylcelluloses (CM52):

A column of 1.8 x 20 cm was used and packed with weak cation exchanger CM-celluloses-52. For the preparation of the resin, CM-celluloses-52 was swelled in Tris buffer pH 7.4 (30 ml/g of dry powder) for 48 h at room temperature without stirring. During the swelling period the supernatant was removed and replaced with fresh buffer several times. The resin was poured into the column down a glass rod with a bed volume of 38 ml. Two bed volumes of TED buffer pH 7.4 were run at a flow rate of 40 ml/h through the column in order to reach equilibration.

(B) Separation procedure:

The concentrated pooled wash fractions drived from DE-ion exchange, were loaded on the column. After an initial pre wash with 70 ml TED buffer. pH 7.4 at flow rate of 40 ml/h. protein was eluted using linear gradient of sodium chloride 0.0 M to 1 M in Tris buffer.

Fractions of 3 ml were collected. The eluate was constantly monitored for its spectrophotometeric absorption at 280 nm and specific binding percentage using ^{125}I-CEA as described in chapter five (5-6). The specific binding percentage for each fraction calculated and plotted against the fraction number. Fractions with high specific binding activity were pooled and concentrated by dialysis against sucrose. The protein content, specific binding activity and purification folds of the pooled fraction were evaluated as described in section (6-4-1).

6-4-3 Gel Filtration of Cytosolic CEA Receptor on Sepharose CL-6B Column:

(A) Preparation of the column:

As described in chapter 3 section 3-1 (Gel filtration chromatography –1), 1x38 cm column has been used.

(B) Purification procedure:

Purification of CEA receptor on sepharose CL-6B Column was performed according to three protocols:

The First Protocol:

The concentrated pooled fraction obtained from CM-cellulose ion exchange, was applied to 6B-spharose column directly, then fraction of 2 ml were eluted with TED buffer pH 7.4 at a flow rate of 33 ml/h. then each fraction constanly monitored for its absorption at 280 nm and the specific binding precentage was estimated as described in chapter five section (5-6). The SB% of each fraction was calculated and plotted against the fraction number, the fractions contain the binding activity were pooled and concentrated by dialysis against sucrose. The protein content of this pooled fraction was determined using lowry. et.al [93]. Also specific binding, total activity, purification fold, and the yield% were calculated as mentioned in section (6-4-2).

The Second Protocol:

Half ml of crude cytosolic homogenate containing approximatly 1.2 mg protein was incubated with 200 µl of ^{125}I-CEA (2 ng CEA; 40000 CPM) for 4 h at room temperature and then 16 h at 4° C with gentel agitation. The resulting mixture was applied to prepared sepharose 6B column and 2 ml samples were collected by elution with TED buffer pH 7.4 at flow rate of 20 ml/h. the radioactivity in each fraction was measured by gamma counter to identify the fraction containing the CEA complex and plotted against the fraction number.

The Third Protocol:

Two hundred µl ^{125}I-CEA alone was applied to prepared sepharos 6B column and 0.5 ml samples were collected by elution with TED buffer pH 7.4 at flow rate 20 ml/h.

The radioactivity in each fraction was measured by gamma-counter and plotted against the fraction number.

6-5 Characterization of Purified CEA Receptor and CEA-Receptor Complex:

6-5-1 Determination of molecular weight by gel filtration:

6B-sepharose column was used for this purpose. The method outlined in Experiment 3-4 was exactly followed to obtain the values of the partition coefficient (K_{av}) of the protein eluted. The values of K_{av} were plotted vs. the values of log M.wt of the proteins eluted. The M.wt of receptor CEA, was calculated from the standard curve obtained as mentioned in section 3-4.

6-5-2 Estimation of stock radius of purified receptor:

The gel filteration procedure was run on 6B-sepharose column exactly as mentioned in section (3-5) chapter three. The partition coefficient (K_{av}) was determined and the values of $(-\log K_{av})^{1/2}$ were calculated, then plotted against the stock's radius of eluted standard proteins. The stock's radiuses of cytosolic CEA receptor were calculated from the straight line obtained.

6-5-3 Analysis of Purified Receptors by Disc SDS-PAGE:

PAGE technique was used to specify the purity of the receptor of CEA and for estimation the molecular weights of receptor.

The experiment was performed as described in chapter 3 section 3-6.

The log M.wt of the standard proteins was plotted against the Rm values and the molecular weight of CEA receptors was calculated from the obtained straight line.

6-5-4 Determination of the isoelectric point (pI) of purified receptors:

Isoelectric focusing technique was used to determine pI of CEA receptor according to Wringley method [99]
Buffer and reagent mentioned in chapter 3 section (3-7) were used in these experiments. Also the method outlined in the same section was exactly followed to obtain the pI values of purified receptor.

6-5-5 Carbohydrate content of purified CEA:

The method of phenol–sulfuric acid that was described by Dubois [101], was used to determine the total carbohydrate in purified cytosolic receptor of CEA.
The same experiment (the steps, solutions, and calculation) mentioned in chapter three in section 3-8 were carried out using purified receptor of CEA.

6-6 The Ultraviolet Spectral Studies:

Buffers, reagent and instruments mentioned in chapter 3 section (3-10) were used in this experiment.

6-6-1 The UV spectra of purified Cytosolic CEA Receptor.

Twenty-five microliters of purified receptors were complete to 0.5 ml with Tris buffer pH 7.2, then placed in a 0.5-cm cuvette in the sample beam and the absorption spectrum was immediately measured against the same buffer in reference beam.

6-6-2 ^{125}I-CEA-Receptor Complex:

1- Forty-five µg of the receptor (protein) were incubated with 50 µls of ^{125}I-CEA (0.5 ng CEA; 40000 CPM) for 4 h at room temperature and then for 16 h at 4° C with genteel agitation. The volume was completed to 1 ml. with Tris buffer pH 7.2 .
2- The reaction was terminated by adding 1 ml of saturated ammonium sulfate at 4° C with immediate vortex mixing. The tube was kept at 4° C for 30 min and was then centrifuged 4000 xg for 15 min. The supernatant was decanted, and the resultant pellets should be drained, and the side of the vessel wiped free of adhering

solution. The content of ^{125}I-CEA-R was determined using gamma counter.

3- The precipitate formed was dissolved to 0.5 ml of Tris buffer pH 7.2, then placed in 0.5 cm cuvett in sample beam against tris buffer pH 7.2 in the reference beam.

The absorption spectrum of the complex solution was measured in the area of (200-350 nm).

Results and Discussion

Ammonium sulphate Fractionation:

Crude extracts are seldom suitable for direct application to chromatographic columns. It is often necessary to use other means for clarification. It simultaneously concentrates the solution and, at the same time, removes most of the bulk proteins. Such an initial fractionation step should also be directed to remove protease's and membrane fragments that some time bind to the protein of interest.

As indicated, ammonium sulphate is the precipitant used most frequently in the salting out of proteins. Its major advantages are:

(1) At saturation, it is of sufficiently high molarity that it causes the precipitation of most proteins.
(2) It does not have a large heat of solution, so that the heat generated is easily dissipated.
(3) Even its saturated solution (4.04 M at 20° C) has a density (1.235 g/cm^3) it is not so large to interfere with the sedimentation of most precipitated proteins by centrifugation.
(4) Its concentrated solutions prevent or limit most bacterial growth.
(5) In solution, it protects most proteins from denaturation. Because of this last property, one often preserves purified protein as suspension in concentrated solutions of ammonium sulfate [198].

There may be good reasons for choosing the initial fractionation stage by Ammonium sulphate, The purpose of this step is to obtain a solution suitable for chromatography. The preliminary test preformed by successive addition of solid ammonium sulphate and to precipitate and remove each step. The results listed in table (6-1) indicated that all fractions contain specific binding but the specific binding increased in precipitation at saturation 60, 70, 80 and 90%. In view of these results, the fractionation procedure for subsequent investigation were carried out by the cytosolic homogenate brought to 50 percent saturation by the addition of solid $(NH_4)_2SO_4$ at 4° C. The supernatant was collected by centrifugation at 6000 xg for 30 min and brought to 90 per cent saturation with solid $(NH_4)_2SO_4$.

The precipitate was then collected by centrifugation, dialyzed against buffer and layered on DEAE ion exchange.

Ammonium sulphate fractionation step increased the specific binding activity (5.1) fold with a yield of 71.2 % (table 6-2)

Ion Exchange Chromatography

The intermediate step in cytosolic CEA receptor purification protocol is Ion exchange when the partially purified receptor obtained by ammonium sulphate fractionation applied on the DEAE-cellulose, The column was washed with 2.4 column volumes of starting buffer to elute the unabsorbed material. The column was developed with 900-ml linear gradient of 0.0 to 1 M NaCl in the Tris buffer.

Anion exchange chromatograph of CEA receptors (Fig 6 -1) revealed five peaks of binding activity (A ⟶ E). Peaks (B ⟶ E) elute from anion exchanger after with an increasing salt gradient. These pooled Fractions (B ⟶ E) represent acidic cytosolic protein (acidic receptor), species with several negative charges are absorbed to the column; separation was due to difference in the surface charge distribution of the protein and the ionic strength. These types of cytosolic receptor of CEA are designated as anionic receptor (B ⟶ E).

Attempts to further purification and characterization of these type of CEA receptor (anionic receptor) failed due to low concentration of these CEA receptors and low binding capacity.

Peak A in fig (6–1) represent the unabsorbed protein; those with no net charge or a net charge of same sign as the DEAE-cellulose pass through the column unretained. The resulting chromatogram in (Fig. 6-1) shows a single peak (A) contained the high binding activity and high concentration of protein, A fraction was collected, lyophilized, dissolved in Tris buffer pH 7.2, and applied on CM-cellulose. The column was washed with 1.6 column volumes of starting buffer, then developed with 160-ml linear gradient of 0.0 to 1 M NaCl.

As shown in fig (6-2), three peaks were observed, the first one represent unabsorbed protein (wash fraction), this is the main peak containing the most of binding activity of CEA. This type of protein (receptors) with no net charge at pH 7.2, pass through the cation and anion exchanger, unretained a pH 7.2 . This is a second form of cytosolic receptor designated as cationic receptor. The active fractions was pooled, and concentrated for next purification method by gel filteration.

The other two peaks (B', C') in (fig 6-2) did not contain binding activity of CEA. These proteins with several positive charges absorbed to the cation exchanger are eluted from the column by an increase in ionic strength.

In general the purification of cytosolic receptors on DEAE-cellulose ion exchange showed 9.3 fold with 51.3 % yield, while on CM-cellulose ion exchange showed 11.76 fold with 18.4 % yield.

Reasons for choosing Ion exchange chromatography as intermediate purification stage include its:
(1) High resolving power.
(2) High protein-binding capacity.
(3) Versatility (there are several types of ion exchangers, and the composition of the buffer and pH can be varied over a mile range).
(4) Straight forward separation principle (primarily according to differences in charge).
(5) Ease of performance.

Gel Filtration Step:

The purpose of the final step purification was used to remove aggregates, degradation products and to prepare a solution suitable for final formulation of purified receptor.

The elution pattern of this experiment revealed as shown in (Fig 6-3) an asymmetrical peak containing CEA binding activity. The pooled peak fractions, which contain binding activity, represent the finally purified cytosolic receptor of CEA (cationic type). In general this step (gel filtration) of purification show 13 fold of purification with 3.14 % yield. The results of the purification protocol were summarized in table (6-2). These data indicate that each step in the process contributed significantly to the purification of final product. The use of gel filtration as final step provided good resolution but poor yield. Therefor it was suggest to remove the gel filtration step from all subsequent experiment of the purification procedure.

Fig (6-4) outline of the procedure employed for CEA receptor. This is the first trial to purify CEA receptor from mammary Tissues.

Generally, the purification of CEA receptor is very difficult process due to the very low concentration of the receptor protein. Also, this procedure gives only a preliminary idea about the presence and type of the cytosolic receptor of CEA.

The gel filtration step of the purification protocol consists of another set of experiment as described in section (6-5). Fig (6-5) show the pattern of radioactivity of elutes obtained when ^{125}I-CEA was separated by chromatography alone on sepharose 6B. The column void volume (Vo) measured with Blue Dextran 2000 was found to be

16 ml. The radioactivity peak was observed at elution volume of 30 ml (fraction number 15) and represent the free ^{125}I-CEA.

Fig (6-6) shows the pattern of radioactivity of elute obtained when crude cytosolic fraction from postmenopasual patient was incubated with ^{125}I-CEA and the mixture was chromatographed on sepharose 6B column. Here, the first radioactive peak appeared at an elution volume of 24 ml and represents ^{125}I-CEA bound by molecular moieties present in cytosolic fraction. The last peak eluted at a column volume of 30 ml represents free ^{125}I-CEA.

From these results it is concluded that the binding of the CEA to their cytosolic receptor induces major changes in the molecular parameter of the CEA. Also these data suggest the presence of more than one type of CEA receptor (cationic and anionic) with identical molecular parameters.

Physicochemical Properties of Isolated Receptor:

The Physicochemical properties of purified cationic cytosolic receptor were investigated using different techniques. Gel filtration and SDS-polyacrylamide gel electrophoresis (SDS-PAGE) determine the molecular weight. The stock's radius of purified receptor was estimated by gel filtration technique. The isolelectric point was evaluated using disc gel of ampholine PAGE.

Determination of molecular weight and stock's radius by gel filtration were carried out using standard protein of known molecular weights and stock's radius. The elution volume (Ve) of each protein, was estimated then Kav value was calculated as described in chapter three in section (3-4). The application of the Kav value to the calibration curve (Fig 3-8 and 3-9) and was led to determine of two molecular parameters. The molecular weight and the stock's radius of cationic cytosol receptor of CEA was 83 KD with 37 A°. Also, the molecular weight of purified cationic cytosol receptor was determined by SDS-PAGE technique. Fig (6-7) illustrated the calibration curve that was obtains in the presence 1% SDS. The relative mobilites (Rm) of the different proteins were determined as described in chapter three in section (3-6). Fig (6-8) shows the disc SDS-PAGE profile for purified receptor. The results indicate a single band for cationic type receptor. The M.wt of this type of CEA receptor was found to be 41 KD.

The collected data concerning molecular weight determination by SDS-PAGE and those obtained from gel filtration chromatography showed great variation. The values of M.wt by gel filtration show 2 fold higher than that obtained by SDS-PAGE. This great variation in M.wt determination was attributed to the receptor structure and may be consisted from two identical subunits. The intact receptor molecule when treated with sodium dodecyl sulfate in the presence of 2-mercaptoethanol completely dissociated into two identical molecules by their relative mobility on acrylamide gel electrophoresis, which revealed single band, fig (6-8).

These results suggest that the activated form of CEA receptors are dimeric proteins. The molecular weight of activated CEA receptors 83KD.

Isoelectric focusing technique was used for the estimation of isoelectric point (pI) of purified receptor using disc polyacrylamide gel containing ampholine 3.5 to 10.5 as described in chapter three in section (3-7). (Fig 6-9) was used to obtain pI of this type of receptor. The pI was found to be 6.8, this result confirms the behavior of this type of receptor against ion-exchange chromatography column through purification procedure.

Previous attempts to measure the molecular weight of CEA-receptor complex and other physicochemical properties has been unsuccessful due to low concentration of the CEA-receptor complex formed.

Carbohydrate Content:

The quantities of carbohydrate in finally purified cationic CEA receptor were approximately 15.8% as determined by phenol-sulfuric acid method as described in chapter three in section (3-8).

UV Spectrum Analysis:

Spectra of the receptor CEA, and CEA-receptor complex formed, revealed that receptor protein was absorbed at 280 nm while CEA-receptor complex formed was absorbed at 241 nm. Table (6-3).

Most types of proteins show an absorbance band at 280 nm in the UV region. The absorbance band of CEA-receptor complex at 241 nm may be attributed to change in conformation as result of the binding.

These changes may affect the chromophores responsible for the absorbance of the complex. Absorbance data of different types of proteins show that absorbance at 241 nm was related to S-S [242].

Thus disulfide linkage in the primary structure of CEA may be involved in the formation of CEA-receptor complex.

Table (6-1)
Amount of CEA receptor precipitated by a stepwise increase of the ammonium sulphate concentration

(All details are explained in the text)

% saturation of Ammonium sulphate	Total protein (mg)	Specific binding ng/mg protein	Total binding activity ng
0	21.3	10	210
20	2.5	1.6	4
30	0.98	1.5	1.47
40	0.95	1.18	1.12
50	2.14	4.001	8.9
60	2.45	6.68	16.3
70	1.9	8.57	16.15
80	2.5	7.5	11.25
90	3.5	5.56	19.25

Table (6-2)
Purification Steps of CEA Receptor from Malignant Breast Tumors
(All details are explained in the text)

Purification step	Total protein (mg)	Specific activity ng/mg	Total activity (ng)	Yield %	Purification fold
Crude homogenate	114.6	5	573	100	1
$(NH_4)_2SO_4$ fraction (50-90%) saturation	16	25.5	408	71.2	5.1
DEAE-cellulose ion-exchange (wash fraction)	6	49	294	51.3	9.3
CM-cellulose Ionexchange wash-fraction	1.8	58.8	105.8	18.49	11.76
Sepharose CL-6B gel filtration	0.28	65	18.2	3.14	13

Table (6-3)
UV Spectral Data of the Cytosolic Receptor, and CEA-Receptor Complex (All details are explained in the text)

Protein	Absorption maxi (λ_{max}) (nm)
Purified cytosolic receptor cationic type	211.2, 280
^{125}I-CEA-receptor complex	241

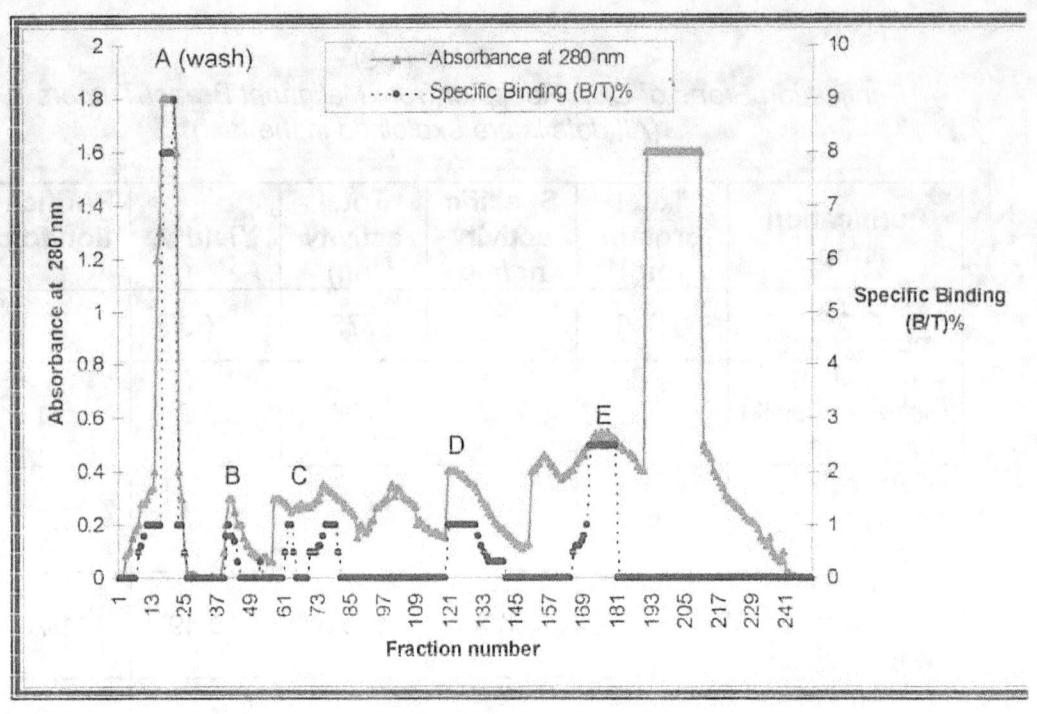

Fig: (6-1) Ion exchnge chromotography of CEA receptors on DEAE-cellulose columns using stepwise gradient NaCl (0.0 - 1M) in tris buffer pH7.2.
  (A): Wash fractions, pooled, contain binding activity against CEA
  (B): Elution fractions, pooled, contain binding activity against CEA, designated as anionic receptor type 1.
  (C): Elution fractions, pooled, contain binding activity against CEA, designated as anionic receptor type 2.
  (D): Elution fractions, pooled, contain binding activity against CEA, designated as anionic receptor type 3.
  (E): Elution fractions, pooled, contain binding activity against CEA, designated as anionic receptor type 4.
       (All details are explaind in the text)

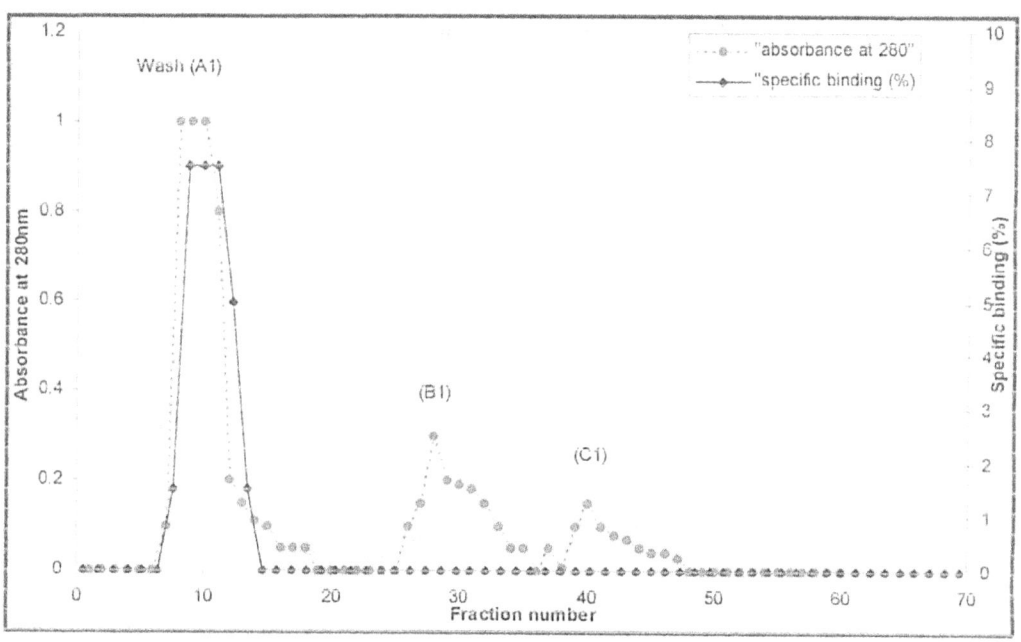

fig.(6-2):-Ion exchange chromatography of CEA receptor on CM_cellulose column using step wise gradient NaCl 0.0 to 1 M NaCl. (A1)=wash fraction pooled with binding activity against CEA ,(B1 and C1)= elution fraction which not contain binding activity against CEA.
(All details are explained in the text)

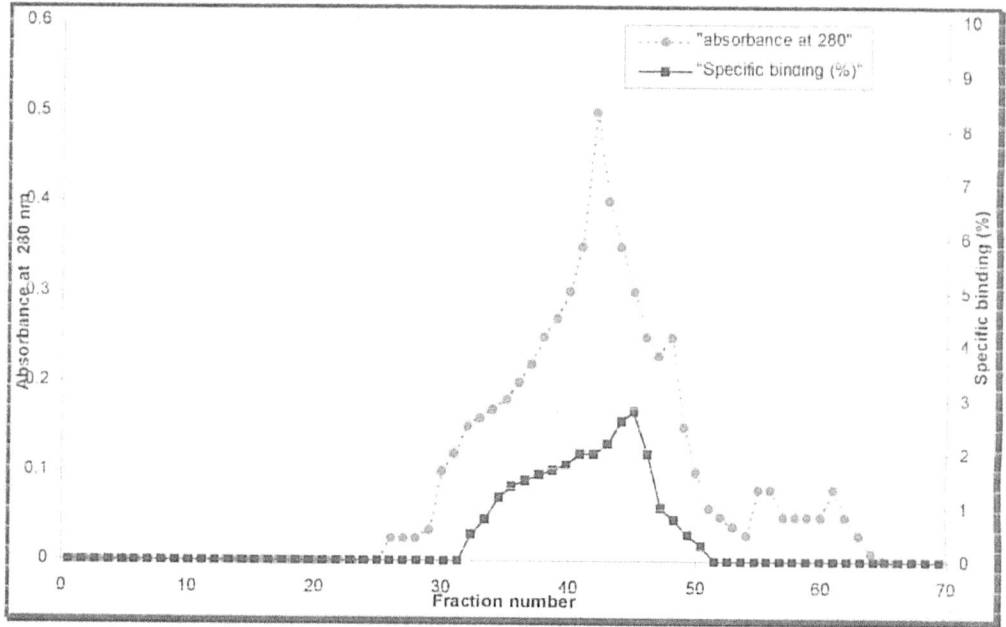

Fig (6-3) Gel filtration profinle of cytosolic receptor of CEA on Sepharose CL-6B column
(All details are explained in the text)

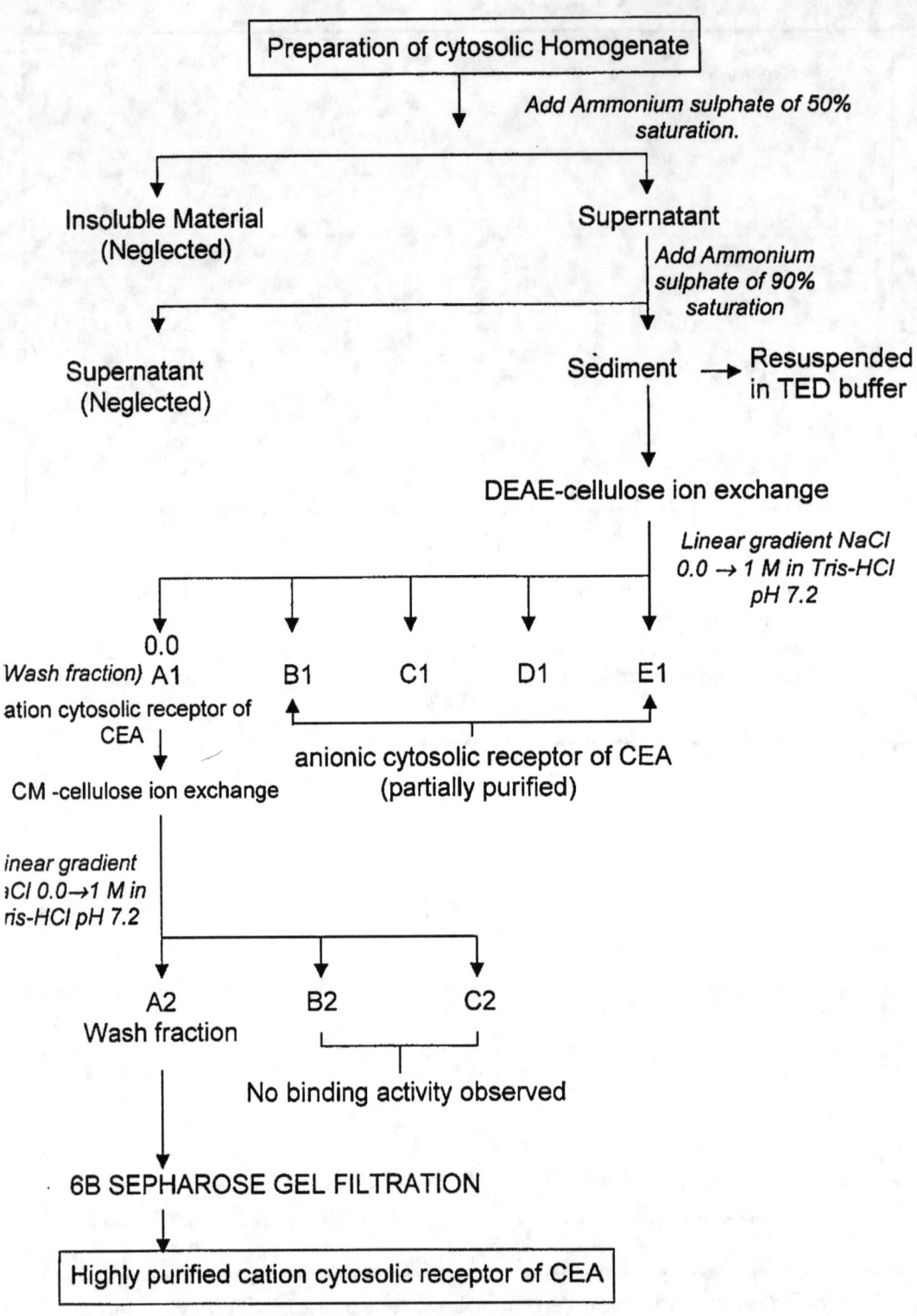

Fig (6-4) Outline of a Suggested Method to Obtain Purified CEA Receptor Isolated from Mammary Adenocarcinoma Tissues.
(All details are explained in the text)

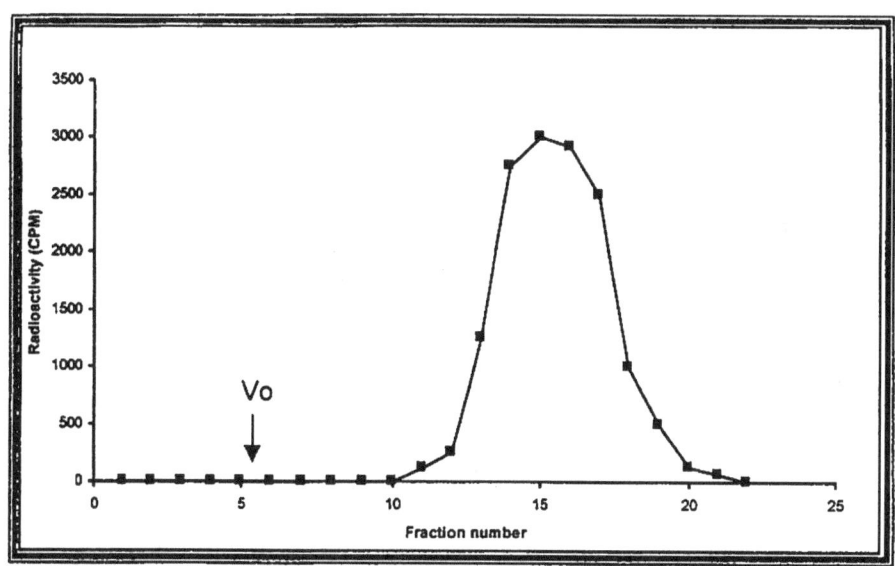

Fig 6-5: Column chromatography of ^{125}I-CEA on Sepharose 6B. Vo=11 ml
All details are explained in the text

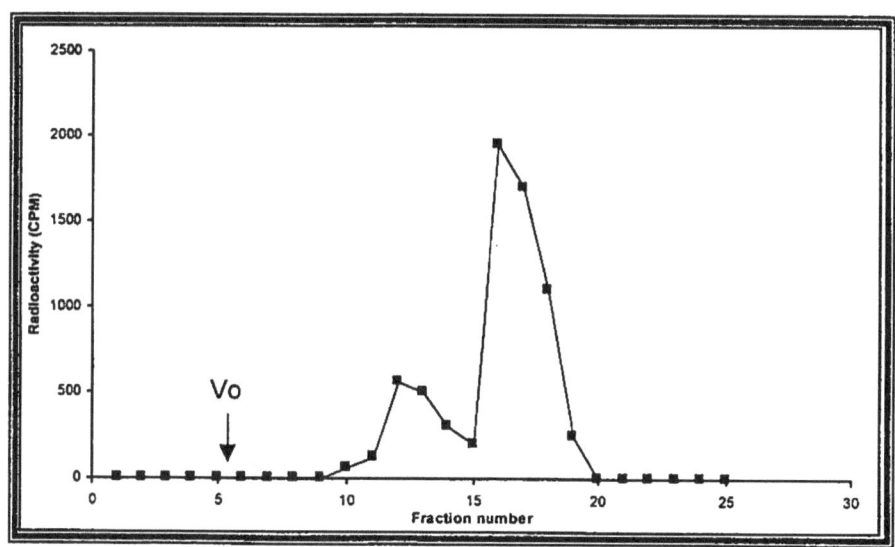

Fig 6-6: Column chromatography on sepharose 6B of mixture of ^{125}I-CEA and crude cytosolic containing receptor capable of binding CEA. Vo=11 ml
All details are explained in the text

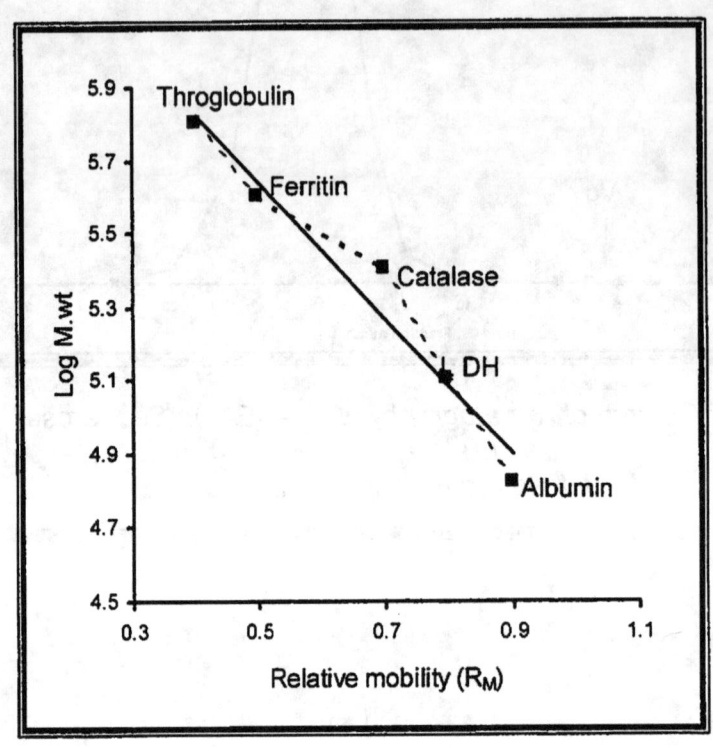

Fig.(6-7): Calibration curve for determination of M.wt by SDS – Polyacrylamide gel electrophoresis

(All details are explained in the text)

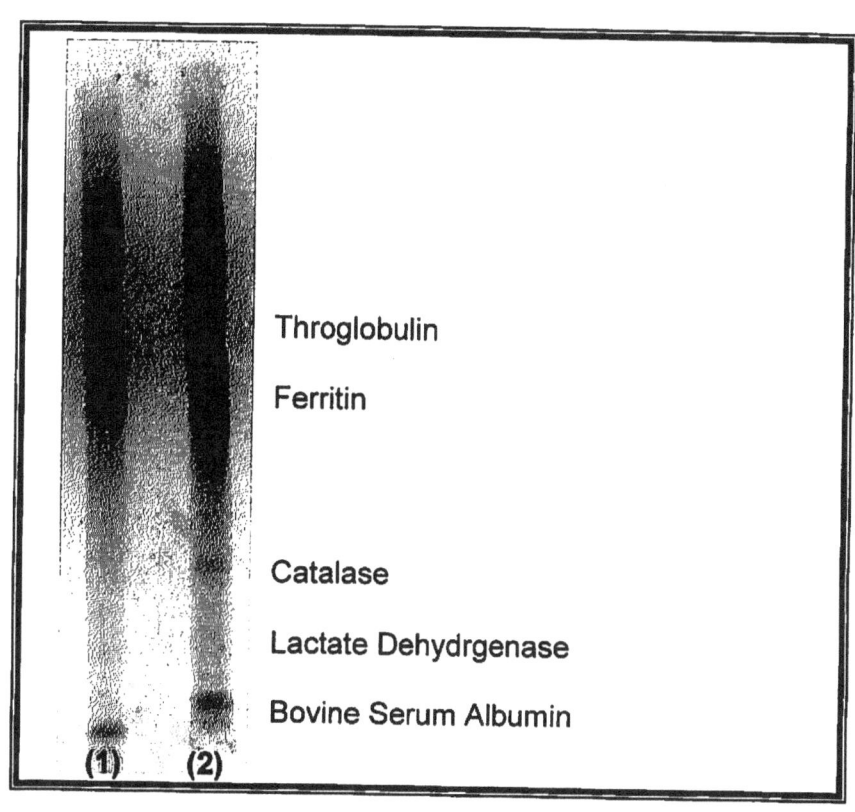

Fig (6-8): SDS polyacrylamide gel electrophoresis profile of purified cationic receptor of CEA.
  Line 1 : purified cationic receptor
  Line 2 : High molecular weight of standards protein
    (All details are explained in the text)

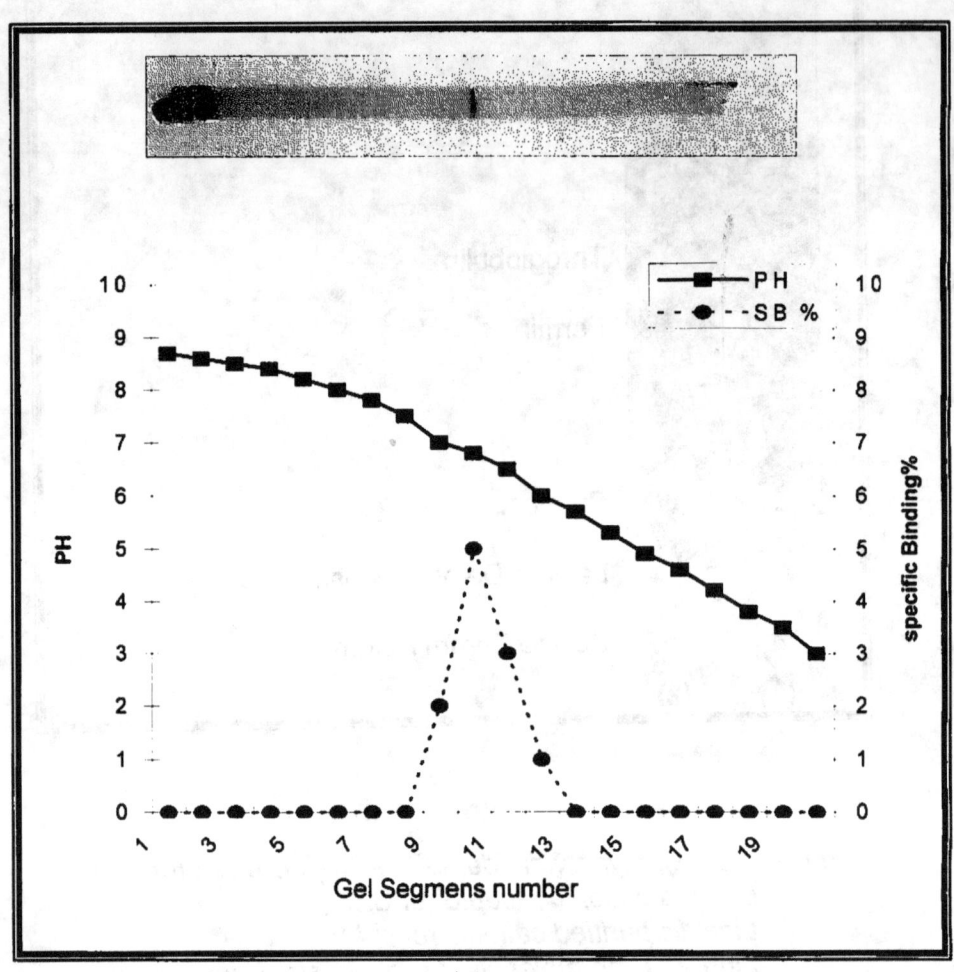

Fig. (6-9): Isoelectric profile for purified cytosolic receptor CEA

(All details are explained in the text)

Chapter seven

Evaluation of the Biological Activity of CEA -Cytosolic Receptor

Abstract

(1) DNA was isolated from whole blood of breast cancer patient and purified on sephadex G-25 column. A column of DNA-affinity chromatography was prepared by coupling the purified DNA to CNBr-activated sepharose. The biological activity of the purified CEA receptor, the crude preparations of cytosolic receptor-CEA complex and purified CEA alone to bind the DNA-affinity column was evaluated. It appeared that CEA-receptor complex, and CEA have the ability to bind the DNA-affinity column while the free receptor did not bind to the affinity column used in this study.

(2) A simple, rapid method for isolating human DNA from tissue has been developed, which can be routinely used in clinical laboratories. The entire procedure take less than 3 h. The nuclear pellet was treated with Triton x-100 urea and phenol/chloroform to remove contaminating protein, then the crude DNA extract was purified by sephadex G-25 spin-column. Typical, 260 /280 absorbence ratio used to assess purity was 1.84 Electrophoresis on a garose gel showed a single DNA band.

Fourier-transform infrared (FTIR) spectroscopy in the 4000-250 cm^{-1} region was used to characterize high molecular weight gnomic DNA from whole blood and mammary adenocarcinoma tissue of same patient.

Introduction

The problem of the biological role of CEA was sharply raised in 1963 [77]. It was then investigated that this protein might be involved in a number of proliferation phenomena, such as fetal and neoplastic growth. Thus, the following questions were asked: when, how and where does it acts during cellular and tissular development?

The function and regulation of the CEA receptor also remains unknown. It is possible that one of the many biochemical changes associated with cancer contribute to this phenomenon or to the inhibition of a negative regulatory element.

It is now apparent that the abnormality of the malignant cell lies at a more fundamental level in the genes that control cell growth and communication. Cancer develops as a result of multiple genetic alterations, occurring over a long period of time, which disrupt the cell cycle, differentiation and growth control.

Generally, Genes that participate in the neoplastic cell transformation fall into three broad category, oncogenes, and tumor suppressor genes and DNA repair genes.

Oncogenes are mutated forms of normal cellular gene called proto-oncogenes [245,246].

Proto-oncogenes are genes, which code for protein that, regulate normal cellular growth processes such as proliferation, differentiation and programmed cell death, and disruption of their normal function has profound consequences for the cell.

Tumor suppressor gene is inactivated in human cancers. Most tumor suppressor gene function directly in cell growth regulation pathways and the mutation in these genes behave recessively in somatic cells. To contribute to tumor formatting, both copies of the particular gene must be inactivated.

Many genes have been identified that play a part in the progression of breast carcinoma. These included P_{53}, HER_2/neu, and cyclin D_1. P_{53} is a tumor suppressor gene that regulates cellular response to DNA damage and other stresses. HER_2/neu and cyclin D_1. are protoncogenes that are found and overexpressed frequently in breast carcinomas [246].

The genetic changes demonstrate the complex interplay of tumor suppressor genes, oncogens and DNA mismatch repair genes during the progression, over years or even decades, from benign to carcinoma.

The discovery of the role played in cancer development by oncogenes and tumor suppressor genes over the past decade has greatly increased our understanding of cancer and has led to new diagnostic approaches. The tools of molecular biology are increasingly available in the routine laboratory and the opportunity exists for detecting many of the genes discussed above [247,248].

The value of IR spectral analysis comes from the fact that the methods of vibration of each group are very sensitive to changes in chemical structure, conformation, and environment. Therefore, there are many applications of FTIR spectroscopy in researches of biochemistry and molecular biology, like; identification of number of hydrogen bounds and the function groups and measurement of their breakage during denaturation, identification of tautomeric forms, interaction between small molecule, such as Riboflavin and Adenine, and determination of ratio of AU to GC pairs t RNA [88].

In this chapter the biological activity of CEA receptors, CEA-receptor complex and CEA alon have been evaluated. Moreover DNA was isolated from whole blood of breast cancer patients and from tumor and benign tissue of each patient, then characterized by FTIR studies in the vibrational region between 4000 and 250 cm^{-1}.

Materials and methods

7.1 Chemicals:

All laboratory chemical and reagents were of annular grade.

Material	Company (origin)
Isoamylalcohol, Ascorbic acid	Analar (England)
Titron x-100, phenol, EDTA, Na_2HPO_4, NaH_2PO_4 glacial Acetic acid, chloroform, SDS, NaCl, HCl, H_2SO_4, urea and sodium hydroxide NaOH	Fluka (Switzerland)
Ethanol, Sucrose	Merk (Germany)
Ethedium bromide	Sigma (USA)
Sephadex G-25	Pharmica
Tris (hydroxy methyl amino methane)	Hopkin & Williams
Ammonium acetate	Difco
Proteinas K	B.D.H / U.K
Boric acid, glyceriol, potassium hydroxide (KOH), $Mg(NO_3)_2$, ammonium molybdate	BDH (England)
Activated CNBr sepharose	Chemical Sweden

7.2 Equipment and Apparatus:

The following equipment and apparatus were used throughout the study.

Equipments	Company (origin)
Cooled centrifuge	International equipment Co.(USA)
Fourier-transform infrared spectrophotometer (FTIR-8300)	SHIMADZU
Quick press	Perkin-Elmer
Electrophoresis content powersupply	Pharmacia fine chemicals (Sweden)
Microwave oven	National (Japan)
pH-meter	Consort C_{832} (Belgium)
Sensitive balance	A&D (Japan)
Vortex mixtur	Griffin & George Ltd (Britain)
Polypropylene column	Pharmacy
Autoclave	AMSCO (USA)
Gamma counter	LKB-Sweden
Homogenizer	Japan-National
Spectrophotometer	Behring-Germany

7.3 Buffers and reagents:

7.3.1 Buffers:
A: Phosphate buffer was prepared by mixing certain volumes of stock solutions:
Solution I: 0.2-M solution of monobasic sodium phosphate (31.2 g of $NaH_2PO_4 \cdot 2H_2O$ in 1000 ml)
Solution II: 0.2-M solution of dibasic sodium phosphate (28.39 g of $NaH_2PO_4 \cdot 2H_2O$ in 1000 ml)

B: 5X Tris-Borate EDTA (TBE) buffer, pH 8.0:
- Tris base   54g
- Boric acid   27.5 g
- EDTA 0.5 M   20 ml
- Distilled water   1000 ml

C: Loading buffer 6X:
- Xylene   0.25%
- Sucrose   40%(W/V) in water
- Bromophenol blue   0.25%

D: TED buffers (pH 7.4):

Tris (0.01 M) buffer containing 0.15 M EDTA, 1.2 mM dithothreitol and 10% glycerol pH 7.4

7.3.2 *Reagent:*

Ethedium Bromide solution (10 mg/ml):
Prepared by dissolving 100 mg of ethedium bromide in 10 ml of distill water.
Other solutions or reagent used were indicated in each experiment.

7.4 Collection of Specimens:

7.4.1 *preparation of Tumor tissue:*

Tumor tissue and corresponding benign breast tissue specimens were obtained from patients with untreated primary breast cancer who underwent mastectomy. The tissue samples were immediately immersed in ice-cold isotonic saline solution. They were collected individually in plastic receptacle and stored at -20° C until homogenization.

7.4.2 *preparation of Blood samples:*

Five milliliter of blood samples was obtained from patients undergoing mastectomy or lumpectomy by venipuncture just before surgery.
Blood sample into EDTA-tube was used immediately or stored at -20° C until use.

7.5 Isolation and purification of human DNA from whole blood of breast cancer patients[249]:

Preparation of crude DNA:

5 ml of EDTA treated whole blood were mixed with two volumes of buffer A and centrifuged at 1800 xg for 15 min, and the supernatant plasma was discarded. The pellet which contains the nuclear fraction was suspended in 2 ml of buffer B by gentle pipetting and mixing, then the suspension was extracted with one volume of solvent A. after centrifugation at 10000 xg for 10 min the aqueous phase was collected, then again with an equal volume of solvent B. the aqueous phase removed after centrifugation and placed on ice until further purification.

DNA purification:

Sephadex G$_{25}$ column was prepared by adding 2 ml of the swollen gel to a (4x0.6) cm polypropylen column, and equilibrating with buffer C. the crude DNA was applied to the column, then the elution was achieved by buffer C. after collection of several 0.5 ml fractions was measured the absorbance for each fraction at 260, 235 and 280 nm.

The absorbance of the DNA preparation was recorded spectrophotometrically, at 260 nm and at 280 nm, to check the purity of the DNA preparation. The concentration of DNA sample was measured according to the equation:

Concentration of DNA (µg/ml) = O.D$_{260}$ x 50 µg/ml

Since a DNA solution with a 0.D260 of 1 contains approximately 50 µg/ml DNA.

The purity of DNA sample was checked by spectrophotometry, the ratio between the reading at 260 and 280 nm (A260 / A280) was used to provide an estimate for the purring of the DNA sample (250).

Solutions:
1. Buffer A: 10 mM Tris hydrochloride, pH 7.5, containing 300 mmol of sucrose and 10 ml of Triton X-100 per liter.
2. Buffer B: 10 mM Tris hydrochloride, pH 7.2, containing 10 mmol EDTA, 8 mol urea and 10 g SDS per liter.
3. Buffer C: 10 mM Tris hydrochloride, pH 7.2, containing 1 mmol EDTA per liter.
4. Solved A: Phenol-10 mM Tris buffer pH 7.2 (6:2 by vol).
5. SolvedB: Phenol-chloroform-isoamyl alcohol (25/24/1 by vol).

7.6 DNA coupling to CNBR activated sepharose:

DNA was covalently linked to insoluble CNBr activated sepharose according to the method of Arndt. Jovin et.al., [249]. CNBr activated sepharose was suspended in potassium phosphate buffer (10 mM) pH 8 and washed with the same buffer 3 times. A solution of purified human DNA (20 µg/ml) from whole blood of breast cancer patients were mixed with CNBr-activated sepharose (8 mg/ml) at a ratio of 1:1 (v/v). the mixture was left to react by gentle agitation on a rotary shaker at 20° C overnight. The DNA-sepharose was washed on a fritted funel with the following solution until no further absorbency at 260 nm was released; 10 mM K-phosphate pH 8, 1M K- phosphate pH 8, 1M KCl and Tris buffer pH 7.4 .

7.7 DNA affinity chromatography:

DNA sepharose obtained in section (7-6) was suspended in Tris buffer pH 7.4 and washed 3 times with this buffer. The gel was packed into 1x8 cm column to a bed volume of 4 ml. The column was equilibrated with TED buffer pH 7.4 . Tracer CEA receptor complexes (1 ml) prepared as described in section 6-4-3 (second protocol), or ^{125}I-CEA alone or receptor alone were loaded separately to the column at 4° C. the samples were passed through the affinity column 4-6 times before washing with 4-6 column volumes of homologous buffer at a flow rate 0.5 ml/min. receptor fraction retained were eluted with TED buffer containing 0.4 M KCl. The eluted fractions of CEA receptors alone were tested for the binding activity, while those consisted of the ^{125}I-CEA and complexes were counted using gamma counter.

7.8 Determination of organic phosphate:

in order to assess the amount of DNA reacted with CNBr activated sepharose , the concentration of phosphate in the original DNA solution and in the prepared solid matrix were measured .phosphate was estimated according to the method of Fiske and Subbarow [252] with the following modified ashing procedure .A sample volume (0.2 ml) of sepharose suspsension was ashed quickly with shaking over a strong flame after addition of 0.12 ml of 10% $Mg(NO_3)_2$ in alcohol . When all brown fumes had disappeared, 0.6 ml of 1N HCl was added, the tubes capped with a marble to reduce evaporation .The solutions were heated in a boiling water bath for 15 min. The mixture was colled and dilluted to 0.4 ml with distilled water then mixed with 0.4-ml perchloric acid (60%), 0.4-ml ammonium molybdate (5%) and 0.2-ml ascorbic acid (1%). The solution was shaked and the absorbance was read after 10 min at 700 nm. A standard solution of phosphate (4 mg/l) was treated as mentioned for sample .The concentration of phosphate was calculated according to the following formula:

$$P(mg/l) = \frac{Au}{As} \times 4$$

Au= Absorbance for unknown sample
As= Absorbance for standard sample

7-9 Isolation of DNA From tissue Samples:

This method based on the methods of Gross Bellard .et.al [250], Blin & stafford[252] and .Adell & ogbonna[247], this procedure was modified from all above method.

1. The frozen tissues were weighed, sliced finely ascalpel in petri dish standing on ice bath. The slices were thawed and furter minced with scissors then homogenized in PBS with a ratio of 1:5 (weight: volume) by using a manual homogenizer. The homogenate was filtered throug two layers of cheestcloth to eliminate fibers of connective tissues, then centrifuge at 200xg for 10 min at 4°C. The supernatant was discarded and the sediment was rehomogenized in ice-cold PBS about 3ml using a manual homogenizer, then centrifuge at 2000 xg for 10 min at 4° C.The supernatant was discarded and the sediment was used in the experiments involved isolation of DNA.
2. Into suitable tube :
   - 500 µl of buffer A
   - 500 µl of sterile distilled water
   - Mix contents of tube thoroughly.
3. Add the pellet, which contains the nuclear fraction, to the tube and vortex vigorously.
4. Add 20 µl proteinas K solution (2mg/ml) to the tube and vortex.
5. Incubation for 1 h at (37° C) with moderate horizontal shaking (300 rpm).
6. Then the solution was cooled at room temperature, an equal volume of solvant A was added and the two phases were gently mixed slowly turning the tubes end over end for 10 minutes.
7. The two phases were separated by centerifugation at 5000 g for 10 min.
8. Remove aqueous layer with a wide – bore pipet and transfer to a fresh tube. Reapeat extraction twice.
9. The supernatant contains the crude DNA.

DNA purification using spin column:

Spin columns can be made in 1-ml syringe or in 0.6ml microcentrifuge tubes.
1. Add about 2 ml of the swollen gel to the (4 x 0.6) cm polypropylene column, and let it settle for approximately 5-10 min, Nest it inside a 1.5- ml tube see fig (7-1).
2. Add 500 µl of buffer c; this mount should reach the top of the suspension.

3. Blance the spin column with that of another group and spin the tubes at 1000 xg
4. Remove the flow through and discard.
5. Repeat steps 2-4.
6. Carefully add crude DNA sample to the column and centrifug for 1 min at 1000 xg then the elution of DNA was achieved by centrifuging several portions (0.5 ml) of buffer c trough the column.
7. After collection of several 0.5-ml fractions in this way, their absorbencies at 280, 260 and 235 nm were measured.
8. The DNA can be quantitated by spectrophotometry, and the quality assessed by running it out on 0.7% agoras gel electrophoresis.

Solution:

Buffer and reagents as mentioned in section (7-4)

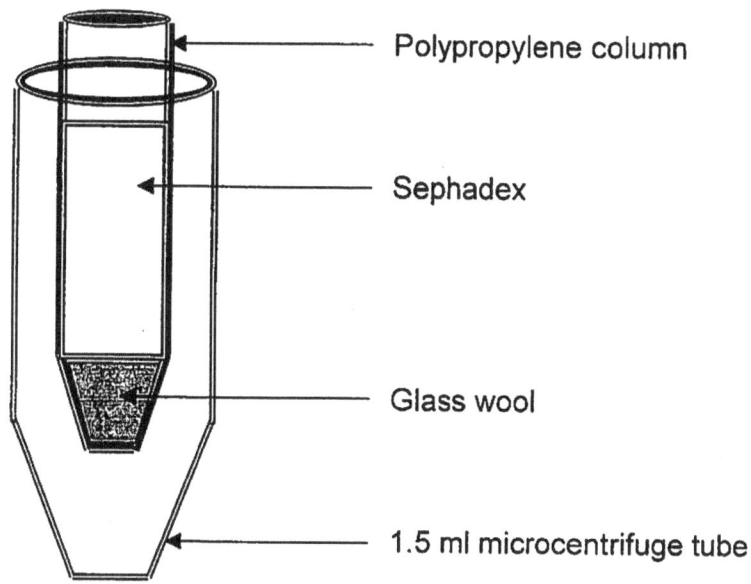

Fig 7.1 Spin column made from microcentrifuge tube

7-10 Gel Electrophoresis:

A 0.7% agarose gel was prepared in Tris – Borate (diluted 1:5 of stock solution), and boiled for 2 min in microwave oven, cooled to 60 c, then ethedium bromide of 10 mg /ml was added to a final concentration of 0.5 µg/ml and mixed thoroughly. After sealing the edges of the mold with adhesive tape, the position of the comb was 0.5 mm above the plate so that a complete well can be fromed when the agarose was added. The remainder of the warm agarose solution was poured into the mold. The gel should be between 3 mm and 5 mm thick, After the gel was completely set (30–45 min at room temperature), carefully the comb was removed and the tape and mount the gel in the electrophoresis tanks. Adding just enough electrophoresis buffers to cover the gel to a depth of about 1mm.

DNA samples were mixed with (1/5 volume) the desired gel-loading buffer and added to the wells on the gel. Generally, gels were run 2-3 h at 70 vol.

DNA bands were visualized by UV. Illumination on UV. transilluminator. Gels were destined in distilled water for 30-60 min to get rid of the background before photographs were taken.

7-11: Spectrophotometric studies by Fourier–transform infrared spectra:

Purified DNA samples with concentration (50µg /ml) and Lyophilized. FTIR spectra were measured from 4000 to 250 cm^{-1} spectra of the four samples of purified DNA were obtained from samples prepared as 7-mm diameter KBr pellets with approximately a 1:200 weight ratio of sample to KBr. pellet were prepared using a Perkin – Elmer model 15 quick press.

The experiment was performed for the following samples:
1. Purified DNA Extracted from mammary adenocarcinoma tissue.
2. Purified DNA isolation from whole blood of breast cancer patients.
3. DNA coupling to CNBr –activated sepharose.
4. CNBr- activated sepharose alone.

Results and Discussion

Isolation and purification DNA from whole blood:

DNA was extracted by phenol chloroform solution then purified by G25 column chromatography. Generally, 5 ml of whole blood was mixed with a lysis buffer to lyse the cells. The fraction that contains the nuclei of leukocytes obtained from this mixture by centrifugation was suspended in buffer containing the strong protein denaturing agents, SDS and urea. The dissociative DNA was extracted twice with phenol / chloroform to remove most of proteins, the sample was rich in DNA at this stage but still contained some proteins. The average A260 /A280 ratio was 1.25±0.06, the crude DNA was purified by sephadex G-25 column. The sample was applied to the column and purified DNA was recovered in the first two fractions .DNA prepared by this method had an even higher A_{260}/A_{280} ratio (1.75±0.085) and a yield of DNA equals to 14.5±4.3 μg /ml. The DNA prepared by this rapid procedure is essentially pure and could be used for the preparation of the DNA-affinity column .the average yield of DNA is lower than that obtained by proteinase K digestion method [252].

Coupling of DNA to CNBr activated sepharose:

DNA has been covalently linked to insoluble matrix of CNBr-activated sepharose, the yield of coupling as indicated from the absorbance at 260 nm and the concentration of incorporation phosphate was 3.75 mg DNA/ml swollen gel.

The coupling of DNA to CNBr–activated sepharose at pH8 involves multipoint covalent attachment of the aromatic groups of the bases rather than merely the single –point attachment of the terminal 5-phosphate described by Manager et.al[253]. This view is supported by the experiments of Berridge and Aronson with CNBr activation of sepharose for RNA coupling[254]. Since DNA is not coupled successfully to activated sepharose in bicarbonate buffer at pH 9.5 –10 the mechanism involving enolate ions for coupling poly (u) proposed by pharmacy firm in their sales literature cannot be the preferred pathway[255]. Coupling large amounts of undenatured leukocytes DNA to sepharose it can be react with the activated gel without single – stranded tails or large single stranded regions from these result we conclude that the coupling for native DNA result from ability of the native to penetrate the gel matrix.

Evidence for the reaction described is provided by the results of FTIR spectroscopy (fig 7-2 and 7-3). These show that on coupling, C=O stretching doublet of DNA at about 1720 cm^{-1} is considerably reduced whilst two new bans corresponding to C=N and aromatic stretching frequencies at 1605 cm^{-1} and 1525 cm^{-1} respectively appear.

Analysis of CEA, receptor and CEA–receptors complex on affinity column:

The receptor protein of CEA which have been obtained from gel filtration (cationic receptor) and ion exchange chromatography was investigated for its ability to bind DNA isolated from whole blood of breast cancer patients. DNA has been coupled to the solid matrix (Sepharose 4B) as described in section (7-6). The receptor proteins were applied and passed through the affinity column (4-6) washed with TED buffer, receptor fractions were eluted with TED buffer containing 0.5 M KCl, then the test was carried out for their binding activity.

The evaluation of biological activity consists of set of experiments in which CEA-receptor complexes prepared as described in chapter 6 section (6-4-3) (second protocol) and native ^{125}I-CEA alone (unliganded to receptor) separately were applied to the column and treated exactly as mentioned for native receptor, then collected fractions were detected by radioactivity measurement.

The results indicate that ligand receptors, which have been obtained from the reaction of the cytosolic receptor and ^{125}I-CEA can bind to DNA. Affinity column fig. (7-4) while the free receptor did not bind to the affinity column used in this study.

A similar investigation of unliganded CEA (^{125}I-CEA) illustrated that these molecules had very low ability to bind DNA affinity column (fig 7-4 a,b) these results agree to certain extent with that obtained by Eaman. et al[112]. Who showed that purified CEA was biologically active.

In vitro and in vivo biochemical studies stated that the binding of estrogens to their receptor lead to receptor activation and increasing its affinity for nuclei, DNA and artificial nuclear matrices [257].

Isolation of DNA from Tumor cells:

The objective of DNA isolation is to obtain useful samples of DNA that are free from some or all contaminating molecules. In practical terms, is translating into separation of the cells of interest from their environment and then separating the DNA from other cellular components. In addition, undesired additives used to facilitate these separations may also need to be removed.

The starting point for most DNA isolation procedures is with harvested cells. In this method, cells are lysed by incubation at 37° C for 1 h in buffer that contains a detergent, proteinas K and EDTA .The detergent serves to dissolve the cell membrane and denatures the proteins. EDTA chelate divalent cations that are required for the activity of nucleases. The basis for this method is that proteinase K .an enzyme that degrades proteins .is highly active in this mixture, whereas DNA, degrading nucleases are greatly inhibited. This incubation is followed by series of organic extractions generally employing mixtures of phenol, chloroform and isoamyl alcohol. The organic solvents are mixed with DNA – containing sample, creating an emulsion to dissolve hydrophobic contaminants and further denature and remove proteins. Since the organic phase are not cosoluble with the aqueous sample, are separate from each other into two phase .The aqueous phase is less dense and thus can be removed from a top the organic phase.

In the final step, the crude DNA sample was applied to a Sephadex G-25 column and the purified DNA was eluted by centrifugation. Most of DNA was recovered in the first four-fraction DNA prepared by this method and had even higher A_{260}/A_{280} ratio (1.8±0.05). Electrophoresis on agarose gel showed a single DNA band (Fig 7-5).

These experiments show that this procedure produced DNA with good quality and is suitable for restriction enzyme digestion.

DNA is a typical slow migrating, high molecular weight and undegraded species in an ethidium bromide-stained agarose gel (Fig 7-5). Also DNA is free of RNA, protein and degrading enzymes. Therefore, DNA prepared by this method is suitable for southern blot analysis, restriction fragment length polymorphism (RFLP) studies and for the polymerase chain reaction (PCR).

Characterization of DNA structures by FTIR spectroscopic:

In this study the DNA isolated from whole blood of breast cancer patients are considered as normal cell DNA sample while those derived from mammary malignant tumor tissue as transformed cell DNA.

The spectrum of purified DNA From mammary adenocarcinoma tissue (transformed cell DNA) and purified DNA isolation from whole blood (normal cell DNA) from the same patient are presented in (Fig 7-5, 7-6 and 7-7)

Based on the infrared spectra data, several important differences may be noted between the spectrum of DNA extracted from mammary

Adenocarcinoma tissue and that taken from whole blood (considered normal cell DNA). The differences detected are:

1. The strong band of normal cell DNA at (3450-2800) cm^{-1} reflects stretching vibrations of hydrogen bands of absorbed water molecule and its peak at 3200 cm^{-1} reflect stretching vibration of NH2 group for adenine, guanine and / or cytosine residues [258]. This band was appeared as a broad band in the case of transformed cell DNA from mammary adenocarcinoma tissue.
2. The strong band of transformed cell DNA from mammary adenoma tissue at (2098.4) cm^{-1} have been assigned to C=N stretching [257]. It was appeared as a shoulder in the normal cell DNA.
3. The band (1739-1500) cm^{-1} appeared as medium and sharp in normal cell DNA while the transformed cell DNA of mammary adenocarcinoma tissue appeared as broad or overlapping bands. Generally, this region contains the following bands according to their relation with nitrogen bases [258,259].

a) Adenine: (1665-1573) cm^{-1} reflect NH$_2$ bending and C=N stretching vibration.
b) Thymine: (1660-1575) cm^{-1} reflect C4=O stretching vibration and ring stretching vibration.
c) Guanine: (1630-1690) cm^{-1} reflect C=O stretching and NH$_2$ scissoring vibration.
d) Cytosine: (1700-1588) cm^{-1} reflect NH$_2$ scissoring vibration and in-plane ring vibrations.
4. The bands (927,887) cm^{-1} appeared as a medium band in normal cell DNA infrared spectrum, while it disappeared in the spectrum of transformed cell DNA isolated from mammary adenocarcinoma tissue. This band reflects symmetric stretching vibration of the group $C{\begin{matrix}\diagup O \\ \diagdown O\end{matrix}}$ [259].

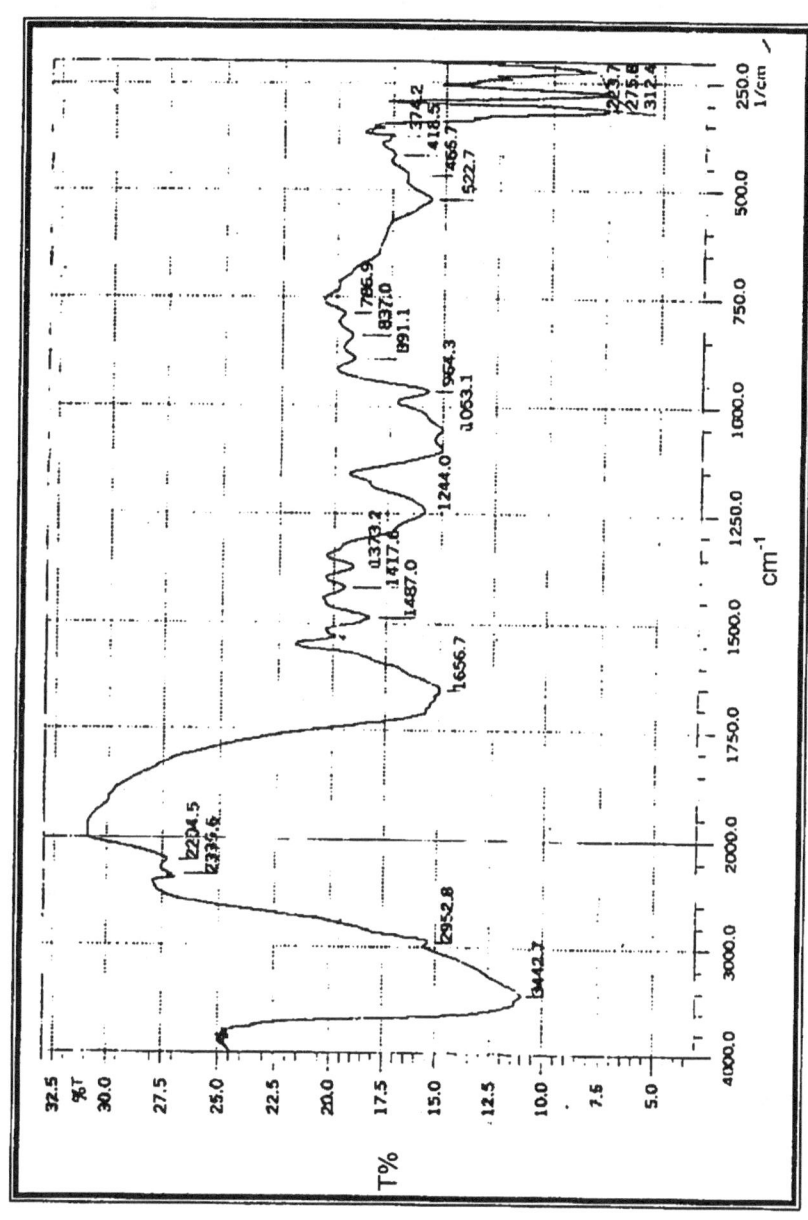

Fig. (7-2): FTIR Spectra of coupling DNA to activated Sepharose
(All details are explained in the text)

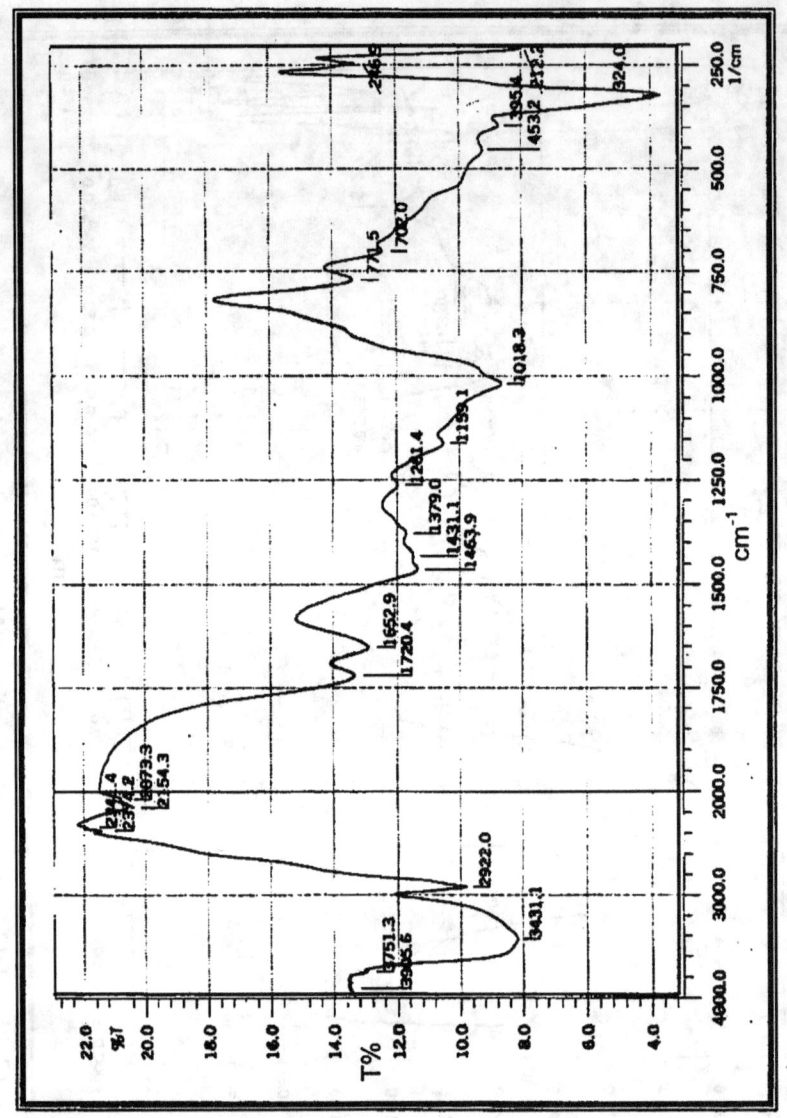

Fig. (7-3): FTIR Spectra of CNBr activated sepharose
(All details are explained in the text)

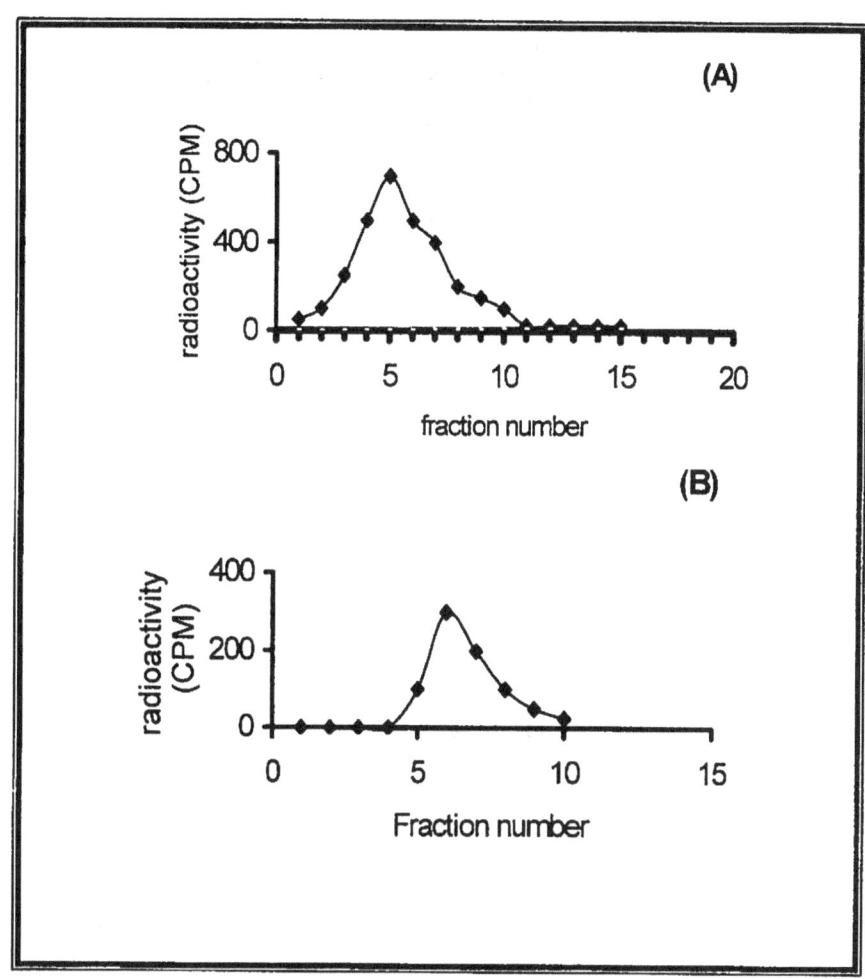

Fig.(7-4): Chromatography of CEA-receptor complex (A), and ^{125}I– CEA alone (B) on DNA-Sepharose column.

(All details are explained in the text).

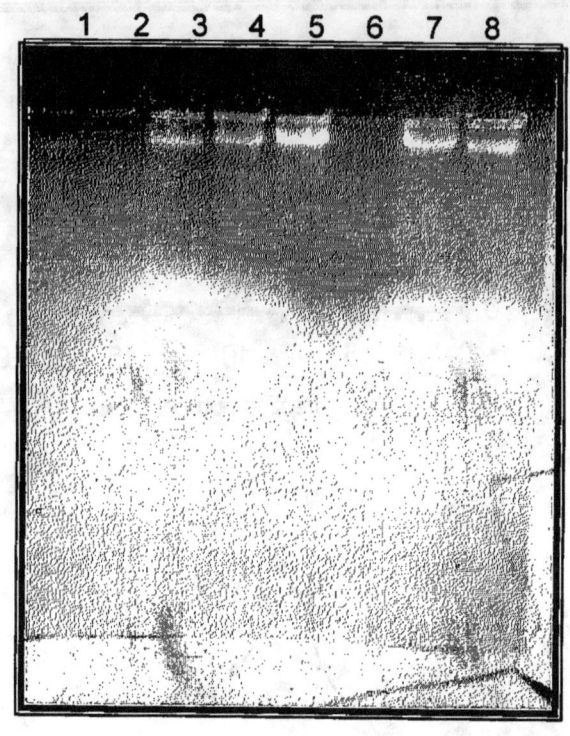

Fig 7-5
Gel electrophoresis of high molecular weight DNA isolates from human

1,2: DNA isolate from benign breast tumor
3,4: DNA isolate from mammary adenocarcinoma tissue of postmenopausal patient
5,6: DNA isolate from mammary adenocarcinoma tissue of premenopasual patient
7 : DNA isolate from whole blood of postmenopausal patient
8 : DNA isolate from whole blood of premenopausal patient
(All details are explained in the text)

CHAPTER EIGHT

GENERAL DISCUSSION

The results of this thesis reveal the role of protein engineering in CEA stability, the energetic of CEA binding receptor, antigenticiy (the number and nature of the antigenic sites). Other studies refer to the difficulty of designing CEA with a specific function[263,264,265]. Considerable amount of efforts had led to some notable successes in this field, such as engineering stability by adding disulfide-bond forming cysteine residues, increasing antigenicity by selective modification of residues at their antigenic sites (epitomes), and using engineered monoclonal antibodies as therapeutic agent [266]. Protein engineering for antigen molecule requires understanding its structure, function and stability. For instance, the precise three-dimensional structure of the protein must be known before engineering can begin[267,268]. This structure requires time-consuming techniques such as x-ray crystallography, NMR, FTIR, ESR and ultraviolet spectroscopy [269,270]. Finally, the parameter affecting CEA structure must be well understood; this must be compensated in the folded protein by chemical interactions such as the burying of hydrophobic amino acid chains into the interior of the molecule.

Number of successes have been achieved in this field in chapter three of this thesis, UV and FTIR spectroscopic have studied the structure and molecular analysis. Fig. (3-18, 3-20 and 3-21). Also the physicochemical studies figures (3-3, 3-5 and 3-12) and stability studies figures (3-13, 3-15, 3-18, 5-8 and 5-9) have proved successful in designing CEA with greater stability, better binding energies and change the Pka values.

The results in chapter three and four give ideas about the role of tyrosine in the antigenicity of CEA figures (3-18, 4-1, 4-8, 4-9 and 4-10), these data suggested that inactivation or modification in tyrosine will change the antigenicity of CEA.

The thermodynamic parameters in chapter five tables (5-4), (5-5) and energy diagram model fig. (5-14) indicate that the binding of CEA to their specific receptor involves formation of multiple non covalent bonds between CEA and amino acid of the binding site. The attractive forces (hydrogen bonds and hydrophobic forces) are weak by comparison with covalent bonds. However, the large number of interactions results in large total binding energy.

The suggested model for bond formation between CEA molecule and its receptor is shown in fig. (8-1). As shown in this fig. the strength of a non-covalent bond is critically dependent on the distance (d) between the interacting groups which must be close (in molecular term) before these forces becomes significant.

In order for an antigenic determinant (epitope) and the receptor-combining site to combine, there must be suitable atomic groupings on opposing parts of the CEA and their specific receptor molecules, the shape of the combining site must fit the epitope fig. (1-3 and 8-1), so that several non-covalent bonds can form. If the CEA molecule and the receptor-combining site are complementary in this way (complementary determine regions), there will be sufficient binding energy to resist thermodynamic disruption of the bond. However, if electron clouds of the CEA and receptor overlap, steric repulsive forces come into play which have a vital role in determine the specificity of receptor molecule for CEA, and its ability to discriminate between molecules [263,264].

Also figures (8-1 and 5-14) reveal the general geometrical requirements for bond formation between CEA and their specific receptor and refer to the probability that CEA is located at a certain distance and angular orientation relative to their specific receptor when the CEA ~ R bond has been formed. The closer CEA and their receptor are held by the molecular geometry, the greater probability of the bond formation, and the less entropy loss when the CEA~R bond is Joined. In principle, knowledge of the lengths and rotational angles and potential energies for all the skeletal bonds in the path CEA~R would permit one to calculate S an T accurately (results of chapter five tables (5-4 and 5-5)). These data will permit the level of theoretical understanding to keep pace with development of new structure for CEA or their receptor molecules. Also, the results of this thesis provide framework for the degree of improvement in affinity and / or removal of unwanted residues surface, from each both molecules (CEA or their receptor). These molecular geometry changes is feasible by protein engineering technology, but in the present instance, one problem for engineering change in CEA or their receptor molecules, there are little concrete information on actual site distribution. In this thesis attempts have been achieved to formulate a rational framework by which the interaction of CEA with various classes of receptor can be explored.

It is not yet possible, However, to make precise numerical change by protein engineering approach because the structure especially the flexible parts or complementary regions of these molecules is not yet well enough understood. Further physiochemical studies of CEA and various classes of receptor – particle with antibody preparation–may eventually yield the requisite data.

A better understanding of such binding phenomena may in turn help to clarify the role of CEA in certain critical steps in the immune response; the affinity of binding site can also modified by protein engineering technology such as point mutation of DNA [265].

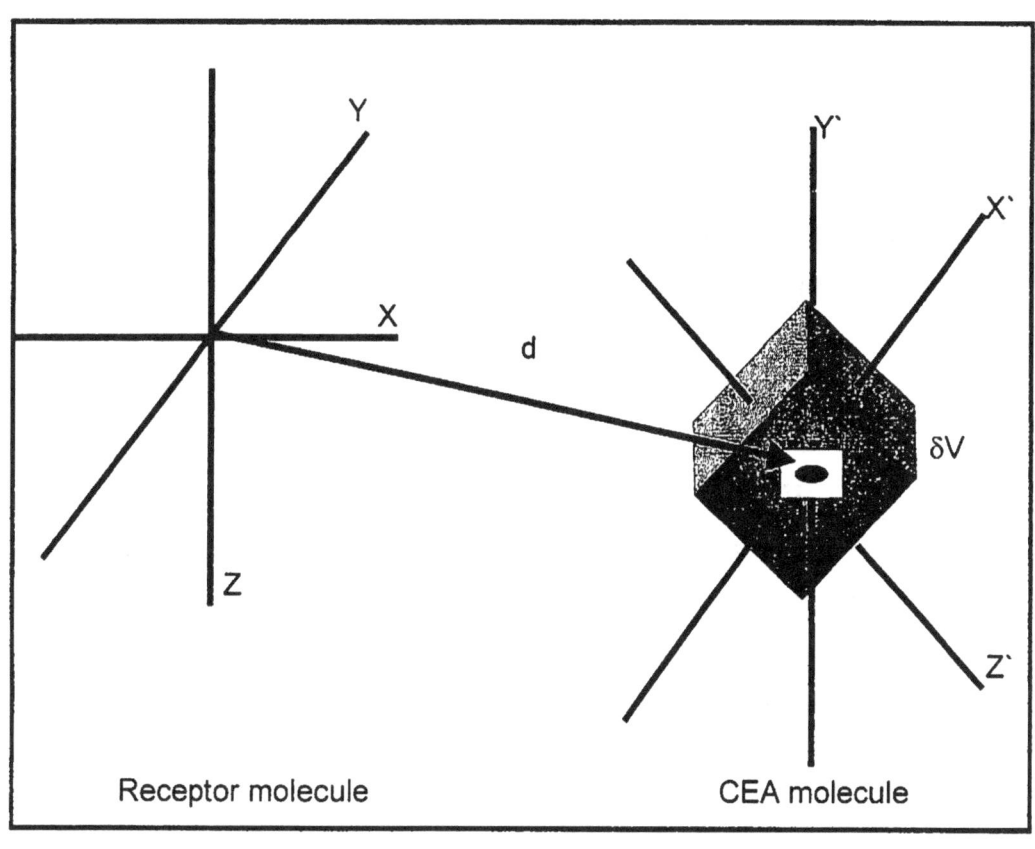

Fig (8-1):
Schematic representation of geometrical requirements for bond formation between CEA and various classes of receptor (R), d= the distance between CEA and the receptor
(All details are explained in the text)

Conclusions

1. The observed elevated levels of CEA in sera of malignant breast cancer patients than in benign breast tumors, and in malignant breast cancer pre-operative than those post operative indicate progression of the tumor. The magnitude of elevation in CA15-3 is more than CEA in the same sera of patient with breast tumors. This indicates that CA15-3 as tumor marker is more specific than CEA.
2. Purified CEA can be labeled with radioactive iodine by chemical oxidation (chloramine. T) without reducing immunologic reactivity and physicochemical properties. Monospecific antibodies obtained from rabbits are suitable for radioimmunoassay.

    Solid phase RIA and IRMA enhanced the potential sensitivity, precision and specificity of measurment as well as improving practicality.
3. The developed protocol of RRA for the assay of CEA receptors is capable to analyze these receptors in cytosolic and nuclear fractions of mammary adenocarcinoma tissues.
4. Kinetic studies for the binding reaction of ^{125}I-CEA with their cytosolic and nuclear receptors in mammary adenocarcinoma tissues were temperature and time dependent. Pseudo first order kinetic at (4,10,20,35 and 45) °C was observed in all cases.
5. Thermodynamic studies of binding reaction of ^{125}I-CEA with cytosolic or nuclear receptor in mammary adenocarcinoma tissues occurs spontaneously ($\Delta G° < 0$), the reaction is entropically – driven since $\Delta S° > 0$. Thermodynamic parameter calculated for the standard state and activated complex specified the role of hydrophobic forces in stabilizing the complex formed.

6. UV spectral of CEA-receptor complex is attributed to conformational changes associated with the binding.
7. Evaluation of biological activity of CEA receptor complex, free receptor and unliganded CEA using DNA affinity chromatography could increase the accuracy of selection of CEA dependent tumors.

Future work:

According to the results obtained in this work, the following works are suggested for the future:

1. Further studies are required for detection and quantitation of CEA-receptor complex in sera and other fluid of breast cancer with different stages.
2. More clinical studies are needed to determine the role of CEA-receptor and utility for diagnosis of patients with cancer.
3. Spectroscopic studies are needed (NMR, ESR, x-ray Fluorescence) to have more information about the DNA of transformed cell.
4. Further studies are required for the humoral immune responses to CEA correlated with the development of breast cancer.
5. The application of the developed method of IRMA and RRA for the assessment of CEA and CEA receptor in the other tumor tissues.
6. Isolation of the messenger RNAs encoding CEA and cloning the $_c$DNA of it, then comparison the purified CEA obtained in this study with that produced by $_c$DNA technology to elucidate the actual native species of CEA with in the breast tumors.

References

References

(1) De vita, V. T., Hellman, S., and Rosehberg, S.A., 1997. Cancer **(Principle and Practice of Oncology).** (5th ed). Lippincott - Ravan Puplishers. New York. P: 1024 – 1156.

(2) Hossfeld, D.K., Sherm, C.D.; and Love, F., 1992. **"Manual of Clinical Oncology".** (5th ed.). Springer – VerLag USA. P: 257 – 275.

(3) David, L., Richhard, L., Frankie, A., et al. 1999. J. **Clini. Oncology**, 17. (3): P 855 - 861.

(4) Ministry of Health., 1998. Result of Iraqi Cancer Registry.

(5) Ministry of Health., 2000. Result of Iraqi Cancer Registry, 1999-2000.

(6) Macmhon,B.,1994"**Advance in Oncolojy**" P3-36

(7) Cavallif, F., Hansen, H. H., and Kaye, S. B., 1997. **"Tex Book of Medical Oncology".** (1st ed). Marin Duntiz ltd. P: 53 – 55.

(8) Aghell, N., Therwath, A., 1994. **India Journal of Cancer** 77: P: 218 – 224.

(9) Chen, Y., Chen, C., Riley, et al. 1995. **Science** 27. P: 270 – 289.

(10) Bishop, J. M., 1987. **Science**, 23: P: 305 – 333.

(11) Bioley, J. E., Cannon and King, M. C., 1986. **Gene Epidemology, suppl.** 1: P: 15 – 35.

(12) Rudy,D.R,Kurowsk,1997."**Familymedicin**" (1st ed) Willkins,P: 41-60

(13) Harris, J. R., Lippman, M. E., Veronesive, 1992. **N. Engle. Med.** 327(5): P: 319 – 328.

(14) Hani, A., Nabi, 1997. **Semin. Med.** 27: P: 30 – 35.

(15) Michael, N. B., 1988. Eru. J. **Cancer. Clin. Oncol.** 24 (1): P: 61 – 68.

(16) Nixon, D. W., 1982. **"Diagnosis and management of Cancer"** (1st ed.). Addison - Wesley Publishhing Company. P: 167 – 200.

(17) Monsees, B., Destoue, J. M., and Gersell, D., 1987. **Radioloyg**, 163: P: 467 – 470.

(18) Toniglo, P. G., Levitz, M. 1995. J. **Natl. Cancer**. 87: P: 190 – 197.

(19) Pannall, P., and Kotasek, D., 1997.**"Cancer and Clinical Biochemistry**", David Burnat , ACB Vetaure Puplication U.K. Chapter1

(20) Vered, M. D., Hideko, Y., and Daniel, P. H., 1998. **Breast Cancer Research and Treatment**, 52: P: 329 – 359.

(21) Hayes, D. E., Bast, R., Desch, C. E., et al. 1996. J. **Natl. Cancer. Inst**. 88: P 1456-1466.
(22) Hilkens, J., Buijs, F., Hilgers, et al. 1984. Int. J. **Cancer**. 34: P:197 – 200.
(23) Duffy, M. J., 1999. Ann. **Clin. Biochem**. 36: P: 579 – 586.
(24) Gendler, S. I., Spicer, A. P., 1995. Ann. **Res. Physiol**. 57: P: 607 – 634.
(25) Price, M. R., Rye, P. D., Petrakou, E., et al. 1998. J. **Tumor. Biol**. 19 Supppl (1): 1 – 20.
(26) Wesseling, J., Vander, V. S., Hilken, J. A., 1996. **Mole. Bio**. Cell. 7: P: 565 – 577.
(27) Jian, W. G., 1996. Br. J. **Surgry**. 83: 437 – 446.
(28) Gimmi, C. D., Morrison, B. W., Mainprice, B. A., et al. 1996. **Nature. Med**, 2 : 1367 – 1378.
(29) Agrawal, B., Kraniz, M. J., Reddish, M. A., et al. 1998. **Nature. Med**. 4: 43 – 49.
(30) Hilken, J. Ligienberg, M., Vos, H. L., et al. 1992. **Biol. Sci**. 17: 359 – 363.
(31) Delves, P. J., and Roitt, I. M., 1998. **Encyclopedia of Immunology** (2nd ed.). Academic press. Limited. New York. P: 798 – 820.
(32) Krebs, B. P., Lalanne, C. M., Schhneider, M., 1978. "**Clinical Application of Carcinoembryonic Antigen Assay** ". The McGraw - Hill Companies, Inc; New York. P 6 – 16.
(33) Bagshawe, K. D., 1975. "**Medical Oncology**", Blackwell scientific Publication, London. P: 257 – 270.
(34) Vildan, Y., Hankan, C., Ethen, N., et al. 1999. J. **Tumor Marker. Oncology**. 8 (4): 33 – 37.
(35) Vildan, Y., Maktav, .D., Hakan, C., et al. 1997. **Clinical. Biochemistry**. 30: 53 – 56.
(36) Takami, M., Misumi, Y., Kuroki, M., et al. 1988. J. **Biol. Chem**. 263 (25) :12716 – 12720.
(37) Stanners, C. P., De Mart, L., Rojas, M., et al. 1995. **Tumor. Biol** , 16 (1): 23 – 27.
(38) Begen, R. H., Vernaar, M. J., Chester, K. A., et al. 2000. **Biochem**. J: 346 – 519.
(39) Burtis, C. A., Edward. R., Ashwood, E. R., 1999. "**The Text Book of Clinical Chemistry** ". (3rd ed.). Philadelphia, W. B. Saunders. Chap. 23: P: 722 – 742.
(40) Harnmarstrom, s., 1999. **Semin. Cacer**. Biol. 9 (2): 67 – 71.
(41) Gold, P., Freeman, S. O., 1965. J. Exp. Med. 121: 439 – 450.
(42) Boehm, M. K., Mayans, M. O., Thornton, J. D., et al. 1996. J. **Mol. Biol**. 259 (4): 718 – 725.
(43) Frangsmyr, L., Baranov, V., Hannarstron. 1999. **Tumor. Biol**. 20 (5): 277 – 281.

(44) Goron, T., Roger, 1976. **Biochem. Biophys**. Act. 458: 349 – 372.
(45) Abraham, F., Chaim, B., Joseph, S., et al. 1974. **Biochem. Biophys**. Act. 417: 123 – 152.
(46) Weinstein, J. N., Parker, R.J., Holton, O.D., 1985. **Cancer. Invest** 3: 84 –91.
(47) Jager, W., Eibner, K., Loffler, et al. 2000. **Anti. Cancer. Res**. 20 (6D): 5179 – 5182.
(48) Bast, Ravdin, P., Hayes, D. F., et al. 2000. **J. Clin. Oncol**.9 (6): 1865 – 1868.
(49) Hitoshi, K., Yuji, H., Fumio, I., and et.al., 1997. In. J. **Cancer**. 72: 377 – 382.
(50) Hosteiter, R. B., Augutus, L. B., Mankorious, R., et al. 1990. J. **Natl. Cancer Inst**. 82 (5): 380 – 391.
(51) Tanak, A. K., Ivagur, H., Hamada, Y., and et.al., 1990. J. **Surg. onco**l. 34: 106 – 116.
(52) Vose, B. M., 1987. **Immunodulating Agent In, Immunolgy of Malignant Diseases**, Edited by V.s Byers and R. W. Baldwin. MTP Press Limited. P 70 – 90.
(53) Thompson, J. A. 1997. In. J. **Cancer**. 72: 197 – 202.
(54) Bayna, E., Shapere, J. H.; Shur, B. D., 1988. **Cell**. 53:145 – 154.
(55) Medoff, J. R., 1988. **Cancer. Res**. 48:1689 – 1695.
(56) Hakim, A., 1984. **Neoplasma**. 34: 385 – 394.
(57) Hheiskala, M. K., 1988. J. **Immunol**. 28:19 – 25.
(58) Medoff, J. R., Clack, V. D., Roche, J. K., 1986. J. **Immunol**. 137: 2057 – 2065.
(59) Pradol, I. B., Laudanna, A. A., Carnerin, C. R., and et.al., 1995. Int. **J. Cancer**, 61:854 – 864.
(60) Von, Kleist, S., Migule, Halla, B., 1995. **Anticancer Res**. 16:1889 – 1895.
(61) Mc. Clay, D. R., Ettensonhn, C.A., 1987. **Ann. Rev Cell. Biol**. 3: 319 – 325.
(62) Findeisen, R., Albrecht, S., Richter, B., et al. 1998 **Clin. Chem. Lab. Med**. 36 (11): 841 – 846.
(63) Hogan, Ryan, A., Fennelly, J., Jones, M., et at. 1980. Br. **J. Cancer**. 41: 587 – 592.
(64) Duffy, M. J., Oconnell, M., 1981. Eur. **J. Cancer** .17: 711 – 714.
(65) Stevens, D. P., Mackay, I. R., 1973. **Lancet**. 2: 1238 – 1239.
(66) Fleisher, M., Ostign, H. F., Besenfelder, E., et al. 1973. **Clin. Chem**. 19:1219 – 1225.
(67) Bailey, N., 1976. **"Statistical Methods in Biology "**. Hodder and Stoughton. London.
(68) Akel, S., Saber, M., Abdallah, H., et al. 1993. J. Egypt. Nat. **Cancer. Inst**.6 (2): 425 – 436.

(69) El-Sayed, M. S., Afafa, Halim, A., 1994. **The New Egypt**. J. Of. Med. 10 (4): 1821 – 1826.
(70) Mori, M., Mimori, K., Ueo, H., et al. 1996. Int. J. **Cancer**. 68: 739 – 744.
(71) Heinze, T., Schuren, Kamper, P., Minguillon, C., and et.al., 1997. **Anti. Cancer. Res**. 17: 2953 – 2954.
(72) Liufj, F., 1993. **Cancer. Bull**. 45: 55 – 60.
(73) Mansour, E. G., Haster, M., Park, C. H., et al. 1983. **Cancer**. 51: 1243 – 1248.
(74) Kuhadjda, Fb., Offutt, L. E., Mendelos, G., 1983. **Cancer**. 52: 1257 – 1264.
(75) Shousha, S., Lyssiotis, T., Godney, V. M., and et.al., 1979. **Br. Med**. J. 1: 777 – 779.
(76) Glon, M., Mone, R., Dittadi, R., et al. 1986. **Cancer**. 57: 917 – 922.
(77) Gold, P., Freemans, S.O., 1969. J. **Exp. Med**. 122: 467 – 478.
(78) Yamanaka, T., Kuroki, M., Kinugasa, T., et al. 1996." **Protein. Exp. Purfi.**" 7(4): 438 – 445.
(79) Dareg, D. A., Turberrville, C., and James, R., 1973. J. **Cancer**. 28: 1916 – 1925.
(80) Tomita, J. T., Safford, J. W., and Hirata, A. A., 1974. **Immunology**. 26: 291 – 298.
(81) Mech, J. P., and Pusztaszeri, G., 1972. **Immunochemistry** 9: 1031 – 1034.
(82) Krupey, J. E., Wilson, Freedddman, S. O., et al. 1972. **Immunochemistry**. (9): 617 – 622.
(83) Slayter, H. S., Coligan, J. E., 1976. **Cancer Res**. 36: 1996 – 2000.
(84) You, Y. H., Hefla, L. Y., Yazaki, p. J., et al. 1998. **Anticancer Res**. 18(5a): 3193 – 3200.
(85) Fuks, A., Banjo, C., Shuster, J., et al. 1974. **Biochim. Biophhys. Acta**. 417: 123 – 128.
(86) Mossner, j., Fishbach, w., 1988. **Res. Exp. Med**. 188:101 – 105.
(87) Scherage, H. A., 1961. "**Protrin Structure**". New York. Academic. Pressc. P175 – 287.
(88) Freifrlder, D., 1982. "**Physical Biochemistry Application to Biochemistry Molecular Biology**". (2nd ed.). Sanfroncisco. W. H. Freeman Company. Chap.14. P 494 – 591.
(89) Herskovits, T. H., Laskowski, M., 1960. J. **Biol. Chem**. 235: 56 – 60.
(90) Theodore, T. H., Micheal, I., 1962. J. **Biol. Chem**. 237:2481 – 2485.
(91) Herskovits, T. T., Laskowiskim, 1962. J. Biol. Chem. 237: 3418 – 3422.
(92) Herskovits, T. T., Mescantl, 1965. J. **Biol. Chem**. 240: 639 – 643.
(93) Lowry, O. H., Rosebrough N. J., Farr, **L., Randell**, R., 1951. J. Biol. Chem. 193: 265 – 268.

(94) Scopes, R., 1982. **"Protein Purification Principles Practice"** New York. Springer. Verlag. P 162 – 200.
(95) Wester, Meier. 1996. "**Electrophoresis in Practice**" (2nd ed). New York. Awiley. Company. Section II. P 101 – 112.
(96) John, F., Robyt, Bernard, J., White, 1987. "**Biochemical Techniques Theory and Practice** " Brooks/Cole Publishhing Company Monterey, California. Chap. 4. P 73 – 121.
(97) Nils, H., Axelsen, 1983. "**Hand book of immunoprecipitiation in Gel Techniques** ".(3rd ed.). W. A. Banjamin. Inc. London.
(98) Janson, J. C., and Ryden, L., 1998. **Protein Purification Principle High Resolution Methods and Application.** (2nd ed.). Ajohn. Wiley. and Sons. Inc. New York. Chap. 1 & 14.
(99) Smith, I.,1976 . **Chromatographic and Electrophoretic Techhniques**. Vo12. (4th ed.). William. Hheinemann. Medical book. London. P 210 – 230.
(100) Wrigley, C. W., 1971. Meth. In Enzy. C. 22: 5559 – 5565.
(101) Dubios, M., Gilles, K. A., **Hamilton**, J. K., Robers. P. A., and Smith, F., 1956. Annal. Chem. 228 (3): 350 – 356.
(102) Segal, T. H., 1976. **Biochemical. Calculations**. John. Whilly and Sons. Inc. P 327 – 350.
(103) Coligan, J. E., Lautenschleger, J. T., Egan, M. L., et al., 1972. **Immunochemistry**. 9: 377 – 386.
(104) Rosali, J., Tillack, T. W., and Marchest, V. T., 1972. Int. J. **Cancer**. 10: 357 – 367.
(105) Sugono, K., Ohkura, H., Hirohashis, et al. 1989. Jpn. J. **Cancer**. Res. 80:1156 – 1160.
(106) Krupey, J., Gold, P., Freedman, S. O., 1968. J. **Expt. Med**. 128: 387 – 395.
(107) Kohler, N., and Lipton, A., 1974. Exp. **Cell Res**, 87: 297 – 301.
(108) Ross, R., Glomset, J., Kariya, B., et al. 1974. **Proc. Natl. Acad. Sci**. US. 71: 1207 – 1210.
(109) Blak, S. D., Whitfield, J. F., and Braun, A. C., 1973. **Proc. Natl. Acad**. Sci. U. S. 70: 675 – 676.
(110) Leffert, R. L., 1974. J. **Cell. Bio**. 62: 767 – 779.
(111) Hoffiman, R., Ristow, H. J., Veser, J., et al. 1973. **Exp. Cell. Res**. 82: 211 – 218.+
(112) Emane, A. S., 2001. " **Biochemical studies on Som Tumor Marker in oral cancer** " ph. D. Thesis supervised by Al-Modhaffar, S. A., College of Science, Baghdad University.
(113) Turner, M. D., Olivares, T. A., Harwell, L., and Kleinman, M. S., 1972. J. **Immunol**. 108: 1328 – 1339.
(114) Rule, A. H., and Golesky-Reilly, 1973. **Immunol. Commun**. 2: 213 – 226.

(115) Rosai, J., Tillack, T. W., and Marchesi, V. T., 1972. Int. J. **Cancer**. 10: 357 – 367.

(116) Banjo, C., Shuster, J., and Gold, P., 1974. **Cancer**. Res. 34: 2114 – 2121.

(117) Mathews, Ch. K., Holde, K. E., 1990 "**Biochemistry**" Callifornia. The Benjamin/Cummings. Publishing. Co.

(118) Loeb, G. I., and Scherage, H. A., 1956. J. **Phy. Chem**. 60:1633 – 1636.

(119) AL-Kazzaz, F. F., 2000. " **Molecular Characterization of Carcinoembryonic Antigen in Some Colorectal Tumor** " ph. D. Thesis supervised by Al-Mudhaffar, S. A., College of Science.

(120) Yang, J. T., Foster, J. F., 1954. J. **Am. Chem. Soc**. 76: 1588 – 1593.

(121) Tanforel, C., Buzzell, J. G., Rands, D. G., et. al., 1955. J. **Am. Soc**. 77: 6421 – 6425.

(122) Silvestien, R. M., Bassler, G. C., Marril, T. C., 1981. "**Spectrophotometric identification of organic compounds**". New York. John Wiley and Sons. P 181- 200.

(123) Donovan, J. W., 1969. J. **Biol. Chem**. 244 (8): 1691 – 1698.

(124) Lreach, S. J., Scherage, H. A., 1960. J. **Biol. Chem**. 235: 2827 – 2833.

(125) Leach, S. J., 1969. "**Physical Principles and Techniques of Protein Chemistry**" Part A. (5th ed.). London. Academic Press. Chap. 3 : 102 – 125.

(126) Gerasimowicz, W. V., Hicks, B., and Pfeffer, P. E., 1984. **Macromolecules**. 17: 2597 – 2603.

(127) Koenig, J. L., 1984. Adv. **Polymer. Sci**. 54: 87 – 154.

(128) Oakes, D. D., Shuster, J., and Gold., 1972. **Cancer. Res**. 32: 2753 – 2760.

(129) Thomson, D. M., Krupey, J., Freedman, et al. 1969. **Proc. Natl. Acad. Sci**.U.s. 64: 161 – 167.

(130) Logerfo, P., Kvupey, J., Hansen, H. J., 1971. **New. Engl. J. Med**. 285: 138 – 141.

(131) Go, V. L. W., Schutt, C. G., Moertel, et al., 1972. **Gastroenterology**. 62: 754 – 760.

(132) Egan, M. L., Lautenschleger, J. T., Coligan, J. E., et al., 1927. **Immunochemistry**. 9: 289 – 294.

(133) McPherson, T. A., Band, P.R., Grace, M., et al., 1973. **Int. J. Cancer** 12: 42 - 54.

(134) Corey, L., James, W. B., and Michael, C., 1981. **Meth. In Enzy. C**. 74: 272 – 298.

(135) Benjamin, E., Richard, C., Geoffrey, S., 2000. Immunology. **Short. Course**. Ajohlv. Willey and Sons. Inc. Publication. Chap. 20. P 401 – 419.

(136) Dhia, F. J., 1983. M. Sc Thesis. University of Baghdad College of Science.
(137) Charles, W. Parker, 1983. **Meth. In. Enzy**. 182: 700 – 718.
(138) Maysoon, R. R., 1979. Ph. D. Thesis. University of Baghdad. College of Science.
(139) Johnston, A., and Thorpe, R., 1987. **Immune Chemistry in Practice.** (2nd ed.). Blackwell Scientific Publications. London.

(140) Harboe, N., Ingild, A., 1973. **J. Immunol**. 2. (2): 161 – 166.
(141) Harboe Closs, M., Deverill, O., 1976. **J. Immunol**. 5: 861 – 865.
(142) Sela, M., and Mozes, E., 1966. **Proc. Nat. Acad. Sci**. USR. 55: 445 – 450.
(143) Parker, W. C., 1967. **Hand Book of Experiment Immunology**. Back well. Scientific Publication. Oxford. P 423 – 450.
(144) Schreiber and Haimorich, 1983. **Meth. In. Enzy**. F. 147: 164 – 175.
(145) Shrooch, R. K., 1998. Ph. D. Thesis. University of Baghdad. College of Science.
(146) Bonnie, S. D., and Eric, D. S., 1990. **Meth. In. Enzy** 182: 663 – 670.
(147) Shvari, F., and morell, A., 1970. **J. Immunol**. 104: 1310 – 1318.
(148) Wassan, A. A., 2000. " **Biochemical studies on Alpha – Fetoprotein and Some Tumor Marker In Gastric Cancer** " ph. D Thesis supervised by Al-Mudaffar, S. A., College of Science, Baghdad University.
(149) Maysoon, K. H., 2001. " **Molecular Characterization of Testostrone Receptor in Mammary Tissues Effected by Tumors** "M. Sc Thesis supervised by Al- Mudaffar, S. A., College of Science, Baghdad University.
(150) Hunter, W. H., and Greenwood, F. C., 1962. **Nature**. 194: 495 – 501.
(151) Marchalonis, J. J., 1969. **Biochem**. J. 113: 299 – 305.
(152) Morrison, M. G. S., Bayse, and Webster, R. G., 1971, **Immunochemy**. 8: 289 – 294.
(153) Abelw, G. I., Perova, S. D., and Sokolenko, A. A., 1976. Ann. N. Y. **Acad. Sci**. 276 – 282.
(154) Leif, W. and Jerker, P., 1966. **Biochim. Biophys. Acta**. 130: 257 – 260.
(155) Sedlacek, H. H., Grigat. H., Renk. T., and Seiler. F. R., 1981. **Meth. In. Enzy**. C. 74: 87 - 105.
(156) Hendry, R. M., and Herriman, J. E., 1980. **Immunol. Method**. 35: 285 – 292.
(157) Filippussion, H., and Hornby, W. E., 1970. **Biochem**. J. 120: 215 – 219.
(158) Graciela, G., and Sven. E. S., 1981. **Meth. In. Enzy** C. 74: 571 – 588.

(159) Koroulas, A. O., and Moro, L., 1971. J. **Immunol**. 106:1630 - 1640.
(160) Catt, K. and Treger, G. W., 1967. **Science**. 158: 1570 – 1572.
(161) Braford, M. M., 1976. **Anal. Biochem**. 72: 248 – 257.
(162) Morris, B. J., 1976. **Clinica. Chimica.** Acta. 72: 213 – 225.
(163) Foucard, T., Bennich, H., Johansson, S. O., et al. 1975. Int. **Archs. Allergy. Appl. Immun**. 48: 812 – 820.
(164) Nilsson, L. A., 1983. j. **Immunol**. 17 (10): 57 – 68.
(165) Ryley, H. C., and Brogan, T. D., 1973. J. **Clin. Pathol**. 26: 852 – 860.
(166) Folkevson, J., Westergaard, J. G., Hindersson, et al. 1979. "**Carcinoembryonic Proteins**". Vol. II. Elsevier. Amsterdam. P 503 – 512.
(167) Schwartze, M. L., Pizzo, S. V., Hill, R. L., et al. 1975. J. **Bio. Chem**. 248: 1395 – 1402.
(168) Ronald, R. B., Reivfe, A. L., Patricia, et al. 1996. **Clinical. Chem**. 45: 104 - 110.
(169) Harboe, N. M. G., and Ingild, 1983. **Immunol**. 17(10): 345 – 351.
(170) Cinader,R., 1967. "**Antibodies to Biological Active Molecules**". Pergamon Press. Oxford.
(171) Ceska, M. A., Sjodin, V., and Grossmuller, 1971. **Biochem**. J. 121: 139 – 145.
(172) Rosp, U. C., Pennisi, F., Bianchi, et al. 1967. **Biochim. Biophys. Acta**.133: 486 – 494.
(173) Lambert, B., and Jacquemin, 1973. **Biochimie**. 55: 1395 – 1400.
(174) Parish, C. R., and Stanley, P., 1972. **Immunochemistry**. 9: 853 – 860.
(175) Repke, D. W., and Zull, J. E., 1972. J. **Bio. Chem**. 247: 2189 – 2195.
(176) Buckle, R. M., and Potts, J. T., 1970. J. Lab. **Clin Med**. 76: 46 – 53.
(177) Mcpherson, T. A., Band, P. R., Grace, M., et al. 1973. Int. J. **Cancer**. 12: 42 – 54.
(178) Turner, M. D., Olivares, T. A., Harwell, L. et al. 1972. J. **Immunol**. 108: 1328 – 1339.
(179) Dandliker, W. B., and Satussure, V. A., 1970. **Immunochemistry**. 7: 799 – 810.
(180) Farr, R. S., 1958. J. **Infect. Dis**, 103: 239 – 244.
(181) Gallagher, T. S., Voss, Jr., 1969. **Immuno. Chemistry**. 6: 573 – 579.
(182) Rodbard, D., 1971. "**Principles of Competitive Protein-Binding assay**". J. B. Lippincott. Co. Philadelphia. P 204 – 215.
(183) Steiner, A. L., Kipnis, D. M., Utiger, R., et al. 1969. **Proc. Nat. Acad.** Sci. USA. 64: 367 – 373.
(184) Steiner, A. L., Parker, C. W., and Kipnis, D. M., 1972. J. **Biol. Chem**. 247: 1106 – 1112.

(185) Skom, J. H., and Talmage, D. W., 1958. J. **Clin. Invest**. 37: 783 – 791.
(186) Hales, C. N., Randler, 1963. J. **Biochem**. 88: 137 – 143.
(187) Fltschen, W., 1964. **Immunology**. 7: 307 – 312.
(188) Coller, J. A., Circhow, R. W., and Yin, L. K., 1973. **Cancer. Res**. 33: 1684 – 1688.
(189) Yalow, R. S., and Berson, S. A., 1959. **Nature**. 184: 1648 – 1655.
(190) Meade, R. C., and Klitgaard, H. M., 1962. **Nuclear. Med**, 8: 407 – 413.
(191) Parker, C. W., 1972. "**Progress In Clinical Pathology**" Vol. 4. Blackwell Scientific Publication Oxford. P 141 – 160.
(192) Mcphersn, T. A., and Carnegite, P. R., 1968. **Clin. Med**. 72: 824 – 830.
(193) Ratcliffe, J.C., 1974. **Brit, Med. Bull**. 30: 32 – 36.
(194) Grodsky, G. M., and Forsham, P. H., 1960. J. **Clin. Invest**. 39: 107 – 111.
(195) Smith, T. W., Butler, V. P., and Itaber, E., 1969. **New. Eng. J. Med**. 281: 1212 – 1216.
(196) Rehfeld, J. F., and Stadil, F., 1973. **Scand. J. Clin. Lab. Invest**. 31: 459 – 463.
(197) Utiger, R. D., Parker, M. L., and Daughady, W. H., 1962. J. **Clin. Invest**. 41: 252 – 256.
(198) Naval, J., Villacampa, M. J., Goguel, A. F., et al. 1985. **Proc. Natl. Acad**. Sci. USA. (82): 3301 – 3316.
(199) Villacampa,M. J., More, R., Naval,J., et al. 1984. **Biochem. Biophys. Res. Commun**. 122: 1322 – 1327.
(200) Kanevsky, V. Yu., Pozdnyakova, L. P., Aksenova, O. A., et al. 1997. **Biochem. Molecul. Bio,. Int**. 41(6): 1143 – 1147.
(201) Severin, S. E., Moskaleva, E. Yu., Posypanova, G. A., et al. 1996. **Tumor. Targeting**. 2: 299 – 302.
(202) Uriel, J., Trojan, J., Moro, R., et al. Ann. N. Y. 1983. **Acad. Sci**. 417: 321 – 325.
(203) Moro, R., Tamoki, T., Wegmann, T. G., et al. 1993. **Tumor Biol**. 1993. 14(2): 116 – 121.
(204) Suzuki, Y., Zeny, C. Q. Y., and Alpert, E., 1992. J. **Clin. Invest**. 90: 1530 – 1536.
(205) Uriel, J., Villacampa, M. J., Moro, R., et al. 1984. **Cancer. Res**. 44: 5314 – 5319.
(206) Laborda, J., Naval, J., Calvo, M., et al. 1987. **Int. Cancer**. 40 (3): 314 – 320.
(207) Uriel, J., Naval, J., Laborada, J., 1987. J. **Biol. Chem**. 262: 3579 – 3583.

(208) Torres, J. M., Darracq, N., and Uriel, J., 1992. **Biochim. Biophys. Acta**. 60: 1159 – 1160.
(209) Moskaleva, E. Y. U., Posypanova, G. A., Shmyrev, I. T., et al. 1997. **Cell Biol. Int**. 21 (12): 793 – 798.
(210) Weiland, G. A., Minneman, K. P., Molinoff, P. B., 1980. **Mol. Pharmacol**. 18: 341 – 345.
(211) Seely, D. H., Wang, W. Y., Salhanick, H. A., 1980. **Biochem. Biophy. Acta**. 632: 535 – 539.
(212) Burton, K., 1965. **Biochem. J**. 51: 660 – 666.
(213) Scatchard, G., 1949. **Am. N. Y. Acad. Sci**. 51: 660 – 668.
(214) Weiland, G. A., Molinoff, P. B., 1981. **Life Science**. 29 (4): 313 – 318.
(215) Rae-Venter, B., and Dao, T. L., 1982. **Biochem. Biophys. Res. Commun**. 107 (2): 624 – 630.
(216) Freifelder, D., "**Physical Biochemistry**" Trans. By Al- Mudhaffer. S. A. 1984. Baghdad University. Press.
(217) Chamberlain, J., Jargarinec, N., Ofner, P., 1966. **Biocem. J**. 99: 610 – 616.
(218) Thompson, S. A., Johnson, M. P., Brooks, C., 1982. **The Prostate** 3: 45 – 49.
(219) Shiu, R. P. C., Friesen, H. G., 1974. **Biochem. J**. 140: 301 – 306.
(220) Shiu, R. P. C., Friesen, H. G., 1974. **Biochem. J**. 249: 7902 – 7908.
(221) Birkinshow, M., Falconer, I. R., 1972. **J. Endorinol**. 140: 310 – 316.
(222) Melandder, W., Hhovarth, C., 1977. **Arch. Biochem. Biophys**. 183: 200 – 206.
(223) Evans, J. S., Levine, B. A., 1980. **J. Inorg. Biochem**. 12: 227 – 231.
(224) Cox, J. A., Malnoe, A., Stein, E. A., 1981. **J. Nucl. Med**. 14: 695 – 700.
(225) King, R. J. B., and Main, Waring, W. I. P., 1974. "**Steroid Cell interaction**". (1st ed.). The Butter Worth Company. P 10,11,18.
(226) Walent, J. H., and Groski, J., 1990. **Endocr**, 126 (5): 2383 – 2391.
(227) Kosk-Kosicka, D., Bzdega, T., Warzynow, A., 1989. **J. Biol. Chem**. 264 (33): 1949 – 1955.
(228) Malencik, D. A., Anderson, S. R., 1986. **Biochem**. 25: 709 – 713.
(229) Nemethy, G., Scherag, A. J., 1962. **Phys. Chem**, 66: 1775 – 1780.
(230) Waelbroeck, M., Van, Obberghen, E., Demeyts, P., 1979. **J. Biol. Chem**. 254: 7736 – 7741.
(231) Haro, L. S., and Talamantes, F. J., 1985. **Mol. Cell Endocrinol**. 43: 199 – 204.
(232) Ross, P. D., and Subramanian, S., 1981. **Biochemistry**. 20: 3096 – 3100.
(233) Blumenthal, D. K., and Stull, J. T., 1982. **Biochemistry**. 21: 2386 – 2391.

(234) Laport, D. C., Wierman, E. M., and Storm, D. I., 1980. **Biochemistry**.19: 3814 – 3819.
(235) Farber, E., 1973. **Cancer. Res**. 33: 2537 - 2550
(236) Dulbecco, R., 1970. **Nature**. 227: 802 – 806.
(237) Martz, E., and Steinberg, M. S., 1972. **J. Cell. Phsilo**.79. 83.
(238) Stoker, M. G. P., 1973. **Nature**. 246: 200 – 203.
(239) Holley, R. W., and Kiernan, J. A., 1974. **Proc. Natl. Acad. Sci. USA**. 71: 2908 – 2911.
(240) Gold, P., 1971. **Ann. Rev. Med**. 22: 85 – 90.
(241) Murgita, R. A., and Tomasl., 1975. **J. Exp. Med**.141: 269 – 286.
(242) Goeken, N. E., and Thompson, J. S., 1977. **J. Immunol**. 119: 139 – 142.
(243) Gowenlock, A. H., Editor, Varley, S., 1988. " **Practical Biochemistry**". (6th ed.). Heinemann Medical Books. London. P 1018 – 1050.
(244) Bullough, W. A., Wallis, M. J., 1974. **Endocrinology**. 62: 463 – 468.
(245) Karalogiu, D., Yasasever, V., Kizir, A., et al. 1996. **J. Exp. Clin. Cancer**.15 (4): 335 – 342.
(246) Vincent, T., Devita, Jr., Samuel, Hellman, Steven, A., et al. 1996. **Important Advance in Oncology. Lippincott-Raven Puplishers**.
(247) Elldge, R. M., Fugua, S. A. W., Clark, G. M., et al. 1993. **Breast. Cancer. Res. Treat**. 26: 225 – 238.
(248) Muller, M., Volkmann, M., Zenigarf, H., et al. 1994. **New. Engl. J. Med**. 330: 865 – 872.
(249) Adell, K., and Ogbnna, G., 1995. **Clin. Chem**. 36/2: 261 – 266.
(250) Arndt-Jovin, D. J., Jovin, T. M., Bahr, et.al., 1975. **Eur. J. Biochem**. 54: 411 – 416.
(251) Fiske, C. H., Subbarow, V., 1925. **J. Biol. Chem**. 66: 375 – 380.
(252) Gross-Beilard, M., and Chambon, P., 1973. **J. Biochem**. 36: 32 – 37.
(253) Blin. N., and Stafford, D., 1976. **Nucleic. Acid Res**. 3: 2303 – 2308.
(254) Kunkel, L. M., Smith, K. D., Boyer, S. H., et al. 1977. **Proc. Natl. Acad. Sci. USA**. 74: 1245 – 1250.
(255) Wagner, A. F., Bugianesi, R. L., Shen, T. Y., 1971. **Biochem. Biophys. Res. Commun**. 45: 184 – 189.
(256) Berridge, M. V., Aronson, A. I., 1973. **Anal. Biochem**. 53: 604 – 610.
(257) Pharmacia Fine Chemicals AB., 1974. "**Affinity Chromatography Principles and Method**". P 45 - 46. Rahms. Lund Sweden.
(258) Grody, W. W., Schrader, W. T., O'Malley, B. W., 1982. **Endocrin. Rev**. 3: 141 – 150.

(259) Parker, F. S., 1971. "**Application of Infrared Spectroscopy in Biochemistry Biology and Medicine**". Plenum. Press, New York, P 274 – 286.

(260) Taboury, J. A., Liquier, J., and Taillandier, E., 1985. **Con. J. Chem.** 63: 1904 – 1910.

(261) Maniatis, T., Fritschand, E. F., and Sambrook, 1982. "**Molecular Colning A Laboratory Manual**". Cold. Spring. Harber. Laboratory. New York.

(262) Hudson, L., and Hay, F. C., 1978. "**Practical Immunology (2nd ed.). Black Well Scientific Publication**". Oxford/London.

(263) Sunil, M., Salil, D., 1997. "**Molecular Biotechnology**" (2nd ed.). Wiley - Liss Publication. New York, P 109 – 120.

(264) Blundell, T. L., 1994. **Trends in Biotechnology.** 12(5): 145 – 155.

(265) Bernstein, F., Koetzle, T. F., Williams, et al. 1997. **J. Molecular Biology** 112 (3): 535 – 340.

(266) Alton, E. W., 1995. **J. of Pharmacy and Pharmacology.** 47: 351 - 354.

(267) De Vos, A. M., Ultsch, M., and Kossiakoff, A. A., 1992. **Science** 255: 306 – 310.

(268) Dougherty, D. A., and Stauffer, D. A., 1990. **Science** 250: 1558 – 1565.

(269) Marshall, G. R., and Cramer, R. D., 1988. **Sciences** 9: 285 – 292.

(270) Wu, T. P., Yee, V., Tulinsky, A., et al. 1993. **Protein Engineering.** 6(5): 471 – 490.

PART (B)

Development of some Immunobiochemical Techniques for the study Carcinoembryonic Antigen (CEA) in Colorectal Tumors

Prof.Dr.Sami A. AL-Mudhaffar
Dr. Sahib Ali AL-Atrakchi

Abbreviations

ARA	Arabinos
BSA	Bovine Serum Albumin
CEA	Carcinoembryonic Antigen
CRC	Colorectal Cancer
CR	Colorectal
CRT	Colorectal Tumor
CFA	Complete freund's Adjuvant
GAL	Galactose
GAL NAC	N-Acteyl Galatosamine
GUL NAC	N-Acteyl Glucosamine
GDA	Gluter Dialdehyde
GA	Gluteraldehyde
MAN	Mannose
MBP	Mannose Binding Protein
NSB	Non-specific Binding
NGP	Normal Glycoprotein
NHS	Normal Human Serum
PAGE	Poly Acrylamide Gel Electrophoresis
PEG	Poly Ethylene Glycol
PBS	Phosphate Buffer Saline
PRA	Peroxidase Rabbit anti-CEA Conjugate
HRP	Horseradish Peroxidase
HnRNP	Are a large group of 20 proteins (hnRNP A- hnRNP u) that associate with pre-mRNAs in eukaryotic

Summary

There have been a number of reports concerning the isolation and purification of carcinoembryonic antigen (CEA). Our laboratory has became interested in this problem as a first step in the development of an immunodiagnostic tests which could find application in early diagnosis or in monitoring therapy in digestive system cancer. Also, this research was mainly designed to develop some Biochemical and immunological techniques which could then be assessed for its value in diagnosis and prognosis

1) A method was developed for the preparation of carcinoembryonic antigen (CEA) of human digestive system from large quantities of metastatic tumor tissue. The purification process involves the sequential steps of extraction in perchloric acid, lentil lectin affinity chromatography and immunoadsorption chromatography. The final product shows a high degree of uniformity as determined by both physicochemical and immunochemical criteria.

2) A sensitive and specific non competitive solid phase enzyme immunoassay for detection and quantitation of carcinoma bryonic antigen (CEA) in nanogram quantities was established according to the following that is to measure CEA in sear, filude and tissue extracts. It was characterized to be simple, rapid and suitable for automation.

   a. Peroxidase was isolate from white radish roots and purified to homogeneity as ascertained by polyacrylamide gel electrophoresis. The isolation and purification method was characterized to be a very simple, which was about five times cheaper than the rather expensive commercial preparation and has a significant higher activity.

b. Antiserum to human CEA was obtained from rabbits and guinea pigs by intramuscularly inoculation with highly purified CEA.

Monospecific anti-CEA was isolated and purified from other immunoglobulin subclasses and some serum proteins by ammonium sulfate precipitation at 41 % saturation and DEAE cellulose ion exchange chromatography.

c. The two-step Glutataldehycle method has been used to conjugate white radish peroxidase to rabbit anti-CEA antibody? The conjugation prepared has been used for enzyme immunoassay. The employed method showed high capacity binding of anti-CEA to peroxidase without loss of activity.

d. A process was described for chemical adsorbed of guinea pigs antiCEA antibody on polypropylene tubes treated with glutaradehyde. The coated tubes prepared used in EIA. Also, Quantitve studies on antibody binding to polypropylene tubes have been done with purified anti-CEA antibody. The result show that the binding of anti-CEA IgG, after 1 hr at room temperature occurred and the maximum amount of immunoglobulin (Ig) that can be adsorbed was 1000ng/mm^2.

3) Assay parameters were optimized by investigating the concentration of reagen, temperature, pH, Ion strength and the reaction kinetics in each of the assay steps. The results indicated that the assays can be performed in 3-4 hr with a sensitivity rang of 0.5 to 6 ng in the region of 90 to 10 % binding was obtained under optimal condition included the following 1- temperature:

lower than 30, 2- PH 7.2. 3- Ionic strength, 0.05 M or more phosphate buffer.

4) EIA kit prepared has been applied successfully to measure CEA level in serum samples obtained from healthily donors, colorectal benigh patients and colorectal cancer patients. The results obtained were compared in term of sensitivity, specificity, simplicity, reproducibility, Accuracy. And convenience for use in routine diagnosis with solid-phase RIA. Also, the EIA as good tools for diagnostic and prognostic.

Table of Contents

Subject		Page No
	abbreviation	263
	Summary	264
	Table of contents	267
Chapter one : introduction and literature survey		273
	Abstract	274
1-1	Introduction	275
1-1-1	Definition and Detection of CEA	275
1-2	Physical properties of CEA preparations	276
1-3	Molecular structure and chemistry of CEA	278
1-3-1	Structure of the carbohydrate moiety	279
1-3-2	Origin of Hethrogrneity	282
1-3-3	Protein structure	283
1-3-3-1	Amino acid composition of CEA	283
1-3-3-2	Structure of the protein moiety of CEA	284
1-3-4	Nature of the carbohydrate – protein linkage in CEA	288
1-3-5	The antigenic site of CEA	288
1-3-6	The tumor – specific grouping of the CEA molecule	290
1-4	Purification of CEA	291
1-5	The physiological roles of carcinoemryonic antigen	292
1-5-1	CEA as an adhesive molecule	292
1-5-2	Carcinoembryonic antigen , tumorogenesity and metastasis	294
1-6	CEA receptors	297
1-7	CEA Biology	301
1-7-1	Distribution and tumor specificity of CEA	301
1-7-2	Cellular localization of the CEA	302
1-7-3	Cellular and humoral immune responses to CEA	304
1-7-4	Circulating CEA	305
1-7-5	Metabolism CEA	306
1-8	Bio eassay of CEA	307
1-8-1	Radioimmunoassays for CEA	307

	Subject	Page No
1-8-2	Nature of the circulating substance (s) measured by radioimmunoassay	311
1-9	Immunochemical studies of CEA	312
1-9-1	Binding studies between I-CEA and various antisers	312
1-9-2	Lecin binding capacity of CEA	314
1-9-3	Comparative inhibition studies in the I-CEA – anti – CEA system	316
1-9-4	Materials cross-reacting with CEA	318
1-9-5	Kinetic and thermodynamic studies of binding of I-Ant CEA antibody to CEA	319
1-10	Clinical application	320
1-10-1	Diagnosis of cancer	323
1-10-2	Use of assay for the surveillance of cancer patients	324
	Ami of the study	326
Chapter Two : Isolation and purification of CEA		327
	Abstract	325
	Introduction	329
	Materials and methods	330
2-1	Chemicals	330
2-2	Instruments	331
2-3	Buffer and solution	331
2-4	Patients	332
2-5	Collection and initial preparation of tumor specimens	332
2-6	Extraction of CEA by perchloric acid	333
2-6-1	Solutions	333
2-6-2	Method of extraction	333
2-7	Purification of CEA	333
2-7-1	Solution and Buffer	333
2-7-2	Preparation of purified lentil lectin	334
2-7-2-1	Extraction method of lentil lectin from common lentil seeds	334
2-7-2-2	Purification of lentil lectin by gelfiltration chromatography techniques	335
2-7-2-3	Lectin activity assay	336
2-7-4	Coupling of lentil lectins to CNBr activated sepharose	336
2-7-5	Column packing and purification procedure	337

	Subject	Page No
2-8	Purification CEA by immunoaffinity chromate-graphy	338
2-8-1	Buffers and solutions	338
2-8-2	Preparation of antibody	339
2-8-3	Purification of IgG (anti-CEA)	339
2-8-4	Anti CEA Immunoadsorbent preparation	340
2-8-5	Colum preparation sample application and elution	340
2-8-6	Estimation of CEA by IRMA method	341
2-9	Analysis of the purified	343
2-9-1	Solutions used	343
2-9-2	Procedure	344
2-10	Result and discussion	345
2-10-1	Preparation of tumor specimens and partial purification of CEA by PCA	345
2-10-2	Lentil lectin affinity chromatography techniques for purification of CEA	346
2-10-3	Immunoaffinity chromatography techniques for purification of CEA	348
	TABLES	352
	FIGURES	353
Chapter Three : Preparation of EIA kit		356
	Abstract	357
	Introduction	359
	Material and method	360
3-1	Chemical and solution	360
3-2	Instrument	360
3-3	Preparation of peroxidase from whiteradish roots	360
3-3-1	Extraction and purification of peroxidase	360
3-3-1-1	Solution and materials	360
3-3-1-2	Procedure of purification	360
3-3-2	Measuring of peroxidase Activity	363
3-3-2-1	Reaction mixture	363
3-3-2-2	Enzyme Assay calculation	364
3-3-3	Analysis of purified peroxidase by polyacrylamide gel electrophoresis	364
3-4	Antisera generation to CEA	364
3-4-1	Preparation of experimental animals	364
3-4-2	Immunization of animals	365

	Subject	Page No
3-4-3	Isolation and purification of specific antibodies to CEA	366
3-4-4	Methods used for identification of pure anti-CEA immunoglobulins	366
3-4-4-1	Cellulose acetate electrophoresis	366
3-4-4-2	Immune electrophoresis (IEP)	367
3-5	Preparation of peroxidase anti-CEA conjugate for enzyme Immunoassay	370
3-5-1	Material	370
3-5-2	Methodology for performing the PRA	371
3-6	Preparation of antiCEA-Coated polypro-ylene tubes	372
3-6-1	Material solution and Appartus	372
3-6-2	Coating methodologies	372
3-6-3	Calculation	373
3-7	Binding capacity assessment of anti-CEA to polypropylene tubes	373
3-7-1	Material reagent and apparatus	373
3-7-2	Assessment methodology	373
3-7-3	Calculation of binding capacity	374
3-8	Assay condition for EIA experiments	374
3-8-1	Amount of CEA (antigen)	375
3-8-2	Amount of anti-CEA conjugate peroxidase (rabbit anti-CEA conjugate peroxidase (PRA)	376
3-8-3	Incubation temperature effect	377
3-8-3-1	The first protocols : temperature of first incubation	377
3-8-3-2	The second protocol: second incubation temperature effect	377
3-8-4	Effect of incubation time	378
3-8-4-1	The first protocols: time of first incubation	378
3-8-4-2	Second protocol: time effect of second incubation	379
3-8-5	Effect pf PH	379
3-8-5-1	First protocol: PH effect on binding between guinea pig anti CEA which coated polypropylene tube and CEA molecule	379
3-8-5-2	Second protocol: PH effect on second binding	380
3-8-6	Ionic strength effect	381
3-8-6-1	First protocol: effect of ionic strength in first incubation	381
3-8-6-2	Second protocol:effect of ionic strength in second incubation	382

	Subject	Page No
3-9	Preparation of standard curves	383
3-9-1	Solutions	383
3-9-2	Procedure	383
3-9-3	Calculation	384
3-10	Result and discussion	385
3-10-1	Extraction and purification of peroxidase enzyme	385
3-10-2	Antibody productions	387
3-10-2-1	The choice of animal species	387
3-10-2-2	The route of injection	389
3-10-2-3	Collection and storage of immune serum	392
3-10-2-4	Isolation and characterization of anti-CEA	393
3-10-3	Enzyme antibody conjugate	394
3-10-3-1	Types and mechanism of coupling	394
3-10-3-2	Choice of enzyme	397
3-10-4	Preparation of antibody coated-polypropylene tubes	398
3-10-4-1	Mechanism of antibody coated tube	399
3-10-4-2	Tube selections	401
3-10-5	Nonspecific absorbents measurement and other factors interfering with the binding of CEA to anti – CEA	403
3-10-6	Maximum binding capacity of antibody to polypropylene tube	405
3-10-7	Assay condition results	408
3-10-7-1	Effect of CEA concentration	409
3-10-7-2	Effect of rabbit anti-CEA conjugate peroxides (RAP)	410
3-10-7-3	Effect of temperature	410
3-10-7-4	Effect of time	411
3-10-7-5	Effect of PH	412
3-10-7-6	Influence of ionic strength	412
3-10-8	The standard curve	412
	TABLES	415
	FIGURES	417
Chapter Four : Evaluation and clinical application of EIA kit		426
	Abstract	427
	Introduction	428
	Materials and methods	429
4-1	Chemicals	429

	Subject	Page No
4-2	Instrument	429
4-3	Solutions	429
4-4	Patients	430
4-5	Blood sampling	431
4-6	Collection of specimens and preparation of tissue homogenate	431
4-6-1	Tissue preparation	432
4-7	Protein Assay	432
4-8	Estimation of CEA by IRMA method	432
4-9	Determination of CEA by EIA method	432
4-10	Statistical analysis	433
4-11	Results and discussion	433
4-11-1	Reference and measuring range	434
4-11-2	Reproducibility	434
4-11-3	Correlation of RIA and EIA	434
4-11-4	Sensitivity specificity accuracy and efficiency of EIA kit	435
4-11-5	Recovery assay	436
4-11-6	Result of tissue determination of CEA colorectal tumors cancer and normal specimens	436
4-11-6-1	Normal specimens	436
4-11-6-2	Benign colorectal tumor	437
4-11-6-3	Colorectal cancer tissue	437
4-12	General discussion	438
	TABLES	440
	FIGURES	443
	References	445

Chapter One

Introduction & Literature Survey

ABSTRACT

Single measurement of the two-biochemical tumor markers (CA 15-3) and CEA were carried out in serum samples obtained from 40 healthy donors, 22 breast benign patients and 122 breast cancer patients. Mean values of these tumor markers in breast cancer patients were significantly higher ($P<0.05$) than that found in healthy normal or patients with benign breast tumors.

CA15-3 shows the best sensitivity (54%) for detecting preoperative breast cancer patients, than CEA, which gave (44%) sensitivity. Also, CA15-3 gave the highest specificity (100%) for discriminating non-malignant patients while CEA had specificity of (77%).

The cytosolic CEA concentration was determined in the tumor, benign and normal tissue of breast cancer patients. Significant differences between values from the tumor and normal specimens were found. There was no correlation between the preoperative levels of serum CEA and cytosol level of CEA in the patients with carcinoma. Also, CEA in cytosols did not correlate with either stage or histology. It was concluded that the test might provide calculable information for the evaluation and planning of treatment.

Chapter One

Carcinoembryonic Antigen (CEA)

1-1 Introduction:

The term carcinoembryonic antigen (CEA) was first used by Gold and Freemdam[1,2] to described atumor associated antigen found in the cellular membrane of adenocarcinomas from entodermally derived digestive system epithelia, It is a macromolecular glycoprotein with molecular weight of approximately 200 and with beta electrophoretic mobility. It is also present in foetal gastronintestinal tissue and with alphafetoprotein has been one of the most widly studied oncofetal antigens. Extensive studies using radioimmunassay have now shown that CEA is present in serum and associated with many form of cancer[3] and also with various non- malignant diseases and it can also be detected in low amounts in various normal tissues[4]. Although many years have clasped since the initial work of Gold and Freeman it is only in the last ten years that preparations of CEA have been widely examined with regared to their purity, heterogeneity of molecules carring the antigentic group and relative potencies, despite the fact that such studies promis to provide data which may enable the reproducibility and agreement of CEA radioimmunoassay to be improved and may also provide a way of assessing whether some molecules with CEA activity are more cancer specific than others.

1-1-1 Definition and Detection of CEA

In view of the heterogeneous nature of the glycoprotein it is impossible to define CEA precisely in terms of physical and chemical properties. A definition of CEA at the present time has to be based on its specific immunological reaction with a monospecific anti-CEA antiserum which has been shown to be identical in specificity to the original antiserum prepared by Gold and Freedman[1]. This is important since it has been clearly established that CEA possesses at least two different immunogenic groups: a unique group which defines CEA-like molecules and a second determinant which is common to CEA and the glycoprotein NGP which is also found in normal and tumoural tissues [5,6,7]. Double diffusion studies have shown that antibodies to both the groups can easily be obtained by inoculating animals with purified CEA preparations[8,9]. NGP has a smaller molecular weight than CEA and can be substantially separated from the latter by Sephadex G-200 chromatography[10] but it is still often a contaminant of CEA and antisera raised to conventionally prepared CEA could contain antibodies which react specifically with NGP[8]. In addition antisera raised to current CEA preparations could also contain other antibodies which react with non-CEA contaminants, even after extensive absorption, indicating the presence of other cancer with beta electrophoretic mobility.

1-2 Physical properties of CEA preparations

1. Molecular size

Using molecular sieve chromatography, an approximate molecular weight of 200 000 daltons was obtained for CEA[10,11]. Furthermore, sodium dodecyl sulfatepolyacrylamide electrophoresis, using a mixture of glycoproteins of known molecular weight as standards, suggests a mean molecular weight for CEA of 200000[10-13]. Each preparation of CEA obtained from colon cancer tissue has given rise to a single peak upon ultracentrifugation, with a sedimentation coefficient of 7-8 S, which is in keeping with the results of molecular sieve chromatography and sodium dodecylsulfatepolyacrylamide gel electrophoresis[13]. However, without the availability of a shape-dependent parameter, partial specific volume, and other physical data, an exact molecular weight cannot as yet be calculated for any given CEA preparation.

2. Molecular charge

CEA has been reported to migrate in the β- globulin region upon immunoelectrophoresis in agar gel at pH 8.6[13]. Polyacrylamide gel electrophoresis of purified CEA preparations has yielded a single, but somewhat diffuse band[13]. Heterogeneity of mobility was particularly notable upon comparison of the products of tumor tissues which had arisen in different sites within the gastrointestinal tract[4].

Neuraminidase treatment of CEA resulted in a narrow, more homogeneous electrophoretic band, and decreased the variation noted between the different preparations.

The Isoelectric focusing of purified CEA revealed isoelectric points of 3.0 and 3.75. However, following neuraminidase treatment of purified CEA a single homo-geneous zone of activity was obtained with an isoelectric point of 5.0[14,15]. Other investigators have observed that a characteristic feature of all purified CEA samples which they examined was a double peak of CEA activity in the range of pH 2-3[11,12,13]. They also noted CEA activity with isoelectric points of 3.5, 4.0, 4.25 and 4.5. On the other hand, observations of CEA preparations with single isoelectric points of 4.8[13] and 4.7[14] have been reported. Isoelectric focusing of crude tumor extract yielded peaks of CEA activity at pH 2.4, 3.0, and 4.5 through 6.4[15].

3. Miscellaneous physical parameters

The CEA molecule has been showm to be soluble in water, perchloric acid and half-saturated ammonium sulphate but is insoluble in ethanol[16]. It is relatively resistant to boiling[16,17]. The properties of solubility in both perchloric acid and half- saturated ammonium sulphate form the basis of a number of the radioimmunoassays for serum CEA presently being employed [17]. (Table 1-1).

TABLE (1-1): Physical properties of CEA

- Soluble in perchloric acid
- Soluble in 50% saturated ammonium sulfate
- Insoluble in ethanol
- Heat stable
- Sedimentation coefficient of 7-8 S
- β-mobility on agar electrophoresis at pH 8.6
- single polydisperse band on polyacrylamide gel electrophoresis
- Molecular weight of 200 000 ± 20 000
- Isoelectric points of < 3 and 3.75 ± 0.25

1-3 Molecular Structure and Chemistry of CEA

CEA as a glycoprotein was evident from its solubility and apparent stability in perchloric acid[15]. The difficulties encountered in studying CEA are therefore those encountered in general glycoprotein chemistry. Biosynthesis of the carbohydrate moiety of a glycoprotein is believed to be a post-ribosomal event in which the enzymic assembly of the saccharide Chains taken place after the protein has been completed[16]. Glycoprotein structure is therefore only partly under genetic control and considerable variation in structure is possible. This variation often takes the form of micro-heterogeneity of the intermediate and peripheral sugar residues whereas the innermost carbohydrate residues are relatively homogeneous in structure. CEA appears to be no exception to this and the physical and chemical properties of a CEA preparation will be the properties of the "average" molecule of CEA found in the mixture. Since the enzymic activity for the biosynthesis and possible breakdown or modification of a glycoprtein may vary in different individuals and in the malignant state[17,18,19] it is not surprising to find variations in the

Chapter One

carbohydrate content and composition between different CEA preparations.

1-3-1 Structure of the carbohydrate moiety

Glycoproteins are complex macromolecules consisting of a variable number of oligosaccharide subunits and one or more polypeptide chains. Those glycoproteins studied to date have revealed structures consisting of linear and/or branched oligo-saccharide chains of variable length attached to the polypeptide chains via O-glycosidic linkages to serine or threonine, or via a peptide bond to asparagine. A number of different analytic approaches can be used to elucidate this type of structure.

a. **Acid hydrolysis of CEA:** Partial acid hydrolytic cleavage of oligosaccharide chains to obtain low molecular weight fragments is an established technique for the elucidation of the structure of glycoproteins[20]. The release of monosaccharides or oligosaccharides at defined time intervals provides information on the sequence of the various components within the chain. In addition, the isolation and characterization of such fragments may indicate the mode of linkage between the individual sugars.

On the basis of the foregoing rationale, purified CEA was subjected to controlled hydrolysis with polystyrene sulphonic acid at pH 2.4 at 60°C and 86°C[20]. Heterosaccharide fragments were released which contained either mannose and N-acetylglucosamine or N-acetylglucosamine alone. Further structure elucidation was not possible since only trace quantities of the purified fragments were obtained.

b. **Enzymatic hydrolysis of CEA:** Although numerous glycosidases are available which can degrade isolated glycopeptide fragments, only a few such enzymes will degrade the native intact molecule. However, these latter enzymes are not readily available in a highly purified form and their enzymatic specificities have not been well characterized.

The action of neuraminidase on sialic acid-containing glycoprotcins has been intensively studied in the last decade. A preparation of neuraminidase from *Clostridium perfringens* was used to remove the sialic acid from CEA[21]. Similar experiments were performed with neuraminidase from *Vibrio cholerae*[22] and both enzymes were able to remove 100% of the sialic acid residues present in CEA, demonstrating the presence of sialic acid in terminal positions in the CEA molecule.

Attempts to remove galactose residues from CEA by β-galactosidase have been unsuccessful[23]. Oxidation of CEA with galactose oxidase with subsequent reduction with NaB^3H_4 indicates the presence of at least 2 residues of galactose at terminal positions, and 10-12 galactose residues in penultimate positions of the putative carbohydrate branches of the CEA molecule[23-29]. Attempts to remove sugars other than sialic acid from CEA with exoglycosidases have not been successful[25]. Nevertheless, the enzymatic approach, using combinations of appropriately purified endoglycosidases and exoglycosidases to elucidate the carbohydrate structure of CEA,. should be pursued with vigor.

c. **Periodale oxidation of CEA:** Periodic acid and its salts, which cleave carbon-carbon bonds between adjacent dihydroxy positions in sugar moieties of glyco-proteins, have been most useful in the structural analyses of such molecules. Periodate oxidation of CEA has resulted in complete destruction of sialic acid and fucose, the elimination of 25-50% of mannose and galactose, but no destruction of N-acetyl-glucosamine. The CEA preparations so treated showed no loss of CEA antigenic activity[25,26]. It is important to note, however, that since reduction and hydrolysis were not carried out, the hemialdal groups or the aldehyde groups of the sugars were still attached to the oxidized molecule. These modified groups may still be immunologically active despite the absence of the precursor monosaccharides from the sugar analysis.

d. **Carbohydrate components of glycopeptides**: Following neuraminadase treatment, the resultant sialic acid-free CEA was exposed to the non-specific protease nagasc. Six glycopeptides were isolated by sequential chromatography on Scphadex G-25, cellulose powder and the cation exchange resin AG 50W-X4. On the average, these glycopeptides were 92% carbohydrate in composition. The molecular weights of these glycopeptides were estimated to be of the order of 4000 by Sephadex G-25 chromatography. This would suggest that the CEA molecule may be composed of side chains containing approximately 17 sugar residues. Furthermore, the variable monosaccharide content of these glycopeptides suggests that the carbohydrate subunits are heterogeneous in nature[24,25].

Figure (1-1) depicts Schematic model of the general structural features of CEA. It is known that the carbohydrate moiety of CEA exists as multiple side chains attached through asparagine linkages to glucosamine residues[27]. It is also likely that the side chains are distributed asymmetrically although on average there appears to be about seven residues per side chain and a maximum of about 80 chains[28]. Fucose and sialic acid are present at non-reducing ends and the latter residues are attached to the 3-position in galactosc[29]. Galactosc and mannose constitute the intermediate portion of the carbohydrate moiety where branching occurs[29-30]. Concanavalin A binding is abolished by a single Smith's degradation[31] indicating that this lectin binds to mannose residues present in the outer chains. The protein moiety of CEA is stabilized by six disulphide bonds[32]. The

Chapter One

available evidence[30-33] suggests that the antigenic site in CEA is situated in the innermost carbohydrate chains or in the protein and activity is abolished if the three dimensional structure of the protein is destabilized by cleavage of the disulphide bonds.

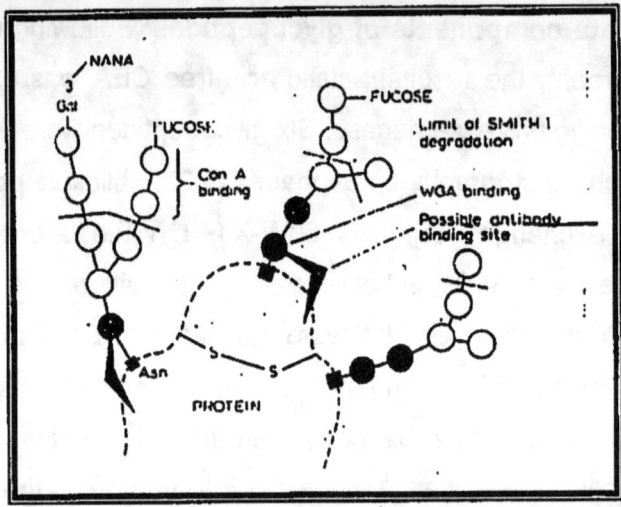

Figure (1-1): Schematic model of the general structural features of CEA.

○ Intermediate chains mainly MANNOSE and GALACTOSE

● N-ACETYLGLUCOSAMINE
WGA-wheat germ agglutinin
(All details are explained in the text)

1-3-2 Origin of Hethrogrneity

Examination of glycoproteins by techniques such us electrophoresis, ion-exchange chromatography and isoelectri focussing have demonstrated heterogeneity with respect to charge density and net molecular charge[34]. A major contribution to this is micro-heterogeneity in the form of variation in the number of terminal sialic acid residues and this can be distinguished from charge variation originating in the protein structure. Treatment of a glycoprotein with neuraminidase will remove sialic acid and an increase in its cationic eleclrophorctic mobilily and a considerable simplification in its isoelectric focussing pattern can be

Chapter One

expected. Residual heterogeneity observed by the above techniques can be attributed to charge variation on the protein[35]. It is known that heterogeneity in the carbohydrate structure of a glycoprotcin can result through variation at the genetic level as well as to variations in post-ribosomal biosynthesis[34,35]. It may therefore be important to distinguish between heterogeneity occurring at a single locus due to post-ribosomal events and variation generated in carbohydrate chains as a result of being attached to different positions on the peptide chain depending on variation in the structure of the protein. Aspects of post-ribosomal biosynthesis of glycol-proteins which may have a particular bearing on the tumour specificity of a potential marker substance arc tissue specificity and developmental differentiation. Identical polypeptide chains have been shown to be glycosylated differently in different tissues. For example, hen scrum transferrin synthesised in the liver has an asparagine-linked carbohydrate group of different composition to a similarly linked group in ovo-transferrin syn-thesised in the hen oviduct[34,35]. Furthermore developmental changes, possibly associated with changes in glycosyl transfcrase activity have been detected in other types of glycoprotcins[36]. These aspects of heterogeneity are particularly interesting as they provide a biochemical basis for studying components of oncofoetal antigens produced in various malignant and non-malignant conditions of various tissues, in order to find out if these components vary in structure.

1-3-3 Protein Structure

1-3-3-1 Amino acid composition of CEA:

Approximately 50% of the protein portion of CEA is composed of ammo acids with a terminal carboxyl and hydroxyl group in their side chains (Table 1-2). The other amino acid residues are usually present in lower proportions and the sulfur-containing amino acid methionine is

Chapter One

usually absent. The presence of 12 residues of cysteine in the CEA molecule has been reported[37].

Although a significant degree of variability may be observed in the amino acid composition of different colonic CEA preparations when the amino acid content is expressed on the basis of total weight of material, the apparent variability in amino acid content of such CEA preparations is reduced when the content of any amino acid residue is calculated on the basis of the total protein portion of the molecule[38,39]. A comparison of nine different colonic CEA preparations from different laboratories similar results with respect to most of the amino acid residues Table (1-2). However, a degree of variability was observed in the chemical composition of CEA derived from a gastric tumor when compared to colonic cancer preparations[38-44].

1-3-3-2 Structure of the protein moiety of CEA.

The N-terminal amino acid in CEA purified from liver metastases of colon cancer has apparently been shown to be lysine by different investigators[38-51]. The identity of the C-terminal amino acid has not been established as yet.

Amino acid sequencing of five different CEA preparations from colonic tumors shows identical sequences of the first 20 to 30 amino acid residues[46,47]. Similar sequences were obtained upon analysis of CEA produced by a human colonic tumor line maintained in hamsters and from CEA isolated from human serum[47]. However, oikawa., et.al., have reported the primary structure of CEA deduced from the cDNA sequence, demon-strating that CEA is synthesized as a precursor with a single peptide followed by 668 amino acid of the putative mature molecule; the first 108, N- terminal residues with lysinein the N-terminal position are followed by three very homologous repetitive domains of

178 residues each and than by 26 mostly hydrophobic residues at the C-termenal, which are suggested to comprise a membrane anchor(48).

TABLE (1-2): Amino acid composition of CEA

Results of amimo acid analyses of CEA obtained in four different laboratories. Samples of CEA were purified from hepatic metastases of colonic carcinomas. The data are expressed as follows: (weight of amino acid/weight total protein of sample). 100%. n.d., not done; a, Banjo et al.(40), means of results of six different preparations; b, Hansen, H. J. as reported by Kupchik et al.(41); c, Coligan et al.(42), Terry et al.(43); d, Westwood, J.(44)

Amino Acid	a	b	c	d
Aspartic acid	14.1	16.6	15.0	14.7
Glutamic acid	11.3	12.4	11.6	10.6
Serine	8.4	10.5	8.1	10.4
Threonine	8.0	8.6	7.9	9.6
Isoleucine	6.0	5.8	5.0	4.7
Leucine	10.3	9.4	9.0	8.2
Proline	6.5	4.6	10.0	8.4
Glycine	3.3	4.2	3.1	5.5
Alanine	3.8	3.9	4.1	6.2
Valine	5.8	6.6	6.3	7.3
Tyrosine	3.6	5.8	5.6	3.6
Phenylalanine	3.3	2.7	3.8	2.2
Lysine	2.9	2.9	3.4	2.8
Histidine	2.0	1.8	2.4	1.8
Arginine	4.6	4.2	4.9	3.3
Cysteine*	0.0	0.0	0.0	0.8
Methionine	0.0	0.0	n.d.	Trace
Tryptophan	n.d.	n.d.	n.d.	n.d.

*In a, b and c, determinations of cysteic acid were not performed. Hence, cysteine converted to the cysteic acid form during hydrolysis would not have been detected. In d. the content of cysteine was determined as cysteic acid after oxidation of the molecule by performic acid[45].

Chapter One

Most recently study showed that CEA consists of 34-amino acid processed leader sequence, 108 amino acid N domain three very similar pairs of internal domain of 178 amino acid each, denoted A_1B_1, A_2B_2, and A_3B_3, terminated by a 27 amino acid C terminus[48-51] Fig(1-2).

Furthermore the previous investigations using site-directed mutation have implicated many different subdomains in N-domaine of CEA. Maryam et.al. suggested that at least three different regions in the N-domainedonated GYSWYK, region1, NRQII, region2 and QNDTG, region 3 as depicted in Figure (1-2). These three region are exposed, adjacent and play a major role in CEA- mediated homotypic adhesion[49-51].

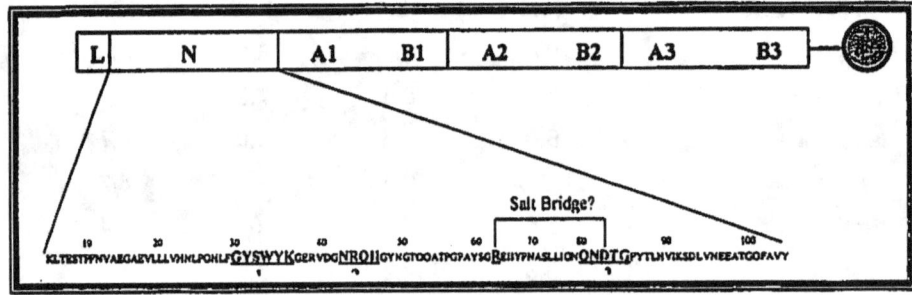

Figure (1-2): Schematic diagram of the structure of CEA showing the amino acid sequence of the CEA IgV-like domain (N-terminal domain). The N-terminal residue of the mature protein is assigned 1 and potential homotypic binding subdomains (1,2,3) are *bold* and *underlined*. The position of a putative salt bridge from Arg-64 to Asp-82, suggested by Bates et al.[51] from computer modeling is indicated.

Three Dimensional structure studies by Beta et.al[51] and other[50] suggested that CEA has considerable amount of antiparallel B sheet. This B sheet has been some what twisted and deformed from the idealized structure shown in Fig. (1-3). The tertiary structure of CEA as predicted by computer modeling depicted in Fig.(1-4). This modles imply that the protein face of beta- sheet in neightboring CEA domains lie on alternate side of the CEA structure, such a modle has implication for the adhesion interactions between CEA molecule on adjacent cell or for the antibody targeting of CEA[50-53]

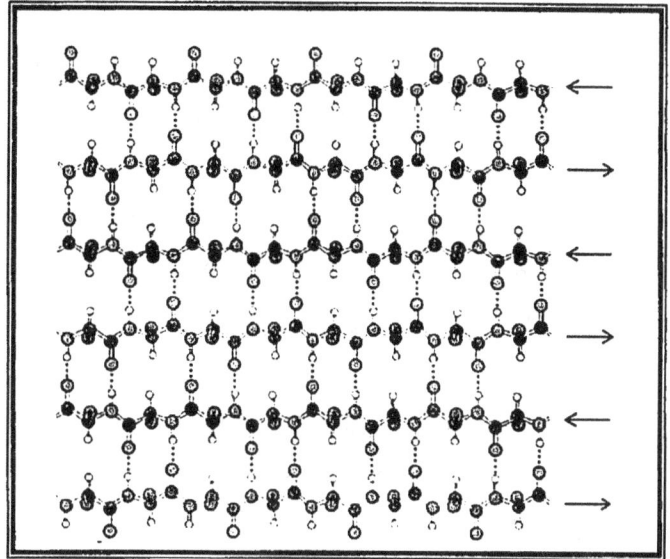

Figure (1-3): Antiparallel β pleated sheet. Adjacent strands run in opposite directions. Hydrogen bonds between NH and CO groups of adjacent strands stabilize the structure. The side chains are above and below the plane of the sheet.

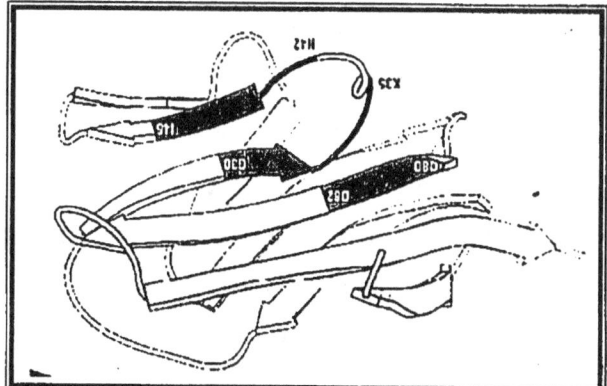

Figure (1-4): A hypothetical three-dimensional structure for the N-terminal domain of CEA obtained by molecular modeling, all details are explained in the text.

Chapter One

1-3-4 Nature of the carbohydrate-protein linkage in CEA

The elucidation of the carbohydrate-protein linkage(s) in the CEA molecule requires knowledge of both the amino acid and monosaccharide residues which are involved, and the nature and position of the functional groups forming the bond(s). The most commonly described carbohydrate-protein linkages involve the amino sugars. The glycosylamine linkage of some glycoproteins has been found to involve the amide group of asparagine and the glycosyl group of N-acetylglucosamine[53]. A second type of bond involves N-acetylgalactosamine linked, O-glycosidically, to serine or threonine residues[54]. Studies of the glycopeptides obtained from CEA have provided indirect evidence for the involvement of N-acetylglucosamine in the carbohydrateprotein linkage[53,54]. It is also of interest that asparagines N-acetylglucosamine, displays weak inhibitory activity in the CEA radioimmunoassay[17]. The absence or the low content of N-acetylgalactosamine in CEA, and the inability to remove heterosaccharides from CEA upon mild alkaline treatment, make it unlikely that N-acetylg-alactosamine is involved in the carbohydrate-protein linkage[53-55].

1-3-5 The antigenic site of CEA

Degradation studies[20-36] have shown that 85% of the carbohydrate residues in CEA can be removed without appreciable loss of antigenic activity, showing that the immunodeterminant is present in the innermost carbohydrate residues or in the protein sub-structure. The predominant sugar residue in the degraded material is N-acetylglucosamine and this is consistent with its strong reaction with wheat germ agglutinin. Some studies[23,24] had indicated that carbohydrate is involved in the immunological activity of CEA and that N-acetylglucosamine[53], or an asparaginelinked N-acetylglucosamine[54], may play a role in the determinant. These studies involved measuring the activity of CEA

Chapter One

fragments obtained either by acid hydrolysis using polystyrene sulphonic acid or proteolysis using the enzyme nagase. Many of the fragments appeared to be predominantly carbohydrate enriched in N-acetylglucosamine relative to neutral sugars, but the activity was always considerably less than that of untreated CEA. More recent studies[37] have shown that integrity of the protein sub-structure of CEA is important for high immunological activity. Thus the activity is abolished by treatment of CEA with 0.5 M NaOH at 20 °C and reduced to 3-5% of the activity of untreated CEA on cleavage of the disulphide bonds. The tentative conclusion reached[30] was that the carbohydrate moeity of CEA does not contain the immunodeterminant. This however may be an oversimplification since particular residues in the innermost part of the carbohydrate may be involved in the antigenicsite but require to be held in a particular conformation by the protein sub-structure for full activity as suggested by some investigators[30-33]. This may explain why a variety of N-acetylglucoscimine-rich heterosac-charides failed to inhibit ^{125}I-labelled CEA-anti-CEA binding[17]. Variation in the affinity of different CEA glycoproteins for anti-CEA antibodies may be accounted for by heterogeneity of carbohydrate residues in or adjacent to the antigenic site or by direct perturbation produced by varuation in the protein substructure.

In view of its association with non-malignant disease and also its presence in normal tissues, the CEA determinant usually described cannot be strictly termed a tumour specific site[35]. However the possibility exists that tumour specificity may be conferred on structure of intermediate or peripheral sugar residues in some molecules which also possess CEA activity. Similarly there is no evidence ruling out possible cancer specificity residing in the protein structure of some CEA molecules.

1-3-6 The tumor-specific grouping of the CEA molecule

The results of studies described earlier[40-47] using polystyrene sulphonic acid for the partial hydrolysis of CEA strongly suggested that a heterosaccharide grouping consisting solely, or largely, of N-acetylglucosamine was of major importance in the tumor-specific antigenic site of the CEA molecule[40]. However, the monosaccharide N-acetylglucosamine was not able to inhibit ^{125}I-CEA-anti-CEA binding[30-33]. Nevertheless, the central role played by this amino sugar was further illustrated when the proteolytic enzyme nagase was used to prepare a variety of immunologically active glycopeptides from the CEA molecule[39]. These fragments were of various molecular weights, between 1000 and 5000. Different fragments retained tumor-specific antigenic activity in the absence of one or more of the monosaccharides, sialic acid, mannose, galactose, fucose and N-acetylgalactosaminc. In all instances, N-acetylglucosamine was present in relatively high concentrations in the small immunologically-active fragments.

Studies of the intact CEA molecule have revealed that upon removal of all the sialic acid residues of CEA by neuraminidase, no loss of activity results[37,44,45,54]. Further-more, upon periodate oxidation of CEA, all of the sialic acid and fucose, and 20-25 % of the mannose and the galactose residues are destroyed without any decrease in the inhibitory activity of the CEA molecule[25,26,44]. It is worth noting that there was, however, no destruction of any N-acetylglucosamine residues during periodate oxidation.

The glycopeptide fractions obtained by the nagase degradation of the CEA molecule each contained 7 or 8 amino acid residues. In every instance, aspartic acid or asparagine and glutamic acid or glutamines were the major amino acid constituents. Hence, it may well be that either one or both of these residues may be covalently bonded to the carbohydrate moiety of CEA. Recently, most study showed that a molecule consisting of aspartic acid bound to N-acetylglucosamine via an N-acetylglycosylamine-type linkage is capable of weak inhibition of ^{125}I-CEA-anti-CEA binding (Table 1-5)[53,54]. This observation suggests that the immunodominant grouping of CEA may not be present at the terminal non-reducing end of the complete heterosaccharide chain of CEA, as it is in other glycoprotein and polysaccharide antigens[45]. It is still, however, possible that the determinant group is present in the terminal position of an incomplete heterosaccharide chain Fig (1-1). Although the results strongly suggest that the carbohydrate moiety is intimately involved in the immunodo-minant tumor site of the CEA molecule, the protein moiety may make an important contribution to the conformation of the tumor-specific site.

Recent data[50,51] indicate that reduction and alkylation of the CEA molecule may markedly diminish its binding activity to anti-CEA. This would support the possibility that protein conformation is of some importance in the binding activity of the CEA determinant.

1-4 Purification of CEA

CEA has been purified by a variety of different techniques. In our laboratory metastatic tumor lesions have been used whenever possible in order to obtain large quantities of cancer tissue from a single source. Purification of the CEA has been-achieved by a sequence of procedures including perchloric acid extract, column chromatography on Sepharose 4B and Sephadex G-200, and poly acrylamid gel preparative electrophoresis[11-13]. Recent modify-cations in this purification procedure have included removing the perchloric acid by column chromatography on Sephadex G-25 (coarse), and concentration of the eluate by ultrafiltration through an Amicon PM-30 membrane. Alternatively, perchloric acid can be removed by rapid dialysis through an artificial kidney. This eliminates

Chapter One

the need for a lengthy dialysis step. In addition, the CEA preparations have been rechromatographed on Sephadex G-200 following block electrophoresis[56].

Other methods of CEA purification have been reported. These have included: lithium diiodosalicylate for CEA extraction and ion exchange chromatography for product separation[56,57]; perchloric acid extraction, pevikon electro-phoresis, Sephadex G-200 chromatography and isoele-ctrofocusing[58]; perchloric acid extraction followed by sequential column chromatography on a mixed bed resin of DEAE-cellulose and CM-cellulose, Sepharose 6B, and Sephadex G-200[59]. Thus, different investigators have employed different techniques for the isolation of CEA. It is still uncertain if the products obtained by the various methods are identical.

1-5 The Physiological Roles of Carcinoemryonic Antigen:

The physiological roles of CEA family members are largely unknown[60], but being Ig super-family members suggested that might play some important roles in cell-cell or cell-substrate recognitions or they might work as receptors for the effecter molecules.[61] Adhesive cell-cell and cell-substrate interactions plays, as one component of the morphogenetic process, a key role in the life history of an organism[62,63], and cellular invasion and metastasis of malignant cells[64].

1-5-1 CEA as an Adhesive Molecule:

Adhesive molecules are morphoregulatory molecules whose genes expression effect cell patterning and tissue signaling through mechano-chemical effects on cell linkage, shape and movement[65].

Recent studies strongly support the idea that adhesive molecules are crucial for the segregation of different cell types. The observation suggest a primary role for adhesive molecules and in linking cells in a proper sequence during morphogenesis and in stabilizing formed structures. Benchimol,S. et.al., Present evidence obtained with CEA. c-DNA transfectants of cells not previously producing CEA that CEA indeed functions as a homotypic intercellular adhesion molecule[66].

Adhesion is an essential mediating event in the evolution of metazon life, and in present day it plays a central role in development and meta morphogenesis[62,64].

Adhesion molecules determine the specificity of cell to cell and cell to substrate associations and have provided molecular in sights into embryonic development[64] cellular invasion and metastasis.[65] The successive production of different types of adhesion molecules during embryonic development and the consequent inductive interactions in the resultant cell collectives have been postulated to be responsible for the execution of the three dimensional body plan in higher organisms[67].

At the molecular level, CEA contain one or more Ig-related domains that share a common folding pattern displaying multiples of a sandwich structure of two antiparalle B sheets, with each B-strand consisting of 5-10 amino acid[67]. In mediating a diversity of intermolecular binding interactions, this stable Ig-fold serves as a general structural platform for presenting specific functional determinants on the faces of B-sheets or at the loops connecting these B-strands[68]. CEA protein- protein interactions can be either homophilic or heterophilic and occur either between the faces of the B-sheets or at the loop regions of the Ig-fold[60]. The intermolecular contacts common to crystals of both rat and human CEA, for example, are head-to-head interactions between the GFCC'''C B-sheets of domain1[23,69].

The ability to disrupt self interactions of CEA represents a valuable experimental and clinical tool, because such interactions are required for many of their signaling and other biological functions. CEA self

Chapter One

interactions are considered to be relatively week[67,68]. At the level of individual interacting molecule, CEA often bind over relatively extended surfaces[68,70]. Within the binding interface there are nonetheless binding points of greater significance. Zhou et al[71] suggested a double reciprocal antiparalle binding model for CEA- mediated intercellar adhesion involving two bonds between the N- terminal domain of one molecule on the surface of apposite cells. Although peptides representing the entire N and A_3B_3 domains of CEA could specifically block CEA-mediated intercellular adhesion between cells, parallel interactions between CEA types of interaction would have the effect of clustering of molecules on the cell surface.

More recent results indicate[50,51] that the three N domain regions, GYSWYK, NRQII and QNDTG Fig. (1-2), are all involved in CEA – mediate adhesion.

1-5-2 Carcinoembryonic Antigen, Tumorogenesity and Metastasis:

The liver is a common site for metastasis from various forms of primary malignancies. Both experimental and clinical results reveal that the presence of carcinoembryonic antigen (CEA) enhances liver metastasis from colorectal carcinoma cells[17,72]. CEA is a highly characterized, cell surface glycoprotein overexp-ressed by various tumor cells and provides a tool for tumor tissue-specific targeting. Increasing amounts of CEA in the serum correlates with high degree of specificity for the rat 80-kDa protein by both fluorescein isothiocyanate analysis and Western blotting[84,85,86].

In more recent study Olga v. et. Al.[85,87,88], suggested Fig (1-5) that CEA interacts with hn RNp M_4 (hnRNps are large group of 20 protiens hnRNp A- hnRNP-U that associate with pre-mRNAs in the eukaryotic cell[86]) on the surface of Kupffer cells through the PELPK –binding site.

The CEA hnRNp complex is endocytosed by kupffer cell and initiates the signaling cascade that stimulates production of IL-1α, IL-6, IL-10, and tumor necrosis factor-α cytokinase. Upon stimulation the CEA –hnRNp M_4 complex dissociates, CEA is modified by removal of sialic acid residues and is recycled by the hepatocytes asialo-glycoprotein receptor. The further path way for the hnRNA M_4 is unknown.

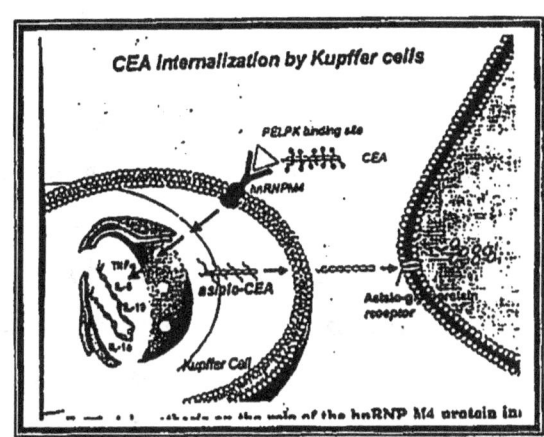

Figure (1-5): A hypothesis on the role of the hnRNP M4 protein in CEA Tumorogensity and metastasis. The suggestion that CEA interacts with hnRNP.

The development of metastatic recurrence after surgical removal of the primary tumor[73]. Earlier the investigators have shown that CEA production of human colorectal cancer cell lines directly correlates with the metastatic potential[74]. Poorly metastatic colon cancer cell lines become highly metastatic when transfected with the cDNA coding for CEA[75,76]. As a member of the immunoglobulin supergene family, CEA is involved in intercellular recognition and may facilitate attachment of colorectal carcinoma cells to sites of metastasis. In an experimental metastasis model of colorectal carcinoma in athymic nude mice, systemic injection of CEA enhanced experimental liver metastasis and implantation in liver by weakly metastatic tumor cells[77,78].

Chapter One

To successfully treat cancers, it is necessary to prevent the development of metastasis after the treatment or removal of the primary malignancy. Therefore, it is important to elucidate the mechaism by which CEA enhances metastatic potential. The molecular basis by which CEA can influence metastasis is only partly understood. As a Olga. V. et al have shown that CEA is rapidly cleared from the circulation of experimental animals, accumulates in liver, and is endocy-tosed in vitro by Kupffer cells. This initiates a series of signaling events that leads to tyrosine phosphorylation on at least two intracellular proteins[79] and is followed by induction of IL-1α,IL-6,IL-10, and tumor necrosis factor-α cytokines[80,81]. CEA uptake by Kupffer cells is independent of its carbohydrate composition and is mediated by an 80-kDa binding protein[82,83]. CEA is recognized by this binding protein through a 5-amino acid sequence, Pro-Glu-Leu-Pro-Lys(PELPK), located at the hinge region (amino acids 108-112)between the N- terminal and the first immunoglobulin loop domain[84-85]. Molecular modeling studies have suggested that this region is exposed on the surface of the molecule. Olga.v.et al have recently shown in a subset of colorectal cancer patients that mutations in the PELPK region of CEA results in the accumulation of large amounts of CEA in the serum[83,86,87]. To further study the interaction between the peptide sequence, PELPK, and rat Kupffer cells, the CEA–binding protein was purified using a combination of gel filtration, preparative polyacrylamide gel electrophoresis, and affinity chromatography on CEA-Sepharose[84,88,89]. A polyclonal antibody to the rat 80-kDa protein was produced in mice that blocks uptake by isolated rat Kupffer cells of both CEA and PELPK peptide conjugated to albumin. This antibody shows a high degree of specificity for the rat 80 kDa protein by both fluoreciein isothiocyanate analysis and wester bloting.

Chapter One

1-6 CEA Receptors[11,12,13,89,90,91,92]

Little is known about the physiological roles of CEA and very little attention on CEA receptors. These receptors to be found on the surface of embryonic and tumor cells while they are absent on the surface of normal mammalian cells[89,90,91,92].

The first trails to isolate purified and characterized of CEA receptor from mammary adenocarcinoma tissues. The purification procedure included Fractionation with ammonium sulfate, ion exchange chromatography (DEAE and CM-cellulose) and gel-filtration in sepharose 6B. The first type Acidic cytosolic receptor, while the second type designated as cationic cytosolic receptors.

Characterization experiments show that cationic receptor has molecular weight 83000 dalton, stock radius 37^0 A and it contains 15.8% Carbohydrate. In isoelectric focusing one band was observed with isolectric points (pI) 6.8.

UV spectral studies showed that ^{125}I –CEA- receptor complex absorption maximum occurs at 241 nm whiles the absorption of the receptor at 280 nm.

The thermodynamic parameters studies and energy diagram model figure(1-6) indicate that the binding of CEA to their specific receptor involves formation of multiple non covalent bonds between CEA and amino acid of the binding site. The attractive forces (hydrogen bonds and hydrophobic forces) are weak by comparison with covalent bonds. However, the large numbers of interaction result in large total binding energy.

The suggested model for bond formation between CEA molecule and its receptor is shown in figure (1-7). As shown in this fig. the strength of a non-covalent bond is critically dependent on the distance(d) between the interacting groups which must be close (in molecular term) before

Chapter One

these forces becomes significant.

In order for an antigenic determinant (epitope) and the receptor-combining site to combine, there must be suitable atomic groupings on opposing parts of the CEA and their specific receptor molecules, the shape of the combining site must fit the epitope Fig. (1-1,1-5, and 1-7), so that several non-covalent bonds can form. If the CEA molecule and the receptor-combining site are complementary in this way (complementary determine regions), there will be sufficient binding energy to resist thermodynamic disruption of the bond. However, if electron clouds of the CEA and receptor overlap, steric repulsive forces come into play which have a vital role in determine the specificity of receptor molecule for CEA, and its ability to discriminate between molecules[43,94].

Also figures (1-7 and 1-6) revealed the general geometrical requirements for bond formation between CEA and their specific receptor and refer to the probability that CEA is located at a certain distance and angular orientation relative to their specific receptor when the CEA ~ R bond has been formed. The closer CEA and their receptor are held by the molecular geometry, the greater probability of the bond formation, and the less entropy loss when the CEA ~R bond is Joined.

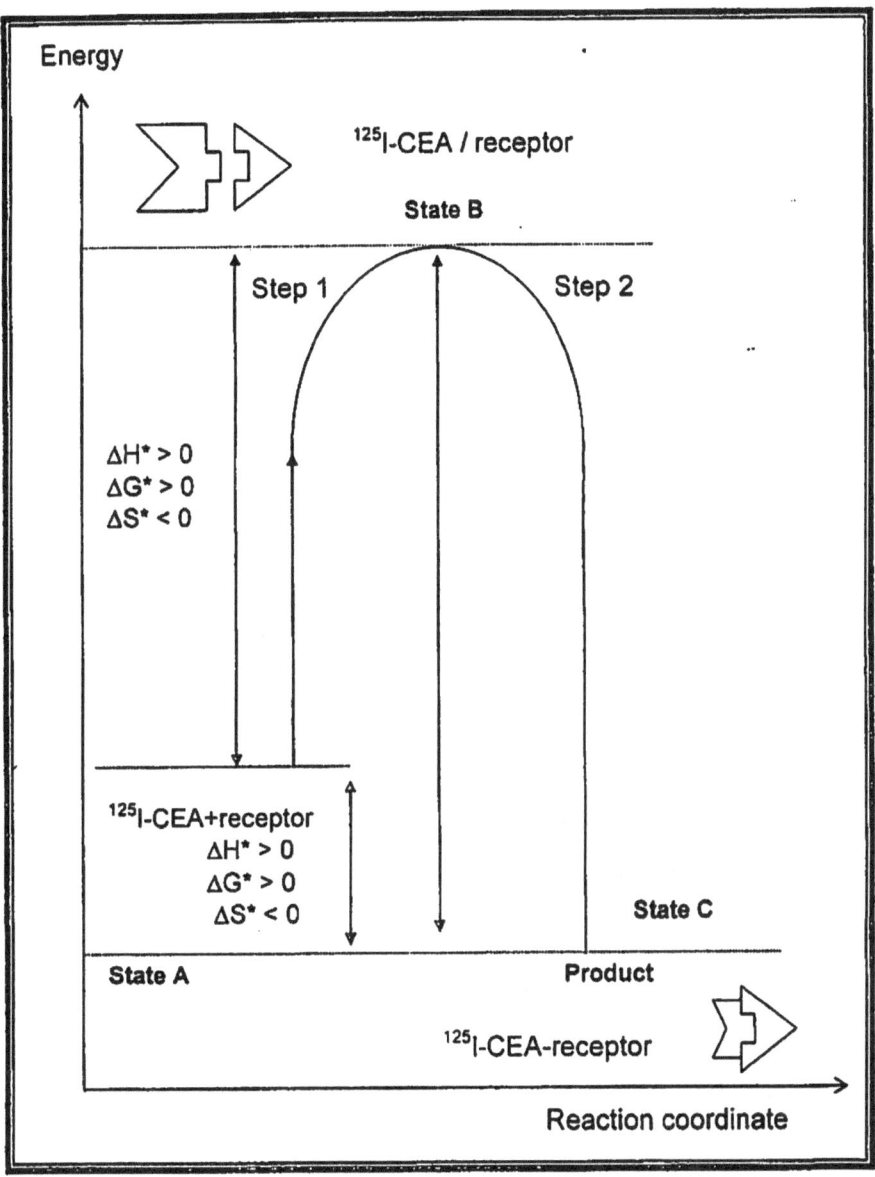

Figure (1-6): General energy diagram and thermodynamic model applied to the complex formation between ^{125}I-CEA and receptor

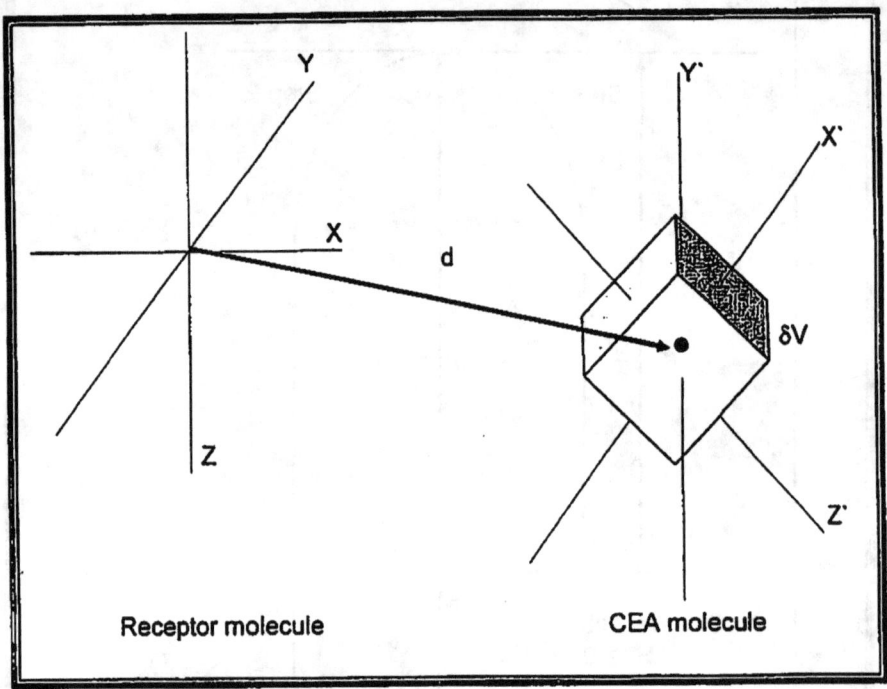

Figure (1-7): Schematic representation of geometrical requirements for bond formation between CEA and various classes of receptor (R), d= the distance between CEA and the receptor (from Ref 12)

1-7 CEA Biology
1-7-1 Distribution and tumor specificity of CEA

Utilizing the colon cancer system as a model, a study was undertaken to determine whether comparable components are present in other human tissues. Approximately 3000 tissue specimens from all parts of the human body. Encompassing both normal and a variety of histopathological states, were examined by direct precipitation and precipitation inhibition in agar gel. It was found that the same constituent was detectable in all test specimens of primary and metastatic cancerous lesions arising from the entodermally-derived digestive system epithelium. The concentration of the tumor antigen was greater in lower bowel malignancies than in those of the upper gastrointestinal tract. It should be emphasized that this antigen was apparently absent from primary cancers in all other tissues, including those of the entodermal portions of the mouth. Benign tumors of the bowel and metastatic lesions of other organs to various parts of the digestive system were also devoid of these components. This would indicate that the presence of the tumor antigen in the cancers in which it was found was dependent upon the tissue of origin; rather than the tissue of growth, of the tumor[45,46].

The marked localization of the tumor antigen to entodermally-derived digestive organ cancers suggested the possibility of some relationship between this component and the embryonic development of the human digestive system. Hence, a number of embryonic and fetal tissues were examined by gel precipitation. These studies revealed that the antigen, which in the adult was localized to digestive system cancers, could be detected in embryonic and fetal gut, pancreas, and liver in the first two trimesters of gestation[96]. This component was, therefore, named carcinoembryonic antigen (CEA) of the human

Chapter One

digestive system. This antigen could not be detected in fetal digestive tissues in the third trimester or in any other tissue at any time during gestation.

The very sensitive techniques which have recently been developed for the detection of CEA suggest that this material may be present in very low concentrations in tissues other than those which have been described above(97,98). The problem of whether the material found in these tissues is identical to the CEA isolated from digestive system cancers, or if there are "CEA-like" moieties which may mimic the presence of CEA in sensitive assay systems, will be considered more fully below.

1-7-2 Cellular localization of the CEA

In initial attempts to determine the cellular location of the CEA, unfixed frozen sections of cancerous tissue from the digestive system were treated with fluoresceinconjugated rabbit anti-CEA antiserum. It was observed that staining appeared quite sharply localized to the region of the plasma membrane of the neoplastic cells[99]. Suspensions of viable colon cancer cells were then prepared and incubated with fluoresceinconjugated antiserum. The majority of cells examined by ultraviolet microscopy revealed the pattern of a beaded-necklace or signet ring, typical of immunofluorescent localization of antigens to the surface of the cell.

Suspensions of cells from colon cancer in tissue culture were mixed with specific rabbit anti-CEA antiserum. The reaction was followed by phase-contrast microscopy, and revealed a rapid and massive agglutination of cultured cells[100]. Pretreatment of the antiscrum with minute quantities of purified CEA completely inhibited agglutination, as it did. the immunofluoresccnl reactions described above. Thus, functionally as well as morphologically, the CEA behaves as a constituent of a

Chapter One

plasma membrane or, at least, as a component lying close to the surface of tumor cells.

Subsequently, a study was undertaken to assess the position of the antigen in the ultrastructure of the surface of the colon cancer cell. Viable explants of single cells from colon cancers were incubated with ferritin-conjugated goat anti-CEA antiserum. The suspension of cells was then washed thoro-ughly and processed for examination by electron microscopy. The pattern of localization of the ferritin-antibody conjugate revealed that the plasma unit membrane structure itself remained virtually unstained. However, a heavy ferritin label was found in the glycocalyx or "fuzzy coat", immediately adjacent to the surface membrane[101]. Presumably then, CEA is not an integral structural component of the trilaminar image usually referred to as the plasma membrane, but lies even further to the periphery of the cell. It is not certain, however, whether CEA is an integral part of the glycocalyx, or is a secretory product in transit across the cell surface.

Finally Tanaka, C.A. et.al., were indicated that the pattern of CEA in CRC cells classified into three types:

1. CEA located along the apical surface
2. CEA located in the cytoplasm.
3. CEA located in the surrounding stroma of tumor cells[102].

Furthermore, the plasma CEA level, the extent of tumor invasion, and the degree of tumor differentiation were closely related to these three types[103]. For example, patients in whom CEA existed on the entire surface or on the outside of the cancer cells tended to have a higher plasma CEA level, more frequent tumor invasion, and lower tumor differentiation than did those in whom CEA was present a long the apical surface or within the cytoplasm of the cancer cells[102].

1-7-3 Cellular and humoral immune responses to CEA

Both humoral and cell-mediated immunologic reactivity against CEA have been assessed. A specific humoral immune response against CEA, primarily of the IgM class of immunoglobulins, has been demonstrated by at least two techniques[104-106]. It has, further, been observed that the methodology employed for antibody detection is of major importance in determining the results which are ultimately obtained. Hence, bis-diazotized benzidine-hemagglutination produced positive results with the sera of patients bearing digestive system cancers only if the tumor had not undergone metastatic dissemination[104]. On the other hand, the techniques of radioimmuno-electrophoresis and radioimm-unochromatography were able to detect anti-CEA antibody in the sera of patients with disseminated cancers[105,106]. The use of a modified Farr technique, even with acid-dissociation for the detection of antibody bound to antigen, was unable to detect anti-CEA antibodies under any circumstances. Hence, it may be that the technologic problems involved, and the reagents employed, have been responsible for the inability of some workers to demonstrate the presence of specific-CEA antibodies in the sera of patients with colon cancer[106]. It is noteworthy that such antibodies have been demonstrated in the circulation of pregnant women[104].

A very elegant in vivo demonstration of anti-CEA antibody production in patients with colon cancer, and the potential pathophysiologic effects of the production of such CEA-anti-CEA immune complexes, has recently been reported in a patient suffering from carcinoma of the colon and the nephrotic syndrome. Employing immunofluorescent techniques to examine the kidney biopsy from this patient, it was found that CEA, immunoglobulin, and complement had been deposited in the glomerular basement membrane[107].

Chapter One

Upon examining the area of cell-mediated immune responsiveness to the CEA, it becomes apparent that no substantial evidence for such a phenomenon has ever been put forward. Although cell-mediated immunity against antigens common to human colon cancers and fetal gut epithelium has been demonstrated by the use of the colony inhibition technique, it was simply suggested that the CEA might be the common factor involved, but no studies to investigate this point were performed[108]. Recent work employing delayed skin reactions to intradermally inoculated antigen prepared from various tissues has shown that patients with carcinomas of the colon generally give a positive skin test to extracts of human fetal intestine and colon cancer tissue, but not to similar extracts of normal adult colon. The skin reactive antigen(s) involved, however, appear to be distinct from purified CEA[106,107]. In addition, purified CEA fails to stimulate lymphocyte transformation in tests of patients suffering from colon cancer[108].

1-7-4 Circulating CEA

The initial observation, by bis-diazotized bernidine hemagglutination, that anti-CEA antibodies were absent from the sera of patients with disseminated bowel cancer, remained to be explained. One possible explanation for this phenomenon was that the CEA in the glycocalyces of the cells of a large tumor mass could serve as an antibody sink, absorbing anti-CEA antibodies as the blood circulated through the neoplastic tissue. A second possibility was that the neoplastic tissue could release CEA directly into the circulation. In the presence of a large mass of tumor tissue, the corresponding concentration of antigenic material in the serum would be relatively high and could lead to CEA-anti-CEA complexes in antigen excess. Under such circumstances then, the anti-CEA moieties would no longer be available for participation in subsequent serologic reactions in vitro.

Chapter One

In order to determine whether or not the CEA could leave the glycocalyx of the tumor cell surface and enter the circulation, a radioimmunoassay for the detection of this material was developed. The technique initially employed was based on the principle of coprecipitationinhibition in half-saturated ammonium sulfate[109]. The initial study performed demonstrated that the assay could detect nanogram quantities of circulating CEA. The results also suggested that the assay was highly specific for CEA in the sera of patients with bowel cancer. A great deal of work along these lines has since been performed, and the theoretical and practical implications of the results obtained to date will be under discussion.

1-7-5 Metabolism of CEA

The question has been raised as to whether CEA is produced by the tumor in situ, or if this material may be synthesized at another site in the body, and then adsorbed onto the tumor cell surface. Data obtained from studies performed both with tissue-cultured colon cancer cells in vitro[110-111] and xenografted human colon cancer tissue in hamsters[110] have demonstrated that CEA is produced by tumor cells in situ.

There is a great deal yet to be learned about the metabolism of CEA. Studies of CEA concentrations in the sera of patients who have undergone apparently complete bowel tumor resection indicate that the CEA is catabolized rapidly, and serum concentrations postoperatively frequently fall to undetectable levels 2-14 days after surgery[112]. The site of CEA breakdown in man remains unknown but animal experiments suggest that the liver is a major site of catabolism of CEA[111,112].

The serum decay of CEA administered to xenogeneic animals has also been studied, and has shown a rapid disappearance comparable to that seen in the human. In fact, these studies suggested a biologic

Chapter One

heterogeneity within any one population of CEA molecules because different rates of decay were observed with time[111,112].

1-8 Bioeassay of CEA

1-8-1 Radioimmunoassays for CEA

The initial experimental work on CEA, summarized in the foregoing discussion, established the existence of a material associated with carcinomata originating from the entodermally derived portion of the gastrointestinal tract and with certain fetal tissues. It is important to note that the original description of this molecule was through its antigenic activity in the heterologous host. Thus, the tumor site of CEA is defined by antibodies that bind specifically to the molecule but cannot be removed from the antiserum by absorption with normal tissues. Subsequent efforts, in our laboratory and other laboratories, led to a physicochemical description of the molecule which bears this tumor antigenic site. The distinctions between antigenic activity, the tumor site, and the CEA molecule are analogous to the operational descriptions of enzymatic activity, the active site of an enzyme, and the enzyme as a molecular unit, respectively[11-13].

The method of measurement of CEA activity thus becomes central to the definition of the molecule and, in current practice, the most important method utilized is the radioimmunoassay. The radioimmunoassay for CEA then becomes important in several respects. (1), It is used, as noted above, to define the immunological criteria for CEA; (2), It is used as the method of identification of CEA during isolation, and of demonstration of increase of specific activity with purification; (3), Chemical manipulations of CEA designed to determine the structure of the tumor site are assessed in terms of their effects on the immunologic activity of the molecule as measured by the radioimmunoassay; (4), The radioimmunoassay, because of its ability to measure small amounts of

Chapter One

material in serum, is the method of CEA measurement which has been applied to the clinical situation[11-13].

Therefore, an understanding of the available radioimmunoassays for CEA, together with an appreciation of some of the difficulties of such analyses, is necessary to a proper examination of the physicochemical and clinical data which are presented in subsequent sections.

The assays employed are based on the general principal of "saturation analysis"[113] or inhibition of binding in which material in the test sample (or serum) "competes" with radio-labelled CEA for binding to an anti-CEA anti-serum. The degree of "displacement" of labelled CEA from the antibody-bound to the non-antibody-bound or free fraction reflects the amount of inhibitory material in the test specimen. This type of assay system can be described in terms of (1) the antigen employed as radiolabelled material and as standard; (2) the antiserum, (3) the method of separation of antibody bound and free antigen in order to determine the distribution of radiolabelled material in these two compartments, (4) treatment of the test sample before' measurement.

Antigens used in the various assay systems available are generally purified from hepatic metastases of colonic carcinomata but the method of purification varies with different laboratories. There are no universally accepted standards available for use as a reference material, Moreover; immunologic and chemical comparisons are available only for a limited number of preparations of purified antigen. Hence, the identity of the antigens used by different investigator has not been clearly demonstrated and variability in the immunologic activity of the purified standards utilized will affect the results obtained from the assay.

The antisera used in the assays are prepared by a variety of immunization schedules in a number of animal species, utilizing different purified preparations of CEA and are absorbed with non-tumor tissue to

Chapter One

a variable degree prior to use[12,114]. In our own experience, using purified CEA preparations as the immunogen, the antisera obtained are polyvalent and require absorption with normal serum, normal bowel, and normal lung to be rendered monospecific. It has been postulated[12,114], that there are at least three types of anti-CEA antisera in use. Some antisera react with the tumor site of CEA, others are directed towards determinants distinct from this site and hence do not distinguish tumor antigen from antigens in normal tissue, while a third group of antisera represent combinations of tumor and normal specifities. The variability that may be introduced by antiserum differences is illustrated by the results of a radioimmunoassay performed on the urine of patients with bladder cancer utilizing anti-CEA antisera obtained from different laboratories. The incidence of CEA positivity in this group was 100%, 50% and 0% depending on the antiserum employed in the assay[114,115,116].

The radioassays for CEA are most often identified by the procedure used to separate the antibody-bound from free fractions of the antigen and by whether a preliminary step of perchloric acid extraction of the serum is employed. This initial step is utilized in a number of the assays in order to separate the carbohydrate-rich, perchloric acid-soluble glycoproteins such as CEA, from the perchloric acidinsoluble serum components which may non-specifically interfere with the assay[17]. Such a preliminary step lengthens the time required to complete the assay procedure, since prolonged dialysis is necessary to remove the perchloric acid after extraction. Other assay designs Table (1-3) have eliminated this pretreatment step and thus shorten the time required to perform the assay to 24-48 hours[117-123].

The original assay procedure[116] referred to as the "Farr" or ammonium sulphate technique, utilizes a perchloric acid extraction step

Chapter One

and takes advantage of the solubility of CEA in half-saturated ammonium sulphate. Thus, separation of anti-CEA-^{125}I-CEA from ^{125}I-CEA is achieved by the addition of saturated ammonium sulphate to the incubation mixture. The Z-gel technique[118]. also utilizes a perchloric acid extraction step and achieves separation of bound and free antigen by precipitating the anti-CEA-^{125}I-CEA complex with zirconyl phosphate gel. A similar procedure, using zirconyl phosphate gel, but omitting the initial extraction step has also been developed[119]. An alternative technical approach to the problem of separation of bound and free antigen has been the precipitation of the anti-CEA-[^{125}I] CEA by a second antibody with specificity towards the anti-CEA antibody[120,121]. For example, a rabbit anti-CEA antibody, together with any bound antigen, can be precipitated by a sheep anti-rabbit IgG antiserum. Two variants of this procedure are in use Table (1-3) neither of which employ a step of perchloric acid extraction. Other less commonly used assay techniques are outlined in Table (1-3)[122-123].

All the factors, alluded to above, which influence the assay procedure suggest that the inhibition observed in the radioimmunoassay may be of three types[111-124].

(1), specific, in which the inhibitory molecule contains the tumor site and thus quantitatively competes with CEA standards purified from colonic carcinomas; (2), cross-reactive, in which a family of-molecules commonly termed "CEA-like", but as yet incompletely defined, compete to varying degrees with colon tumor-derived CEA in the radioi-mmunoassay; (3), non-specific, in which the inhibitory material bears no immunologic relationship to CEA[17]. Further work will be required in order to define the absolute and relative specificities of the various CEA radioimmun-oassays in use, both for experimental and clinical investigations.

Chapter One

A recent study sponsored by the National Cancer Institute[124].examined the results of a number of different CEA assays performed on selected sera from both normal individuals and patients with a variety of diseases. It was shown that although a given serum sample yielded different absolute values in different assays, the overall diagnostic concordance between assays was in the range of 85%. Whether the 15% discordant results indicate different specificities of the various assays or represent technical problems is unclear at present.

A more detailed analysis of the clinical applicability of the various assays described above is presented in Table (1-3).

TABLE (1-3): Radioimmunoassays for the measurement of circulating CEA

Method	Preliminary extraction	Method of separation of antibody-bound CEA from free CEA	Time to complete assay (days)	Upper limit of normal (ng/ml)
Indirect				
Thomson.et al.[117]	1.0 M perchloric acid	half-saturated ammonium sulfate	5	2.5
Hansen et al.[118]	1.0 M perchloric acid	zirconyl phosphate gel	2	2.5
Direct				
Egan et al.[120]	none	second antibody	2	16
McPherson et al.[122]	none	solid phase	5	2.5
Coller et al.[123]	none	radioimmunoelectrophoresis	0.083	not quantitative
MacSween et al.[121]	none	second antibody	2	5.0
Go et al.[114]	none	zirconyl phosphate gel	2	2.0

1-8-2 Nature of the circulating substance(s) measured by radioimmunoassay

To date, the nature of the circulating substance(s) measured by the CEA radioimmunoassay in the sera of normal individuals and of patients with various diseases has not been defined. It has not been possible to adequately purify the "CEA-active" material from sera in sufficient amounts to allow immunologic and physicochemical comparison with colon cancerderived CEA. Thus, it has not as yet been demonstrated that CEA present in the circulation of patients with colon cancers is identical to that purified from the primary or secondary tumors.

Moreover, there are insufficient data regarding the CEA-active materials measured by radioimmunoassay in the sera and tissues of some patients with diseases other than gastro-intestinal carcinomas. Some preliminary work along these lines has been reported. For example, extraction of the CEA-active material from various non-malignant tissues has yielded from 1/20 to 1/5000 of the amount found in colonic tumors[146,147]. There has, however, been no demonstration that these materials show increasing specific activity with purification. It is of interest, in this context, that nude mice implanted with human colonic tumors develop seropositivity for CEA while CEA activity is absent from the circulation of such mice implanted with human breast or lung tumors[127]. Finally, it has been demonstrated that the CEA-positivity of 15 of 17 sera from patients with ulcerative colitis was abolished by extraction with perchloric acid[128].

These data suggest the possibility that the various "CEA-active" and "CEA-like" materials measured by radioimm-unoassay may not be identical to colon cancer CEA and that further work will be necessary both with regard to purification and analysis of these materials and with respect to defining specificity of the radioimmuno-assay.

1-9 Immunochemical studies of CEA

1-9-1 Binding studies between ^{125}I –CEA and various antisers

Antisera against CEA have been prepared in heterologous animals, including rabbits, goats, and horses. In order to render these sera tumorspecific, they have been absorbed with an excess of appropriate normal tissue extracts[125]. These anti –CEA antiserum preparations have been used to established radioimmunosssays for the measurement of CEA activity in human blood and tissues, and in chemically or enzymatically derived fragments of the native CEA molecule. In addition to anti-bodies directed against the tumor-specific site, the sera of cancer patients and pregnant women also bind to CEA[126]. It is unknown if these homologus antibodies bind to the same site as anti–CEA rasied in heterologous species.

Anti-blood group substance antibodies have been reported to bind CEA Table (1-4). Anti-blood group A antiserum was capable of binding up to 11 % of ^{125}I-CEA[129] despite the absence, in many instances, of N-acetylgalactosamine, the immuno-dominant sugar of the blood group A substance. It is of interest in this context that anti-A antibodies react with placental chorionic gonadotrophin even though N-acetylgalactosamine is absent from this molecule[129,130]. Others have shown that anti-blood group B and Lewis-type antibodies react with the CEA molecule[130-133]. However, anti-I, anti-i and horse anti-pneumococcus type XIV antisera do not bind to purified CEA[131-133].

Antiserum produced against fetal sulfoglycoprotein antigen, a molecule found in gastric juice of patients with stomach cancer, was capable of binding to CEA. This suggests the presence of shared antigenic sites with the fetal sulfoglycoprotein molecule[126,129].

Antisera raised in heterologous species to a 60 000 molecular weight constituent found in normal bowel and lung and variously called non-specific cross reacting antigen colonic carcinoma antigen, etc., react with CEA (see section on cross-reactive material).

Chapter One

TABLE (1-4): Binding studies of CEA

The ability of various antiscra and lectins to bind to CEA or ^{125}I-CEA was examined by primary binding techniques (radioimmunoassay) or by precipitation in agar gels. + indicates that significant binding was demonstrable; — indicates that significant binding could not be demonstrated.

Material Tested	Result	References
Antiserum to		
CEA (heterologous antiserum)	+	126,127
CEA (human antiserum)	+	128,129
Blood group A	+	129,130
Blood group B	+	131,132,133
Blood group Le^a	+	131,132,133
Blood group I	-	131,132,133
Blood group i	-	131,132,133
Pneumococcus type xiv	-	139,41
Fetal sulfoglycoprotein	+	139,41
Lectins		
Concanavalin A	+	134
Wheat germ agglutinin	+	135,136
Phytohemagglutinin	+	137,138
Ricin	+	138

1-9-2 Lecin binding capacity of CEA

Several plant agglutinins have been shown to agglutinate tumor cells and transformed cells more effectively than cells derived from the

Chapter One

normal tissue[134-136]. Since CEA is a glycoprotein found on the surface of tumor cells, the ability of several lectins of defined specificity to bind to CEA has been studied Table (1-4). The lectins employed were concanavalin A, wheat germ agglutinin, phytohemagglutinin, and ricin. Concanavalin A binds polysaccharides containing multiple terminal non-reducing α-D-glucopyranosyl, α-D-mannopyranosyl, β-D-fructofuranosyl or α-D-, arabino-furanosyl residues[134-137]. Wheat germ agglutinin reacts specifically with terminal non-reducing N-acetylgl-ucosamine and its disaccharide, di-N-acetylchitobiose[135], and to a lesser extent with N-acetyl-neuraminic acid[136]. Phytohem-agglutinin binds to more complex heterosaccharides such as that found in fctuin[137], while ricin hinds D-galactose[138].

Immunodilfusion in agar gel was used to study the interaction between CEA and lectins. To quantitate the reactions of lectins with CEA, a modification of the radioimmunoassay for CEA was used. CEA was shown to bind to all four lectins to variable degrees as shown by reactions in agar gel and interaction with ^{125}I-CEA[134,135]. Thus, in lectin excess concanavalin A was able to bind a maximum of 50 % of ^{125}I-CEA. This binding was specifically inhibited by α-D-mannopyranosyl and N-acetylglucosamine. The binding of wheat germ agglutinin to 90% of ^{125}I-CEA, was inhibited by N-acetylglucosamine. Phytohemogglutinin bound a maximum of 80% of ^{125}I-CEA. However, in contrast to the other lectins, the binding of phytohemagglutinin to CEA was not inhibited by monosaccharides such as D-galactose, N-acetylglucosaminc or D-mannose. The binding of ricin to CEA has been reported but quantitative studies were not done[136-138,139].

1-9-3 Comparative inhibition studies in the ^{125}I-CEA-Anti-CEA system

Using the radioimmunoassay for CEA, the ability of various macromolecules, oligosaccharides, monosaccharides, and amino acids to inhibit the binding of anti-CEA antisera to ^{125}I—CEA was assessed. The results, shown in Table (1-5), revealed that, on a weight basis, 1000-3300 times more blood group substances, compared to CEA, is required to produce 50% inhibition of ^{125}I-anti-CEA binding. Neither pneumococcal polysaccharide type XIV, a precursor of ABH blood group antigens, nor the carbohydrate moiety of group A streptococci, which contains 11 N-acctylglucosamine residues in terminal positions produced any inhibition. Similar results were obtained with α-acid-glycoprotein and ovomucoid.

Inhibition studies with the monosaccharides, amino acids, and oligosaccharides shown in Table (1-5) showed no inhibition of ^{125}I-CEA-anti-CEA binding. 1.2×10^6 times more asparagine-N-acetylglucosamine than CEA, on a weight basis, was required to achieve 50% inhibition of the CEA-anti-CEA reaction. However, glycopeptides derived from nagasedigested CEA were relatively good inhibitors, requiring 10-330-fold more material, by weight, to achieve comparable inhibition to intact CEA[139,140].

Chapter One

TABLE (1-5): Inhibition studies of CEA-anti CEA system

The following materials were tested for their capacity to cause inhibition of binding of ^{125}I-CEA by an absorbed anti-CEA antiserum. The relative inhibitory weight is derived as follows: (weight of tested material required to achieve 50% inhibition of binding)/(weight of purified CEA required to achieve 50% inhibition of binding). *indicates that no significant inhibition of binding was demonstrable.

Materials	Relative Inhibitory Weight	References
Low molecular weight Materials (see Table 1-6)		
Monosaccharides	*	140, 41
Amino Acids	*	140, 41
Oligosaccharides	*	140, 41
Glycopeptides		
IgM glycopeptide	*	
Asparagines-N-acetylglucosamine*	$1.2 \cdot 10^6$	139
CEA-derived glycopeptides	10-330	139
Macromolecules		
CEA	1	139
Blood group A	$3.3 \cdot 10^3$, $1.3 \cdot 10^3$	129, 130, 131, 133
Blood group B	$2.6 \cdot 10^3$	133
Blood group Le^a	$73.3 \cdot 10^3$	133
Blood group H	$1 \cdot 10^3$	132, 139
Pneumococcus type xiv substance	*	139, 41
Gastric mucosa A substance	$4.6 \cdot 10^5$	139, 41
Streptococcal group A antigens	*	139
α-acid glycoprotein	*	139
Ovomucoid	*	139, 41
Ovarian cyst fluid material	$1 \cdot 10^3$	139, 41

* 2-acetamido-I-N-(4'-L-aspartyl)-2-deoxy-β-D-glucosylamine

TABLE (1-6): Materials devoid of inhibitory activity

The following materials were tested for their capacity to cause inhibition of binding of ^{125}I-CEA by an absorbed anti-CEA antiserum. Each material was tested in amounts ranging up to 10mg or 10μM, and in no case was any significant inhibitory activity demonstrable.

Monosaccharides	L-fucose, D-arabinose, D-mannose, D-glucose, D-glucosamine, D-galactosamine, D-mannoamine, N-acetyl-D-glucosamine, N-acetyl-D-mannosamine, 2-deoxy-D-glucose, α-methyl-D-glucose, α-methyl-D-galactose, α-methyl-D-mannose, β-methyl-N-acetyl-D-galactosamine.
Oligosacchrides	β-D-gentibiose, D-raffinose, α-D-melibiose, stachyose, α-L-fuco-(1-2)-β-D-gal-(1-4)-D-glc(2-fucosyllactose), α-L-fuco-(1-2)-β-D-gal-(1-4)-{α-L-fuco-(1-3)} –D-glc (lactodifucotetraose), β-D-gal-(1-3)-β-D-glcNac(1-3)-β-D-gal(1-4)-D-glc(lacto-N-tetraose) α-L-fuco-(1-2)-β-D-gal-(1-3)-β-D-glcNac-(1-3)-β-D-(1-4)-D-glc(lacto-N-fucopentaose I), β-D-gal-(1-3)-{α-L-fuco-(1-4)} β-D-glcNac-(1-3) β-D-gal-(1-4)-D-glc(lacto-N-fucopentaose II), β-D-glcNac-(1-3)-D-gal-Er, di-N-acetylchitobiose, chitobiose, (N-acetyl-D-glucosamine) (mannose).
Amino Acids	20 common amino acids

1-9-4 Materials cross-reacting with CEA

A series of materials has been identified in various normal and cancerous tissues which show partial identity with CEA in agar gel diffusion against unabsorbed anti-CEA antisera. These substances have been variously termed: non-specific cross reacting antigen[140], normal glycoprotein[141], colonic carcinoma antigen III[142], breast carcinoma

Chapter One

glycoprotein[142], and membrane associated, tissular autoan-tigcn[141,143]. With the exception of breast carcinoma glycoprotein, which has a molecular weight of 200 000, most of these materials have a molecular weight of about 60 000, and exhibit a β-mobility on agar gel. It appears that normal glycoprotein, CEX,[143], and non-specific cross reacting antigen given reactions of identity in agar gel and are in turn partially identical to fetal sulfoglycoprotein antigen. It is not certain if colonic carcinoma antigen, CCEA-2[144] and breast carcinoma glycoprotein arc identical to the other cross-reacting substances of β-mobility noted above. More importantly, except for CCEA-2 none of these materials has been sufficiently characterized to allow direct comparison with CEA. Their biologic relationship to CEA is unknown and it is as yet uncertain whether they arc responsible for some or all of the "CEA activity" detected by. radioimnumoassay in various tissues and sera noted previously.

1-9-5 Kinetic and Thermodynamic studies of binding of ^{125}I-Ant CEA Antibody to CEA[11-13].

Kinetic and thermodynamic parameters associated with the binding of ^{125}I-antiCEA antibody to CEA in both crude colorectal homogenate and partially-purified fractions were investigated. It was shown that the reaction in all cases studied follow pseudo-first order reaction kinetics.

The maximum binding of carcinoembryonic antigen (CEA) in crude premalignant colorectal tumor homogenate, ulcerative colitis (U.C.) occurred at 15 °C then association rate constant K_{+1} decreased from 42.2 to 26.6 $mg^{-1}.ml.min^{-1}$. The values of affinity constant (Ka) also decreased from 50.0 to 27.5 $mg^{-1}.ml$, while CEA in crude colon cancer homogenate stage-C the rate association constant K_{+1} decreased from 53.4 to 19.4 $mg^{-1}.ml.min^{-1}$, also Ka value decreased from 35.0 to 15.0 $mg^{-1}.ml$. On the other hand, the kinetic parameters for the binding CEA in colon cancer stage-B were independent on, temperatures so that, the maximum rate of association constant value occurred at 5°C and the lowest value at 35°C.

Using the partially-purified fraction from benign colorectal tumor homogenate (polyps), the association rate constant K_{+1} increased from 13.4 to 20.8 $mg^{-1}.ml.min^{-1}$ with increasing reaction temperature from 5°C to 45°C. The values of affinity constant Ka also increased from 60.0 to 250 $mg^{-1}.ml$.

On the other hand, the association rate constant K_{+1} for partially purified CEA from colon cancer homogenate stage-B was decreased from 18.1 to 6.4 $mg^{-1}.ml.min^{-1}$, when temperature increased from 5°C to 45°C, also the highest affinity constant was 155 $mg^{-1}.ml$ at 5°C then decreased reaching 100 $mg^{-1}.ml$ at 45°C. However, the time course data for the binding follows the pseudo-first order kinetics in both CEA (partially-purified and crude).

The van't Hoff plot demonstrated a linear relationship between ln Ka and 1/T, using the partially purified benign tumor homogenate as CEA source. Arrheniuns plot indicate that there was a linear relationship between log K_{+1} and 1/T. The transition state thermodynamic parameters for the formation of ^{125}I-antibody/CEA) complex represented by Ea, ΔG^*, ΔS^* were determined. The goal of such studies is to describe the basic mathematical analysis that could be used to explain the mechanism of binding of CEA to its antibody to form ^{125}I-antibody/CEA complex in human tissue.

1-10 Clinical applications

The application of quantitative assays for CEA to clinical medicine may be regarded as clinical "spin-off" from studies directed toward the investigation of a basic problem in human tumor immunobiology. The

Chapter One

utilization of the initial procedure in clinical, studies suggested that the detection of circulating CEA was virtually diagnostic for bowel cancer[117,118]. However, the data obtained from numerous subsequent investigations have required modification of this early view [11,12,13,117,124-160]. Some of these recent data are outlined in Table (1-7) which lists the percentages of positive. CEA tests in normal subjects and in patients with a variety of conditions. The percentages indicated were chosen as being representative of the majority of the clinical data published, and in most instances, are derived from the largest series available. It should be noted, however, that a wide range of positivity has been reported for many of the clinical states listed. The cut-off points for positivity are those designated by the individual authors and no attempt has been made to subdivide the results on the basis of the type of assay employed. As indicated previously, the concordance between the various assays is high and, at least with regard to clinical. Applications, there is no evidence that the available assays differ greatly in their overall sensitivities.

It should be noted that the term "CEA" as applied to the clinical situation refers to immunologic activity as measured by a radioimmunoassay. This "immunoassay-able" activity may be due to the CEA as it has been defined physicochemically to date or to materials that cross-react with CEA and await physicochemical definition.

Chapter One

TABLE (1-7): Circulating CEA in various clinical states

Data are expressed as percentage of subjects within given category with abnormal levels of circulating CEA. The percentages indicated were chosen as being representative of the majority of the clinical data published, and in most instances, are derived from the largest series available. It should be noted, however, that a wide range of positivity has been reported for many of the clinical states" mentioned.

Clinical status	Percent positive	Reference
Normal		
Healthy, unselected	11	158
Smokers	19	158
Non – smokers	3	158
Malignant diseases		
Colorectum	83	11,124,146
Stage A	45	11,126,146
Stage B	54	11,124,146
Stage C	71	11,124,126,146
Stage D	89	11,124,126,146
Stomach	61	148,158
Pancreas	92	148
Liver	63	150-152
Lung	77	114
Breast	47	13,102,130
Bladder	42	149,151
Gynecologic	65	149,151
prostatic	40	154
lymphoid	36	157,158
Non-malignant diseases		
Cirrhosis of liver	45	
Ulcerative colitis	32	158
Chronic lung disease	57	158
Pancreatitis	43	159
diverticulitis	12	160

Chapter One

At present, the ultimate role of the CEA assay in the practice of medicine remains to be completely defined. However, there are sufficient data available to indicate the clinical situations in which the assay is useful and to suggest areas which warrant further investigation.

1-10-1 Diagnosis of cancer

The assay in its present form should not be employed indiscriminately as a tool for screening apparently healthy individuals in the population because negative tests may be obtained in subjects with early carcinomas[11-13,117-124]. On the other hand, there is evidence from clinic which suggests that the study of selected groups of individuals may be of predictive diagnostic value[150]. In such study, 47% of 81 patients with non-specific gastrointestinal complaints and positive CEA assays were found to harbor gastrointestinal malignancies during longitudinal surveillance with repeated radiologic and endoscopic investigations over a two-year period. The assay may thus be useful as a screening tool in a limited sense; e.g., patients admitted to hospital, those attending a gastrointestinal clinic, or patients with non-specific gastrointestinal complaints not readily attributable to a specific cause.

A positive CEA assay does not establish the presence of a malignancy and it cannot be used by itself without recourse to other clinical and laboratory data. There are several studies which have compared the diagnostic value of CEA with other investigative procedures. This type of analysis of the assay with respect to pancreatic carcinoma demonstrated that the CEA assay was more frequently positive than any other diagnostic test used, including upper gastrointestinal barium series, hypotonic duodenography, coeliac arteriography, and percutaneous transhepatic cholangiography[151]. This study, however, did not clearly demonstrate that the addition of the assay to the investigative procedures led to the detection of malignancies which would otherwise have been missed, or altered the clinical outcome. There is evidence to suggest that the detection rate of colonic cancers is highest when the CEA assay and barium enema are used in conjunction than when either test is used alone[152].

The impact of the "false-positive" assays is different when the test is used adjunctively for diagnosis than when it is used for "single-sample" screening. First, a number of the diseases which manifest "false-positive" results are readily distinguishable from carcinoma (severe alcoholic cirrhosis, emphysema) and can be excluded clinically when a specific individual rather than a population is being examined. More important, many of the non-malignant conditions associated with positive assays show transient rather than persistent elevations and are distinguishable from carcinoma on this basis[158]. Finally, most of the false-positive levels tend to be lower than those found in malignant conditions[48,146]. Thus, it is not entirely useful to simply compare the raw incidence of positivity in various diseases. A definite conclusion regarding the diagnostic usefulness of the test will require a prospective study with long-term surveillance, serial sampling, a comparison of the assay with other diagnostic modalities, and an examination of whether use of the assay will lead to the discovery of otherwise undetected malignancies and/or affect the prognosis through earlier diagnosis.

1-10-2 Use of assay for the surveillance of cancer patients

More definitive data is available to indicate that the assay is useful in the management of patients whose diagnosis has already been established. In general, in patients with carcinomas of the colon and rectum stomach, pancreas, bronchus, breast and bladder, very high CEA levels, usually more than 20 ng/ml, indicate the spread of tumor beyond the original site and thus suggest a poorer prognosis[11,12,13,117-124,150,151,152]. It is important to note that a negative test in such a patient

Chapter One

docs not rule out the presence of metastatic disease, but usually suggests resectability of the lesion[152,153,154].

The postoperative decline of elevated CEA levels to the normal range shows good correlation with apparent complete resection of the tumor and potential surgical "cure". This has been demonstrated in patients with gastrointestinal[124,129,146], mammary[131,102,117], bronchogenic[60,61], urothelial[155], and gynecologic[144,154] cancers. Further, the majority of patients studied over long-term periods (up to 3 years) who maintain negative postoperative levels do not show any evidence of recurrence[150-155,156]. On the other hand, the failure of a CEA level to drop to normal during the postoperative follow-up period is usually associated with incomplete tumor resections[146,153,160], and a steadily rising, rather than transient, increase in the CEA level post-resection indicates progression of the disease[117-124,147-156]. More significantly, the reversion to positive of a previously negative test has been shown to be a sensitive and reliable indicator of recurrence of disease[129,130,131,149]. The time interval between "CEA recurrence" and appearance of clinical or other laboratory evidence of tumor recurrence has varied from two weeks to ten months[149-155]. Serial CEA determinations may therefore allow initiation of anti-tumor therapy at an earlier stage of progression of the disease. This approach becomes especially interesting with the advent of immunotherapy and the notion that such intervention, to be successful, must be initiated when the tumor load is very small; i.e., at clinicairy undetectable levels.

Another area requiring further exploration has been suggested by studies showing that CEA levels correlated well with regression or progression during chemotherapy of carcinomas of the gastrointestinal tract[11,146], lung[114] and breast[13,102,130] and that the test may be useful to monitor the effectiveness of such therapy.

Chapter One

Ami of the study:

1- Developing a method for Extraction, purification and identification of CEA from Tumor tissue.

2- Preparation of CEA kit, which is suitable for clinical application.

Chapter Two

Isolation

&

Purification of CEA

Chapter Two

Abstract

A method is described for the preparation of the carcinoembryonic antigen (CEA) of human digestive system from large quantites of metastatic tumor tissue. The purification process is far more rapid than that originally described, and results in higher yield of CEA than that previously obtained. The procedure involves the sequential steps of extraction in perchloric acid, affinity chromatography on lentil lectin-activated Sepharose and immunoadsorption chromatography. The final product show a high degree of purity, the present techniques allows tumor tissue to be processed at a rate about three times faster than other techniques. Moreover the yield of equally active CEA is approximately three times greater than that previously obtained.

Chapter Two

Introduction

The carcinoembryonic antigen (CEA) of the human digestive system is a tissue component which is found in a denocarcinoma of entodermally derived digestive system epithelium m and in embryonic and fetal digestive tissues in the first two trimesters of gestation[192]. It is protein- polysaccharide constituent of the tumor cell glycocalyx[4] and is released into the circulation of the tumor- bearing patient where it can be detected by means of radioimmunoassay[17]. The results of preliminary studies indicate that the detection of circulating CEA may be value as a diagnostic and prognostic tool in patients suffering from digestive system cancer. Although endogenous CEA can elicit the production of specific, humoral anti-CEA antibodies, the functional significance of the immune response remains unclear[6].

In a previous communication from this laboratory, a technique for the purification of CEA from cancer tissues were reported[11,12,13]. Although the final product showed a high degree of purity by both physicochemical and immuno-chemical criteria, the procedures were both tedious and time-consuming. A1kg aliquot of tumor tissue required 10-12 weeks for complete processing, and resulted in a rather poor yield of 10 mg of purified CEA powder from each kilogram of wet weight of tumor tissue, because of the increasing requirement for purified CEA a procedure has been developed which allows the handling of large quantities of tumor tissue more rapidly and with a greater yield of the final product.

Materials and Methods

2-1 Chemicals

All Laboratory chemicals and reagents used in this study of annular grade.

TABLE (2-1): Chemical used and companies supplied

Material	Company
Glycerol, dithiotheritol, glacial acetic acide, sodium hydroxide, sodium chloride, DETA, manganes chloride $MgCl_2$, $CaCl_2$	Fluka (Switzerland)
Glycin, Ammonium thiocynate, Ammonium persulphate, methyl α-D-glucopyranoside, methyl α-D- manopyranoside	Sigma. U.S.A
Tris (hydroxyl methyl amino methane), sodium azide	Merk Germany
Perchloric acid, Bromophenol- blue, conc. HCl, sodium Bicarbonate. Acrylamide, trichloroacetic acid, sulphosalicylic acid, N, N-methylene bisacrylamide, ethanol, glacial acetic acid, DETA, Commassi Brilliant Blue, N, N, N, N, tetramethyl ethylene diamine (TEMED)	BDH / U.K
Dried lentil seeds	Food shops
Complete freund's adjuvant, Sephadex G50, Activated- CNBr- Sepharose	Pharmacia fine chemical - sweden

2-2 Instruments

TABLE (2-2): Instrument used and companies supplied them.

	Instruments	company
1	Gamma counter type 1270- rack Gamma II	LKB
2	Spectrophotometer ultraspect type 4050	LKB
3	UV–210 a double beam spectroph-otometer	Shimadzu
4	pH - meter	Pye- Unicam
5	Cooling centrifuge; with a maximum speed 5000 r.p.m.	Hettich
6	Cooling centrifuge type 202-MK, with a maximum speed13.500 r.p.m	sigma
7	Memmert water bath, memmert incubator	West- Germany
8	SM- shaker	England
9	Sensitive balance	A & D (Japan)
10	Homogenizer	Hapan National
11	Electrophoresis constant power supply	Pharmacia fine chemicals (Sweden)
12	2 x 100 cm column	LKB – Sweden
13	Dialysis tubes	Spectra – USA
14	Lypholyzer	Virtis – USA
15	Buchner funnel	Gallen kamp UK.
16	Vaccum pump	USA- Millipore
17	Blender	Japan National

2-3 Buffer and Solution

Buffer and reagent used are indicated in each experiment.

2-4 Patients

The study was carried out on one hundred twenty two colorectal patients with malignant tumors (122 mals) whom subjected to curative surgery. Their age mean was 44 range (35-85 years).

According to the histopathological examination of the resected pieces. The patients were grouped in the following:

Group 1: contained of 42 patients with colon cancer stage-B

Group 2: Included of 25 patients with colon cancer stage-C

Group 3: consisted of 43 patients with rectal cancer stage-B

Group 4: contained of 24 patients with rectal cancer stageC-D

The patients were admitted for treatment to Baghdad Teaching Hospital), (Al-Yarmook Teaching University Hospital), (Nursing Home Priver Hospital), (Al-Hussany Hospital).

Patients suffered from any disease that may interfere with this study were excluded. All surgical operation of colorectal tumor was done under the supervision of surgeons; Dr. Zuhair Al- Bahrani, Dr. Hassan Al-Sakafi, Dr. Saaeb Sedeq, Dr. Nazar Teha Makky, Dr. Ali Abd Al-Azeezi.

2-5 Collection and Initial Preparation of Tumor Specimens:

The source of tissue in this series of experiments was human colon or rectum. The specimens removed surgically from adenocarcinoma of colon or rectum and rinsed immediately with ice- cold saline solution then placed in labeled clean polystyrene container in normal salin and kept at -20C° until use. The diagnosis was confirmed postoperatively by histological examination in all cases.

In preparation for extraction, an aliquot of tumor tissue was thawed at room temperature and then trimned of fat, weight, minced. The minced was suspended in homogenization buffer (10% glycerol, 10m M dithiotheritol, 10m M Tris, 1.5n M DETA) pH 7.5 with ratio of 1:4 (weight:

volum) using mechanical homogenizer. The homogenate was filtered through a nylon mesh sieve to eliminate fibers of connective tissues then centrifuged at 4000 r.p.m for 15 min at 4C°. the pellet was neglected and the supernatant was centrifuged at 2000 r.p.m for 15 min at 4C°. the sediment was discarded and the supernatant was used in experiments involved CEA extraction and purification.

2-6 Extraction of CEA by Perchloric Acid :

2-6-1 Solutions:

Perchloric acid (PCA 1.2 M) A volume 13.06 ml of 60% PCA was diluted to 100 ml with deionizer water.

2-6-2 Method of extraction:

Equal volumes of the tumor tissue homogenate and 1.2M perchloric acid were mixed, and then stirred for 30 min on an ice bath. The resulting suspension was centrifuged at 4000 r.p.m at 4C° for 30 min. the sediment was discarded and the supernatant dialyzed for 48 hours against frequent changes of distilled water, at 4C° . the non-dialyzable residue was lyophilized.

2-7 Purification of CEA by Affinity chromatography of Lentil Lectin Coupled to Activated Sepharose 4B

2-7-1 Solution and Buffer:-

1. Equilibrium buffer, It was prepared by dissolving 8.766 gm of sodium chloride in 900 ml deionized distilled water. Then the pH was adjusted to 7. The volume was made up to 1 liter with de-ionized distilled water.

2. 0.05M glucose solution. It was prepared by dissolving 9 gm of glucose in 1 litre of deionized distill water.

3. Elution buffer A pH 7: This was prepared by mixing (1:1) of solution 1 and solution 2.

4. 0.001 M HCl was prepared by mixing 160 microliter of conc. HCl with 2 litter of deionized distill water.
5. Coupling buffer pH 8.3: (1M sodium Bicarbonate 0.1M glucose) this solution prepared by dissolving 10.7 gm of sodium Bicarbonate and 9 gm of glucose in 250 deionized distill water.
6. Blocking buffer pH 8.3: This solution prepared by dissolving 150 gm of glycine in 200 ml of coupling buffer.
7. Buffer B: sodium a cetate buffer, 0.1M, pH 6.0 containing 1M NaCl and 10^{-3}M each of $MgCl_2$, $MnCl_2$ and $CaCl_2$.
8. Elution Solution:
    a. 2 % Methyl - α - D – glucopyranoside.
    b. 10% Methyl - α - D – glucopyranoside.
    c. 20% N - α - D - manopyranoside.
    usual conditions for preparation.

2-7-2 preparation of Purified lentil lectin

2-7-2-1 Extraction method of Lentil Lectin from Common Lentil Seeds:

Dried lentils (500 gm), obtained from food shops, are soaked overnight in cold deionized distilled water. The excess water is drained off and the swollen lentils blended with 5oo millliter of chilled 0.15N NaCl for 5 minutes in a high speed blender. The slurry is centrifuged at high speed (10.000) r.p.m., for 30 min and the sediment is discarded. The clear yellow supernatant is dialyzed against several changes of cold distilled water adjusted to pH 5.8. Most of yellow color diffuses out and a heavy white precipitate forms in dialyzed bag. The precipitate contains most of the hemagglutinin activity. Precipitate is centrifuged down at 4C° and wash twic with cold distilled water adjusted to pH 5.8. It is then dissolved in a minimal volum of 0.15N NaCl. and retained for further fractionation.

Chapter Two

2-7-2-2 Purification of Lentil lectin by Gelfiltration Chromatography techniques:

1- **Preparation of Sephadex** G-50 Columns the dimensions of the columns were chosen according to the following equation[161].

$$Diameter = \sqrt{m/10}\, cm$$

where m: is the amount of protein in mg

the leng of column = 30 x diameter.

In view of such calculation a 2x85 cm column was used.

Sephadex G-50 was prepared as suggested by the manufacturer(pharmicia fine chemical). The dry powder of sephadex G-50 (50mg) was swelling in excess of deionized distilled water (500ml) and left to stand for three days at room temperature without stirring, the excess deionized water decanted then the gel slurry was degassed by section and poured carefully into a vertical glass- column down its wall using a glass rode. After the gel has settled the column outlet was opened, continuing packed till the gel reached as a bed height of 85 cm then equilibrated with equilibrium buffer at flow rate 20 ml/hr.

2- **Separation Procedure of Lectin:**

An aliquot of a partial purified lentil lectin (prepared in section 2-7-1-1) was applied to the surface of Sephadex G-50 column, and the gel is washed with equilibrium buffer until the optical density at 280nm of the eluate was zero.

The column is then washed with elution buffer A pH 7 and fractions of 4 ml were collected at a flow rate 20 ml / hours. The protein content of the column effluent was followed with a UV moniter and the hemagglutinin activity measured as described in section (2-7-2-3).

Fractions containing high amount of proteins were pooled and dialysis against frequent changes of deionized water for 24 hours at $4C°$.

The non dialyzable resiude was lyophoilized and stored at 4-8 C° until used.

2-7-2-3 Lectin activity assay

Lentil Lectin activity was measured by a standard dilution titer assay. Typically a 1:2 serial dilution of lentil lectin was prepared in pH 7.2 buffer isotonic saline. A2% suspension of washed red cells (human) A2% suspension of washed red cells (human) is prepared in same buffer. Equal volumes (0.1ml) of red cell suspension and lentil lectin dilution were mixed in small tubes and the cells allowed settling for 30 min at room temperature. The titer is then read from the settling pattern [161-166].

2-7-4 Coupling of lentil lectins to CNBr activated sepharose:

- **Coupling Procedure:**

1. CNBr activated Sepharose was prepared by suspending 10 mg of freeze – dried powder in 200 ml of 1mM HCl.
2. Wash for 15 min on a Buchner funnel, using atotal of 200ml 1mM HCl per gram dry powder, added and sucked off in several aliquats, the final aliquot of 1mM HCl is suck off until craks appear in the cake.
3. lenti lectin solution was prepared by dissolved 200mg of freeze - dried lentil lectin (prepared in section 2-7-2-1) in 40 ml of the coupling buffer.
4. Mix the lentil lectin solution with gel suspension in end – over – end for 2 hours at room temperatire then filtered on Buchner funnel and wash with 40 ml of blocking buffer.
5. Transfer the medium (Mixture of lentil lectin and gel suspension) to 50ml of blocking buffer for 2 hours at room temperatire.
6. Remove excess blocking buffer by alternately blocking buffer followed by distill water.

Chapter Two

7. Store as suspension in blocking buffer at 4C° for next day, Ready to use as lentil-lectin–activated sepharose conjugate to packed the column.

2-7-5 Column Packing and purification procedure:

1. Lentil lectin-activated Sepharose prepared in section 2-7-4 was poured into a (0.9 x 29 cm; bed volume 17.2 ml) column pouring down a glass rod held against the wall of the column with minimize introduction of air bubbles.
2. The column outlet was opened and the gel was allowed to settle under constant flow rate 15 ml / hr.
3. Wash the column with approximately 10 column volume of coupling buffer to remove excess glycine.
4. An aliquot of the lyophilized powder of the perchloric acid extracted tumor tissue (prepared in section 2-6) dissolved in 2 ml of the sample dissolving (buffer B) loaded on the affinity column.
5. The column washed with sample dissolving (buffer B) until no material appear in the eluent (determined by UV absorbance at 280).
6. After elution of the nonaffinity material, elution of affinity material achieved by using sequential elution with :-
    - ❖ 2 % α - D – methyl glucose pyranosidase.
    - ❖ 10 % α - D – methyl gluco pyranosidase.
    - ❖ 20 % α - D – methyl manno pyranosidase.

    The flow rate was 15 ml / hr.
7. The eluate was constantly monitored for its Spectrophotometeric absorption at 280 nm, and plotted against the fraction number.

2-8 Purification CEA by Immunoaffinity Chromatography:

2-8-1 Buffers and Solutions:

1. Phosphate buffer was prepared by mixing certain volumes of stock solutions.
    - Solution I: 0.2 M solution of monobasic sodium phosphate (31.2 g $NaH_2PO_4 \cdot 2H_2O$) in 1000 ml.
    - Solution II: 0.2 M solution of dibasic sodium phosphate (28.39 gm $Na_2HPO_4 \cdot 2H_2O$)

2. Tris / HCl buffer 0.01 M pH 7.4: It's prepared by dissolving 1.2111gm of tris (hydroxyl methyl) amino methan in 900 ml deionized distilled water. Then the pH was adjusted to 7.4 using HCl (0.1M) the volume was made up to 1 liter with deionized distilled water.

3. Ammonium thiocyanate (NH_4CNS 2.5M pH 8.1): This solution prepared by dissolving 190 gm in 900 ml deionized water. Then the pH adjusted to 8.1. The volume was made up to 1 liter with deionized water.

4. Sodium Bicarbonate (0.01M): this solution prepared by dissolving 0.81 gm of sodium bicarbonate in 1000 ml deionized distills water.

5. Sodium chloride 0.5M: this solution prepared by dissolving 29 gm in 1000ml deionized distills water.

6. Buffer A: Included of tris buffer 5 mM plus 0.002% sodium a zide.

7. Buffer B: Consisted of buffer A plus 0.5 M NaCl.

8. Lyophilized CEA used in this study were providing by Bysangetec Diagostica GmbH & co. KG / France.

9. CEA kit.

2-8-2 Preparation of Antibody:

The antisera against purified CEA were prepared as previously described[12]. In brief: Six rabbits were immunized interamuscularly by four injection of purified CEA in complete Freund's adjuvant (CFA), given twice a week for 2 consecutive weeks; 200 μg of the CEA was injected each time, the right and left flanks being used alternately. Three weeks later all animals were boosted with one more intramuscular injection of CEA in CFA and were bled 1 week afterwards.

2-8-3 Purification of IgG (anti- CEA)

The antibody activity detected after initial immunization, followed by one more booster injections, will be largely associated with IgG molecules[12,56]. Purified IgG was prepared as described previously[12]. In brief: serum is rendered 41% saturated in ammonium sulfate (25 gram per 100 ml), and the precipitate was collected and washed twice with 41 precent saturated ammonium sulphate. The resulting protein precipitate was transferred to the dialysis bag by adding a small amount of deionizer distilled water. Dialysis was carried out against three changes of 100 volumes each of 10mM phosphate buffer pH 6-8. the sample was applied to a column of DEAE- cellulose ($DE-5_2$ whatman) previously equilibrated in the same buffer. After sample application, the column was washed with equilibration buffer (10mM phosphate buffer), and IgG, which did not bind to the adsorbent under these conditions, washed through the column and collected. The active fractions were pooled together and concentrated to between 3 and 5mg/ml by dialysis against polyethylene glycol 6000.

The purified IgG (anti – CEA) was stored at 5C° by adding 0.015-M sodium azide at these condition purified anti–CEA was relatively stable[12].

2-8-4 Anti CEA Immunoadsorbent Preparation:

CNBr activated sepharose was prepared as described in section (2-7-step 1,2) and after washing the wet CNBr-Sepharose cake was added to IgG solution (appioximatly 3 mg/ml) which was to be coupled. The sepharose – IgG fraction suspension was mixed at 4°C for 18 hours, after which it was centrifuged and the supernatant fluid collected. The difference in the concentration of 280 nm of absorbing material in the initial uncoupled IgG solution, and this postcoupling fraction was direct measure of the amount of IgG coupled to sepharose. The IgG – sepharose is washed with buffer for subsequent column packing and operation until no more 280 nm- absorbing material is present in the supernatant after centrifugation.

2-8-5 Colum Preparation, Sample Application, and Elution

1. All operations are at 4 C°.
2. The Sepharose immunoadsorbent was prepared as mentioned in section (2-8-4) was poured into (5x 1.6)cm column with bed volume of 10ml. the column outlet was opened and the gel was allowed to settle under constant flow of (8 ml/hr). The column left for 24 hr at 4C° to allow it is packing.
3. The column was equilibrated with buffer A.
4. The concentrated fractions obtained from lentil lectin- spherrose affinity chromatography, containing the CEA activity were loaded to the column and lefted at 4C° for 2 hr's.
5. Then the column was washed with:
    a. Buffer A (until no further 280nm material absorbing was detected).
    b. Buffer B.
    c. 2.5 M NH_4SCN, pH8.

6. The collected fractions were pooled dialyzed, concentrated and CEA activity was monitored by immunoradiometric method using CEA IRMA kit.

2-8-6 Estimation of CEA by IRMA Method:

CEA levels were measured by immunoradiometric assay (IRMA). The method is based on the use of immobilized antibody coated tubes which binds with CEA in the specimen. A second (^{125}I) labeled monoclonal anti CEA antibody was added to the tubes to form a "sandwich" with the bound CEA.

The radioactivity of the bound monoclonal anti CEA antibody is directly proportional to samples CEA content which is interpolated from the standard curve.

Reagent:

1- ^{125}I-Labeled-anti CEA antibody:

This reagent served as the tracer which was diluted in buffer mixture.

2- Anti-CEA monoclonal antibody coated tubes:
    Ready for use.

3- Standard: 5 vials (0.5 ml) and 1 vial of zero standards (6-ml); ready for use the standard vials contain CEA in buffer, in concentration ranging from 0 to ng/ml.

4- Washing solution concentrate (20X); 1 vial.

The concentrated solution was diluted with distilled water before use to obtain a diluted washing solution.

5- Control samples:

It contained cell culture CEA antigen (human at a fixed concentration).

Chapter Two

Procedure:

The assay protocol is described in table (2-3).

TABLE (2-3): IRMA assays protocol of serum CEA ng/ml

	CEA standard (ng.ml^{-1})						Control		Unknown samples	
	0	1	15	50	125	250	Level I	Level II	1	2-etc
Coated tube no.	1,2	3,4	5,6	7,8	9,10	11,12	13,14	15,16	17,18	19,etc.
Standards (µl)	100	100	100	100	100	100	-	-	-	-
Control serum or samples (µl)	-	-	-	-	-	-	100	100	100	100
Incubation buffer (µl)	100	100	100	100	100	100	100	100	100	100

Then the mixtures were gently mixed then incubated for 2h. at 37°C in water bath, aspirated, and rinsed twice with 1.0 ml deionized water.

* Then two hundred µl of ^{125}I-anti CEA antibody were added to all tubes.
* The assay tubes were incubated for 2h. at 37°C, then aspirated the free tracer and washed twice 1.0 ml de-ionized water.
* The radioactivity of tubes was then measured.

Calculations:

1- The mean net count for each group of tubes was counted in gamma counter for 1 min.

2- The (B/Bmax)% ratio was computed for each standard and unknown samples as follows:

$$(B/B_{max})\% = \frac{\text{Standard or samples mean count}}{\text{Mean counts of the 250 U.ml}^{-1}\text{standard}} \times 100$$

3- The standard curve was drawing by plotting the $(B/B_{max})\%$ value for each standard against the corresponding concentration ng/ml^{-1} on log-log graph paper figure (2-1).

4- The resulting concentration of the patient samples and controls can be directly interpolated from the standard curve by the use of their $(B/B_{max})\%$ values.

2-9 Analysis of the Purified fraction by slab conventional Polyacrylamide Gel electrophoresis (PAGE):

PAGE technique was used to test the purity of the CEA.

2-9-1 Solutions used:

A. Tris-glycine solution (pH 8.9): 22.84 gms of Glycine was dissolved in one litter of distilled water. The pH of the solution was adjusted to 8.9 with tris-hydroxyaminomethane. The volume was then completed to 2 liters with deionized distilled water.

B. Electrode buffer: This was prepared by the 1:1 (v:v) dilution of solution (A).

C. Polyacrylamide solution: 22.2 gms of acrylamide and 0.6 gm. of N.N-methylene bisacrylamide were dissolved in 60 ml. of distilled water. The solution was completed to a final volume of 100 ml. with deionized distilled water.

D. Ammonium persulphate (15 mg/ml) 150 mgs. Ammonium persulphate was dissolved in 10 mls. of deionized distilled water.

E. Bromophenol blue solution 0.25 % (W/V).

F. Fixing solution: This solution was prepared by dissolving 57 gms. of trichloroacetic acid and 17 gms. of sulphosalicylic acid in 150 mls. of ethanol (95%), then the volume was completed to 500 mls. With distilled water.

G. Staining solution: 1.25 gms. of coomassie Brilliant Blue R-250 were dissolved in a mixture of exactly 227 mls. ethanol and 46 ml. glacial acetic acid. The volume of the solution was completed to 500 mls. with deionized distilled water.

H. Destaining solution: Volumes of 300 mls. ethanol and 100 mls. glacial acetic acid were thoroughly mixed. The solution was then completed to a final volume of 1 litter with deionized distilled water.

I. Preserving solution: This solution was prepared by mixing 300 mls. of ethanol with 100 mls. glacial acetic and 100 mls. glycerol. Deionized distilled water was then added to a final volume of 1 L.

J. Five protein solution were used at concentration of 1300
1. Protein fraction I: partially purified CEA by perchloric acid as prepared in section 2-6-2)
2. Protein fraction II: after lenti lectin affinity chromatography (pool peak no 5) Figure (2-2).
3. Protein fraction III: pooled peak No 8 Figure (2-2) that was prepared as in section (2-7-4) after lentil lectin affinity chromatography.
4. Protein fraction IV: pooled peaks after Immuno affinity chromatoyraphy prepared in section (2-8-5).
5. Protein fraction V: purified lentil lectin prepared in section (2-7-2-2).

The above purified protein fractions were concentrated to the optimum concentration (1300 µg/ml.) by dialysis against sucrose.

2-9-2 Procedure:

1. Polyacrylamide gel (con. 7.5 %) was prepared by mixing the following solution respectively (According to the application Note 306 issued by LKB Company).
   a. 7.5 mls. distilled water
   b. 33.0 mls. solution (A)
   c. 22.2 mls. solution (C)
   d. 3.2 mls. solution (D)
   e. mls. solution (E)

2. The slab gel was prepared and fixed in an electrophoresis Apparatus type LKB. The optimum conditions fixed in the application Note 306, were exactly followed.
3. The electrophoretic migration continued until the blue stain of Bromophenol blue reached the gel margin.
4. The gel was then divided into two parts. Part one was sliced to 0.5 cm segments, each segment was put in 500ml of TED buffer pH 7.2, then sliced and cracked softy and left for 24 hr. at 4°C. then the CEA binding activity evaluated by IRAM Method as previously described[12,13].
5. Part two of the slab gel was immersed in the fixing solution (solution H) for 1 hr., and then transferred to the staining solution (solution I) for 2 hrs. in order to stain all the proteins separated by electrophoresis. Excess staining was removed by soaking the gel with destaining solution (solution J). It is preferable to replace the destaining solution twice or thrice in order to secure a complete and fast removal of the excess stain and hence getting more clear bands.
6. The gel slab was kept in the preserving solution (solution L) for 1 hr. to preserve it from dryness and tears.

2-10 Result and Discussion

2-10-1 Preparation of Tumor Specimens and partial purification of CEA by PCA:

The tissue sample to be extracted is usually accumulated in batches and frozen to prevent cellular deterioration. Thus, the first problem encountered is estimating the thawing time of frozed tissue. This is usually a trivial problem in laboratory- scale preparation, but large quantities are often packed in drums or containers holding up to 100 mg of tissue. Thawing time increase with mass and also varies considerably with geometry and thawing conditions employed. Also the thawing times depend on the heat transfer coefficient.

After thawing, tissue was removing from unwanted parts, e.g. connective tissue, blood vessels, and fat, is easily carried out in laboratory by manual trimming, However trimming is extremely time consuming.

The purification by PCA was a achieved by denaturation and precipitation most of the tissue proteins while has a few effect on CEA, which remain in the solution[162]. CEA is generally considered to be stable in acid because it is soluble and its immunological properties are not destroyed[161,162].

The homogenization condition are optimized by systematic of parameters such as the extraction medium, time, temperature and type equipment used to reduce major problems[162,163].

Homogenization was carried out in a cold medium (i.e., 4°C) to avoid protein denaturation[162,163].

The filtration of the tissue homogenate through several layers of nylon gauze was used to remove and suspended pieces of unhomogenized fragments and blood vessels, while centrifugation of the homogenate at 4000 r.p.m. remove the unruptured cells and intact nuclei of the ruptured cells[163].

The purpose of this step is to obtain a solution suitable for chromatography.

2-10-2 Lentil Lectin Affinity Chromatography techniques for purification of CEA:

The intermediate step in CEA purification protocol is lectin affinity chromatography, for this purpose lentil lectin were choosing. As indicate, Lentil lectin binds α-D-glucose and α-D-mannose residues and is an affinity ligand used for the purification of glycoproteins including

Chapter Two

detergent – solubilized membrane glycoproteins, cell surface antigen and viral glycoproteins. Lentil lectin is the hanemagglutinin from the common lentil, *Lens Culinnaris*. When compared to conA, it distinguishes less sharply between glycosyl and mannosyl residues and binds simple sugar less strongly. It also retains its binding ability in the presence of 1% sodium deoxycholate. For these reasons lentil lectin is useful for the purification of CEA, giving high capacities and extremely high recoveries[164-166].

The lectins were extracted from the common lentil seeds by 0.15N NaCl solution then dialyzed and fractionated with gel chromatography using sephadex G-50 (Fig. 2-2-A).

Result from polyacrylamide gel electrophoresis under non-denaturing conditions showed that these lectins were pure to homogeneity (gave only a single band) (Figure 2-2-B)

The purified lentil lectins has been covaiently linked to insoluble matrix of CNBr activated sepharose as described in section (2-7-3) and the conjugated are suspended in blocking buffer at pH 8.3 and poured into column (0.9 x 29 cm) as described in section (2-7-4).

Upon the lentil- lectin affinity column chromato-graphy, the PCA extracted from tumor homogenate produce 9 peaks, (Fig. 2-3). Three nonaffinity peaks (Fractions I,II and III). [The difference in their elution volume is thought to be due to differences in particle size] and 5 affinity fractions. Two of the latter fractions (V and VIII) contained the bulk of the CEA of high specific activity.

Fraction V material comprised about 56% of the total dry weight recovered (Table 2-3).

The other main affinity fraction (VIII) which was obtained after soaking and elution with 20% methyl α-D- mannopyranoside, comprised 32.5% of the recovered weight. Approximatly 90% of the recovered material was specifically attached to the lentil –lectin column (Fraction IV to VIII).

The 2nd major affinity fraction was obtained by soaking the column in 20% methylα-D- mannopyranoside for an extended period (usually 48hr) prior to final elution. Elution with 20% methyl α-D-mannopyranoside immediately after the 10% methyl α-D-glucopyranoside elution did not cause significant elution of additional material even after about 2 column bed volumes had passed. This latter observation probably explain why several investigators[164] fall to recovery any material in their 20% methyl mannoside wash when used conA affinity chromatography to purify CEA from a highly impure CEA preparation.

It seems likely that the different in lentil lectin binding affinity between the bound fractions can be attributed to quantitative or qualitative differences mannose and glucose content, which are not unexpected in view of known microheterogeneity of glycoprotein[165]. Lentil lectin is known to bind specifically to terminal α- linked mannose residues and internal α-1,2 linked D- mannose[166]. Also lentil lectin protein bind more strongly to mannosides than to glucosides, and it bind more strongly to α- glycosides than to β- glycosides[164-166]. All of these sugars are present in CEA and account for approximately 25% of total carbohydrate content[165]. Furthermore lentil lectin binds to terminal α-linked N-acetyl-D-glucosamine[166]. Periodate oxidation studies and methylation analysis indicated that little of this residue is present in most CEA-preparation.

2-10-3 Immunoaffinity Chromatography techniques for purification of CEA

Lectin affinity chromatography is rarely sufficient by itself for the purification of glycoprotein. One should consider this approach as part of

Chapter Two

a general strategy for protein purification.

Immunoaffinity chromatography has become a valuable technique. Because of the extreme specificity and potentially high affinity of antibodies for antigens, this method can be highly efficient in the isolation of any protein for which the investigator has specific, high-affinity antibody.

Immunoaffinity media are created by coupling the anti-CEA (pure IgG anti-rabbit) to CNBr-activated sepharose. The coupling procedure has to be performed by dissolving the anti-CEA in 0.01M $NaHCO_3$, pH 8.3, containing NaN_3. This is the most commonly used coupling buffer. In this pH interval the amino group on anti-CEA IgG are predominantly in the unpronated and reactive from. The ideal sepharose to IgG ratio is approximately 30 to 1 (w/w)[120]. The CNBr- activated sepharose-IgG is usually washed and equilibrated with buffer A. These washing steps are mostly easily performed on glass filter funnel fitted on a Buchner flask (connected to a vaccum suction device) reapted until the unwanted soluble components are removed. After each filtration a glass rod can be used to resuspend the matrix of a new of bufferA. Generally about ≥ 90% IgG coupling to CNBr activated sepharose under coupling condition described. Until used, the prepared anti CEA sepharose immunoaffinity can be store as suspensions at 4C° without loss of activity for 4-6 months. The suspension should contain some anti- bacterial substance such as 0.02% sodium azide.

When the coupling reactions were performed in a buffered medium, it was essential to select convenient column. The column size is usually not a critical parameter. Rather the column size is governed by the capacity of the adsorbent and the amount of substance to be purified.

An anti CEA- CNBr sepharose was packed in column with

Chapter Two

dimension 5x1.6 cm (bed volume 10 ml) to obtain rapid separation. Column packing should follow the usual precaution for chromatographic. For efficient adsorption the column equilibrated with buffer A, before application of sample.

After sample application the column lifted at $4C°$ for 2hr (leave a few millimeter of liquid on top of the matrix surface) to make prolonged contact possible to achieve adequate adsorption.

For efficient adsorption the condition of the sample and the column must allow efficient binding and preferably be optimal for binding. This can be achieved by equilibrating the column with several volumes of starting buffer (buffer A) to remove all unbound material. The chromatography was usually monitored by UV-absorbance, and the washing step was finished when the original base line is reached. The column was then washed with buffer B to remove nonspecific ionic binding.

Figure (2-4) show a typical profile obtained when the active eluate from lentil–lectin affinity chromatography was passed through a column of anti- CEA immunoaffinity. The CEA was eluted from the column with 2.5M NH_4SCN pH 8.1 and could not be detected in the preceding elutions.

Elution of CEA from the immunoadsorbent achieved by using thiocyanates that promote disruption of antigen- antibody complex and allow collection of the CEA in a form that is biologically active.

There are a number of different methods for the disruption of the antibody-antigen reaction. Most of these depend upon the ability to disruptionic bonds and include urea, guanidine-HCl, chaotropic ions, salt solutions, and extremes of pH. Since all these conditions are capable of denaturing proteins, it is important that they should only be used to the most limited degree necessary to produce the desired effect and having done so should be rapidly reversible. In practice 2.5M NH_4SCN, pH 8 has proved to be extremely convenient and satisfactory for this purpose.

The procedure results in high degree of purification of CEA with a recovery 76%..

Figure 2-5 shows poly acrylamide gel profiles after each step of purification. The final product appeared homogeneous.

In conclusion, the present results lead to the following:

1. The quantity of purifed CEA isolated from human digestive, each kilogram of metastatic tumor tissue yielded approximately 100 mg of purified CEA (table 2-4).
2. Two peaks of CEA activity was obtained when the PCA- extract of colorectal tumor was fractionated on lentil-lectin sepharose Fig 2-3.
3. The specific activity increased during purification. (table 2-4).
4. The total time required for processing a given aliquate of 1 kg wet weight of tumor tissue was 3 weeks.
5. The totality of these results leads to believe that while CEA may exist in more than one form; these forms represent definable chemical entities susceptible to complete chemical characterization.

TABLES

TABLE (2-4): Representation values for Meterials recovered from tumor tissue after each step of purification:

Steps of purification	Weight of lyophilized powder (mg)	Specific activity mg (CEA/ mg dry weight)	Total activity (Mm CEA)
Perchloric acid Extract	509	0.23	117.07
Lentil Lectin affinity chromatography Pooled Fraction V	60	1.1	66
Pooled Fraction VIII	119	0.32	38.08
Immunoaffinity chromatography 2.5M NH$_4$SCN Fractions were pooled	59	1.511	89.149

% recovery of total weight applied 76.150

- The specific activities are calculated by dividing the radioimmuno-assay antigenic activity by dry weight.

FIGURES

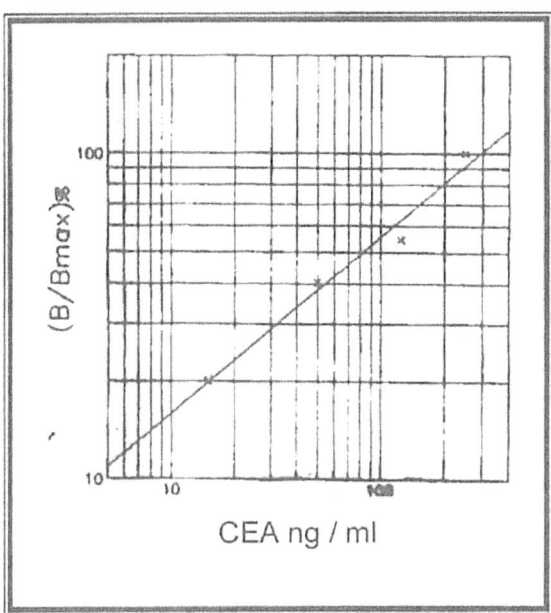

Figure (2-1): The standard curve CEA IRMA (Logarithmic plot)

(All details are explained in the text)

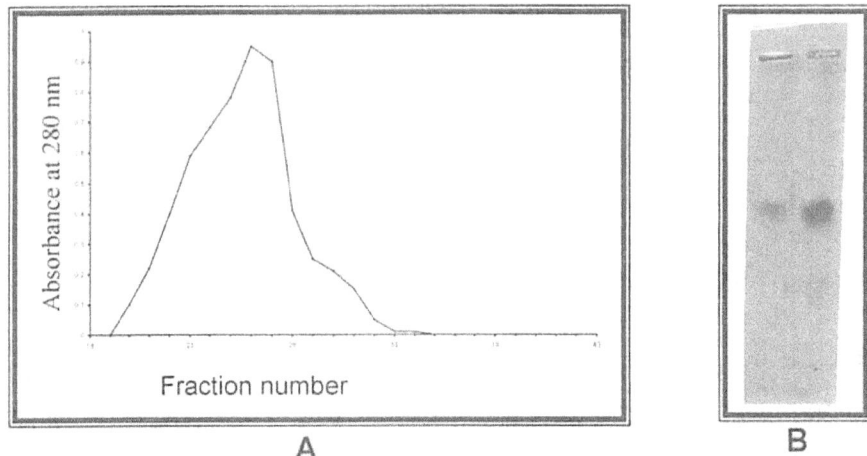

A B

Figure (2-2):

A- Separation of lentil lectin from salin extract of common lentil seeds by using sephadex G-50 gel filtration column.

B- Slab polyacrylamide gel electrophoresis patterns of purified lentil lectins which were present in the sephadex G-50 pooled fraction. The top of the photography is the origin.

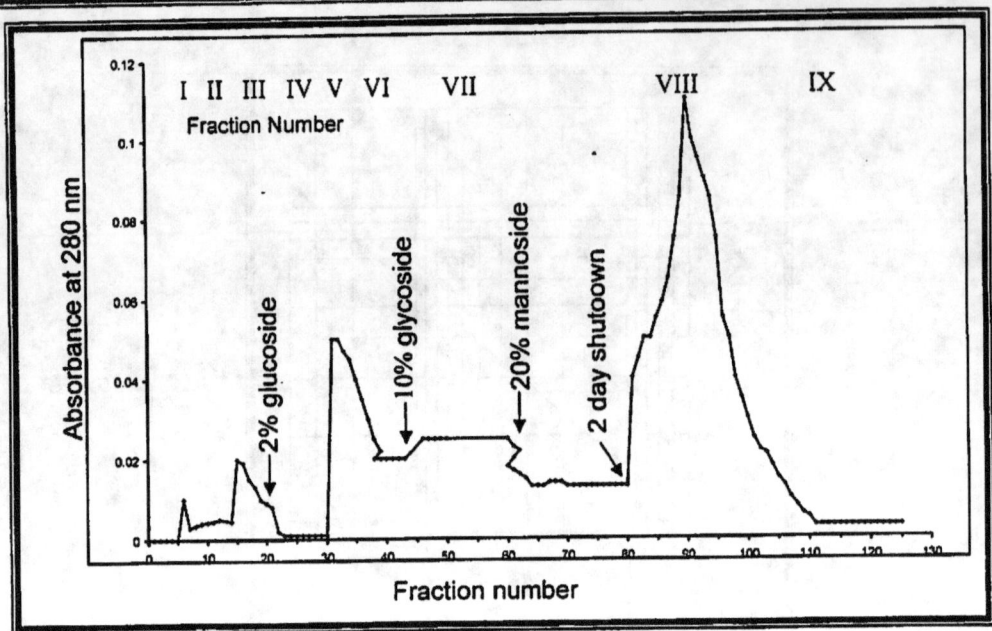

Figure (2-3): Plot of absorbance at 280 nm as a function of fraction number from lentil lectin affinity column. The perchloric acid extracted from colon cancer tumor tissue was applied to a column lentil lectin sepharose 4B°.

(All detail explained in text)

Figure (2-4): The elution profile of human CEA from immunoadsorption chromatography.

(All detail explained in text)

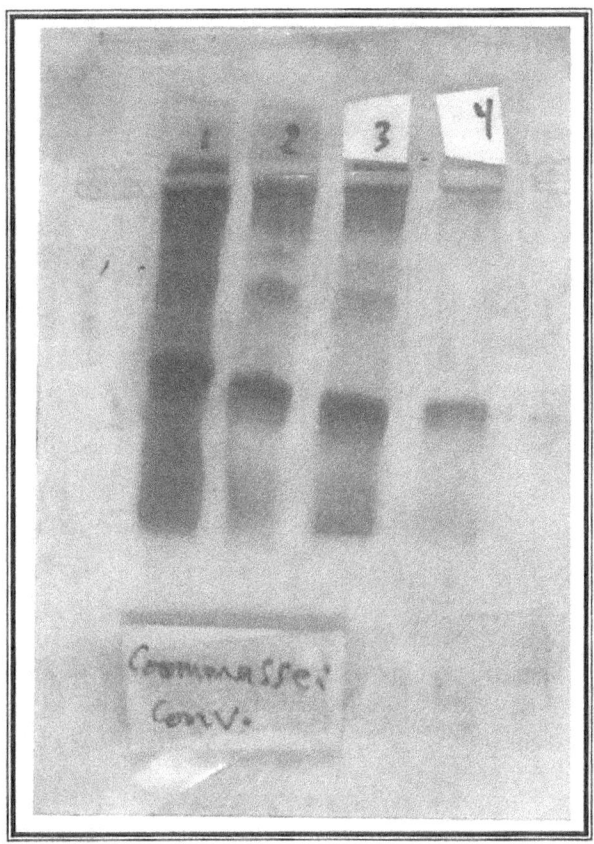

Figure (2-5): Conventional polyacrylamide gel electrophoresis patterns of CEA from various steps of purification as described in table (2-4) the top of the photograph is the origin.

1- Protein components present in PCA exctract from tumor tissue.
2- Protein components present in pooled fractions of peak number affinity pooled peak No V in figure (2-3).
3- Protein components present in pooled fractions peak number VIII in figure (2-3).
4- Protein components present in immunoadsorption chromatography 2.5 NH_4SCN fraction were pooled figure (2-4).

(All details are explained in the text)

Chapter Three

Preparation of EIA Kit

Chapter Three

Abstract

1- peroxidase enzyme was isolated from white radish roots and purified to homogeneity as ascertained by electrophoresis. Purification procedures included ammonium sulfate precipitation, ion exchange chromatography on diethylaminoethyl cellulose and gel filtration in sephacryl S-300 column. Peroxidease activity accounted for 45% of the total activity in the crude homogenate. The method that has been used is very simple, suitable for obtain peroxidase, which is about five time cheaper than rather expensive commercial preparation and has signifycant higher activity.

2- Antiserum to human CEA was obtained from rabbits and guinea pigs immunized with highly purified CEA. Monospecific anti-CEA was isolated and purified from other immunoglobulin subclasses and some serum protein by ammonium sulfate precipitation at 41% saturation and DEAE cellulose ion exchange chromatography.

   The characterization of purified anti-CEA was carried out through cellulose acetate electerophoresis, ouctherlony double diffusion and immunoelectrophoresis, with these techniques, single precipitin line was observed between anti-CEA and CEA.

3- The Two-step glutaraldehyde procedure has been used to couple highly purified white radish roots peroxidase to rabbit anti-CEA. The conjugation experiment showed that the two -step glutaraldehyde method is cirtical for an efficient conjugative and retention of enzyme activity.

4- Pure guinea pig anti-CEA have been used for preparation of antibody coated tubes using glutaraldehyde treated method. The employed technique showed a high capacity for binding antibody on the polypropylene tubes and large proportion of coated antibody

Chapter Three

molecules to retain their ability to bind CEA despite the effect of powerful interaction with tube surface.

5- A sensitive and specific noncompetitive enzyme immuneoassay (EIA) for CEA was developed using glutaraldehyde tube coated with anti CEA, peroxidase conjugated reagent and highly purified carcinoembryonic antigen from several tumors of the digestive trace. Assay parameters were optimized by investigating the concentration of reagent, the reaction Kinetic, reaction temperature, pH reaction and ionic strength of the assay. The assay can be performed at 5hr. A sensitivity range of 30 to 150 ng in region 100 to 10% binding was obtained. The assay proved a useful alternative to radioimmunoassay in those instances where steps involving the use of ^{125}I become limiting, for example, iodination facility and gamma counter availability or prolonge reagent storage.

Chapter Three

Introduction

Enzyme immunoassay (EIA) have been used in immunology to measure the titer and specificity of antisera[167]. In addition, they have used for the detection and quantitation of various antigen[168]. Recently, EIAs have been developed for some pituitary hormones[169,170]. Although radiommunoassay (RIA) is currently the most widely used method for measuring hormones and tumor maker, EIA would appear to offer a number of advantages, for example radioactive isotopes are eliminated in EIA; enzymeconjugated reagents are stable upon storage for prolonged periods, wherease iodinated reagents are not; and finally, analysis time is considerably shorter for EIA as opposed to long counting times for RIA.

The purpose of this chapter to:

1- Preparation enzyme in relatively pure form.
2- Preparation momospecific antibody to CEA.
3- Develop successful EIA technique for the detection, quantification and provide sensitive assay for CEA that is simple and reliable enough for clinical application.

Chapter Three

Material and Method

3-1 Chemical and solution:

1- Most of chemicals and reagent are mentioned in chapter two table (2-1) and other solutions are indicated in each experiment.

2- All buffer solutions were prepared by dissolving the appropriate amount of salts in deionized water and required pH was adjusted.

3-2 Instruments:

Most Instruments used and companies supplied are mentioned in chapter two table (2-2) and other are indicated in each experiment.

3-3 Preparation of peroxidase from white radish roots:

3-3-1 Extraction and purification of peroxidase:

3-3-1-1 solution and materials:

1- Potassium phosphate buffer solution, 0.1M, pH7.

2- Tris buffer, 0.05M, pH7.

3- Phosphate buffer, 0.2M, pH 7.2.

4- O-Dianisidine solution, 0.01 g/ml in absolute of methanol.

5- Hydrogen peroxides solution.

6- Phosphate- buffered saline (PBS), consisting of equal volumes of 0.15M NaCl and 0.15M phosphate buffer, pH 7.2 – 7.3

7- DEAE- cellulose ion –exchange.

8- Sephacryl S-300 gel.

3-3-1-2 Procedure of purification:

The method used was a modification of that employed by Shannon et al.[171] All steps were performed at 4°C.

Step 1. Preparation of Crude Extract:

White radish roots were purchased at local markets. The roots were cut into cubes and homogenized with a minimal volume of 0.4M K_2HpO_4 in a waring Blendor. The homogenate was filtered through

Chapter Three

cheese cloth and centrifuged for 30 minutes at 12,000 xg giving a clear supernatant.

Step 2. Ammonium Sulfate Fractionation:

To the supernatant, saturated $(NH_4)_2SO_4$ solution, pH 7.3, is slowly added with continuous stirring to give 35% saturation. After 30 minutes, the precipitate is separated by centrifuged as above and the supernatant is brought to 90% ammonium sulfate saturation. After standing over night, the residue was collected by centrifugation, redissolved in a minimal volume of 0.05M Tris, pH 7.0, and dialyzed against 0.05M Tris, pH 8.0, containing 0.1M KCl. The dialysate was centrifguge, and the supernatant solution was collected and then concentrated to 5 ml with dialysis against sucrose. The protein content was determined using Lowry et.al method[172] peroxidase content was determined as described in section(3-3-2)[169].

Step 3. Ion-Exchange Chromatography[173,174]:

A. Preparation of chromatography column:

This was conducted on pre-swollen diethylaminoethyl cellulose (DEAE), using 40x2.5 cm column. As suggested by manufacturer and according to the dimensions of the ion-exchanger bed, the required amount of DE52 cellulose was suspended in required amount of acid component (NaH_2PO_4) of 0.5 M phosphate buffer, pH7. the slurry was then degassed using vacuum pressure, along with continuous stirring using a magnetic stirrer.

The slurry was filtered in a Buchner funnel using a 15cm filter paper (Whatman 54) under reduced pressure provided by a venture water pump.

The filtrate was discarded and the ion-exchanger then suspended in the basic component (Na_2HPO_4) of the same buffer.

Chapter Three

The ion-exchanger was then washed once with a 0.1M phosphate buffer pH7.

Equilibration of ion-exchanger was achieved by repeated buffer washing (using the starting buffer which was always a 5mM phosphate buffer, pH 8) until the filtrate had exactly the same pH of the starting buffer.

Fines were then removed by leaving the slurry to stand for about 30 minutes. After this, some of supernatant buffer containing fines was removed. A fresh starting buffer was then added. This final preparation was then packed into the column.

For re-use, the DE52 column was dismantled and the ion-exchanger was washed with strong salt solution (0.5M NaCl), and then with a 0.1M phosphate buffer, pH 7.6. Equilibration, removal of fines and packing of the column was performed as described before.

B. Separation Procedure:

The $(NH_4)_2SO_4$ fractions which were already dialyzed against the starting buffer, were applied in five ml a liquate to DE52 column (with bed dimensions of 30 by 2.5 cm, flow rate 45 ml per hour) This was followed by starting buffer (0.05M phosphate buffer, pH 8). 3ml fractions were collected until absorbace returns to background.

Following the absorption at 280 nm for each fraction and enzyme activity was performed as described in section (3-1-2). Selected fractions containing most of peroxidase activity were pooled, dialyzed against deionized water at 4°C for 48 hr and then concentrated to 5 ml by dialysis against sucrose. The protein content was determined using Lowry-et.al. method[172]. Peroxidase content was determined as described in section (3-1-2).

Chapter Three

Step 4. Gel Filtration on Sephacryl S-300 Column:

A. Preparation of the Column:

The dimensions of the column were chosen as described in chapter two section (2-7-2-2).

The gel was prepared according to the manufacturer's instructions. The pre-swollen gel was swelled in phosphate buffer 0.2M pH 7.2, then settled and excess buffer was decanted. This step was repeated several times. The gel slurry was degassed by suction and left for 24 hr at 4C° to equilibrate with the buffer. The swollen gel was suspended and carefully poured into column (2.8x60 cm) down the wall. After the gel has settled the column outlet was opened, continuing packing till the gel reached a bed height of 60 cm then equilibrated with phosphate buffer 0.2M pH 7.2.

B. Separation Procedure:

The concentrated fractions obtained from DEAE-cellulose ion-exchange, containing the preoxidase activity was loaded to Sephacryl S-300 column. Fractions of 6 ml were obtained by elution with phosphate buffer 0.2M pH 7.2 at flow rate 40 ml/hr. For each fraction, constant monitoring for its spectrophotometeric absorption at 280 nm and peroxidase activity was performed as described in section selected fractions containing high peroxidase activity were pooled, dialyzed at 4C° against several change of deionized water and then lyophilized.

3-3-2 Measuring of Peroxidase Activity:

The method used was modified from Avrameas and Guilbert[170].

3-3-2-1 Reaction Mixture:

The substrate contains 0.2 ml of methanolic solution of orthodianisidine (0.01 g/ml) and 0.05 ml of 30% hydrogen peroxidase added to 20 ml pBS, the substrate solution should be made immediately before used.

Chapter Three

3-3-2-2 Enzyme Assay:

Peroxidase activity was measured by following spectropho-tometrically the change in absorbance at 436 nm due to O-dianisidine oxidation in the present of H_2O_2 and enzyme[170].

3-3-2-3 Calculation:

1- In each fraction, the protein concentration was determined according to Lowry et al.[172],

2- Peroxidase activity $(U / ML) = \dfrac{\Delta A^{\circ}}{\Delta t(\min)} (slop) \times \dfrac{Total\,volum}{Sample\,.vol.} \times \dfrac{1}{\varepsilon}$

Where: ΔA: change in measuring absorbance of time (t).

ε: moler extinction coefficient for O-dianisidine for the assay, the values were as followed:

$$unit/ml = \Delta A / \Delta t(\min) \times \dfrac{3.1}{0.1} \times \dfrac{1}{8.3}$$

3- Total activity = peroxidase activity (unit / ml)X total volume (ml)

4- Specific activity = $\dfrac{\text{peroxidase activity (unit / ml)}}{\text{total protein in assay}}$

5- Purification fold = $\dfrac{\text{specific activity (unit /ml)}}{\text{specific activity of crude}}$

6- Yield % = $\dfrac{\text{total activity of purified peroxidase(unit)}}{\text{total activity of crude extract}}$

3-3-3 Analysis of purified peroxidase by polyacrylamide Gel electrophoresis (PAGE)

This was performed as described in chapter 2 section (2-9).

3-4 Antisera generation to CEA.

3-4-1 Preparation of experimental animals:

The first group of experimental animals male new Zealand rabbits, white, healthy, young adult and with weighting 2.5-3.5 kg at the primary immunization. They were purchased from local market

Chapter Three

Preparation of the rabbit for inoculation:

1- Place the rabbits in a restraining cage (130x70x60cm). They were maintained under the same light period and temperature throughout the period of experiment and received food (green fodder) and water.

2- Shave the rabbit's ear along the vein and apply xylene to dilate the blood vessel.

The second group of experimental animal's guinea pig.

The same preparation and requirement as described above may be applied to the guinea pig.

3-4-2 Immunization of animals:

1- One hundred micrograms of purified human carcinoem-bryonic antigen (CEA) suspended in Freund's complete aduvant (CFA) were injected intramusculary by given twice a week for 2 consective weeks, 25µg of CEA was injected each time, the right and left flank being used alternately. Three weeks later all animal were boosted with one more intramuscular injection of 15µg of CEA and the rabbits were bled twice a week beginning 1 week after the final injection. Starting at this time, blood was collected from ear vein on a regular schedule (twice a week).

2- The collection schedual was discontinued for approximately 3 months and restarted by boosting as described above.

3- The serum may be checked for the presence of antibodies by the double dissfusion method of Ouchterlony test: (Ten microliters of CEA place in the center well of a gar immunodiffusion plate. The satellite wells are filled with undiluted serum. A positive reaction is indicated if the precipitin line becomes visible, usually with 24 hr at room temperature).

Chapter Three

4- The same schedule, using 15μg of CEA, may be applied to second group of experimental animal's are guinea pig.

3-4-3 Isolation and purification of specific antibodies to CEA:

The method for isolation specific antibodies to CEA as described in chapter two section (2-8-3).

3-4-4 Methods used for identifica-ton of pure anti-CEA immunoglobulins:

Both Anti-sera preparations and Anti-CEA immuno-globuline were purified, checked for impurity and specificity by the following techniques:-

3-4-4-1 Cellulose acetate electrophoresis[175,176].

Solutions:

1- Barbital buffer (0.05 M, pH 8.6)

The powder of this buffer was dissolved in 1000 ml deionized distilled water to obtain buffer (0.05 M, pH 8.6) This solution was stable for 2 months at (15-30)°C

2- Staining solution, ponceus S used for

- Trichloro acetic acid (TCA)   30 grams
- Ponceus S   2 grams
- Distilled water   100 grams

The dye dissolved by heating to 60°C following by cooling at room temperature and filtering through filter paper.

3- Acetic acid (5%).

Fifty milliliter of acetic acid was completed with deionized distilled water to 1000 ml.

4- Liquid paraffin.

Procedure:

1- Cellulose acetate paper was immersed for 5 min. in barbital buffer.

2- Cellulose acetate paper was then dried by filter paper and placed on the Instrument Bridge.

3- Microzone cell was filled with barbital buffer and the bridge was placed in the microzone cell.

4- Fifty microliter serum was withdrawn by applicator and laid continuously above the cellulose acetate paper.

5- The cell was connected to power supply and the voltage current was raised gradually to reach 200 volts and 1mA respectively. The electrophoresis was continued for (20-25) min.

6- After the 25 min, the paper was immersed in ponceau S stain for 10 min, in order to fix the band in its position.

7- The paper was washed with acetic acid (5%) and the destining solution was changed several times until the stain has been removed.

8- The paper was dried for 30 min, then immersed in liquid paraffin for 1 min, and the extra paraffin was removed.

3-4-4-2 Immune electrophoresis (IEP)[177,178]

IEP technique was used for immunochemical identity of the purified CEA preparation:

Solutions used:

A) Barbital/barbital- Na buffer, (pH 8.6).

- 5,5 – diethyl barbituric acid (barbital) 30g.
- 5,5 diethyl – sodium barbiturate (barbital –Na)= 155g.
- Sodium azide 10g.
- Calcium lactate 3g.
- Distilled water to make 10 liters.

The barbital was dissolved after a few minutes in 1 litter of boiling distilled water with stirring. Heating is then discontinued and the barbital-Na was added. When this dissolved, sodium azide and calcium lactate were added. Finally, distilled water was added to a final volume of 10 liters[178].

B) 1% agarose in Barbital / barbital –Na buffer, pH 8.6

Two grams of agarose were added to 200 ml of the diluted buffer and dissolved by gentle heating on a magnetic stirrer. The solution was boiled for 5-6 min to ensure that the agarose is completely dissolved. The solution was kept fluid at 56°C in water bath and ready for used after temperature equilibration.

C) Staining solution, ponceus S used for prepared as described in section (3-4-4-1)

D) Destaining solution:

10% glacial acetic acid.

E) Fixing solution:

Picric acid	14 g
Distilled water	100 ml
Glacial acetic acid	200 ml

The picric acid was added to water, which was then heated to 60°C the warm solution was filtered through filter paper and finally the glacial acetic acid was added.

F) Washing solutions: there are two solution

1- 0.1 M NaCl

2- Distilled water

G) Two type of CEA were prepared at concentration of 1300 µg/ml

1- CEA was provided by (CEA IRMA Kit / Byksangetes Diagostic GmbH&Co. KG / France)

2- The purified CEA preparation.

H) The anti–CEA monoclonal solution provided by Byksangetes Diagostic GmbH&Co. KG / France).

Chapter Three

Procedure:

1. An agarose – coated microscope slide (25x75 mm) was used as support for the gel then placed on a horizontal surface, and about 2 ml of buffer 1% agarose was poured onto slides.
2. Holes of 1 mm and longitudinal basin 2 mm wide were made by means of gel puncher; the gel in the hole was removed by a Pasteur pipette.
3. The upper well was loaded with standard CEA and other one was loaded with purified CEA preparation.
4. The plate was then placed in electrophoresis chamber and connected to buffer vessels by filter paper wicks.
5. Electrophoresis was performed with a potential gradient of 3-6 V/cm, corresponding to total of 70-200 v. Initial current was 50 mA/plate.

    Temperature   4°C
    Time about   80 min

6. After termination of electrophoresis, the agarose gel was removed from the trough and 100µl of anti-CEA was introduced into trough.
7. Incubation of the plate was performed in a humid chamber for 24h.
8. Fixing 30 min in fixing solution.
9. Washing: This was done by washing it twice in 0.1 M NaCl and one with distilled water.
10. Drying: the gel was covered with 3 layers of filter paper and place a glass plate and a weight (1 to 2 kg) over them, after 10 min it was removed and finish drying in a stream of hot air in front of a heating fan.
11. Staining: 10 min in staining solution.
12. Destaining: 10% glacial acetic acid till the back ground become clear.
13. Drying: in a stream of hot air in front of a heating fan.

3-5 Preparation of Peroxidase anti-CEA conju-gate for Enzyme Immunoassay:

3-5-1 Material:
1- highly purified white radish peroxidase (prepared as described in section 3-1).
2- Stock solution of glutaraldehyde, 25% in water.
3- Phosphate buffer, 0.1 M, pH 6.8.
4- Sephadex G-25.
5- Isotonic saline.
6- Immunoglobulin preparation, 5 mg/ml in saline (rabbits anti –CEA Immunoglobuline prepared as described in section (3-4)
   Carbonate-bicarbonate buffer, 0.5 M, pH 9.5
   Lysine solution, 1.0 M, pH 7.
   Phosphate-buffered saline, pH 7:5 (PBS)
   Saturated ammonium sulfate.
   Glycerol.

Calculation:
1- In all measurement the spectrophotometer was set to zero with distilled water.
2- The mean value of absorbance for the first set tubes (coated tubes with guinea pig anti-CEA) refered to total binding TB (specific and nonspecific binding)
3- The mean value of absorbance for second set of tubes (untreated polypropylene tubes) referred to nonspecific binding (NB).
4- The value of specific binding is difference between the mean of total binding and the mean value of nonspecific binding.

Specific binding(SB)= Total binding(TB)-nonspecific binding(NB)

$$SB\% = \frac{SB}{TB} X\ 100$$

5- The value of SB% was plotted Vs concentration of CEA.

3-5-2 Methodology for performing the PRA

Peroxidas Rabbit antiCEA conjugate performing by modified from sternberger[179] method.

1- Dissolve 10 mg of peroxidase in 0.2 ml of a freshly prepared 1:25 dilution of the stock glutaraldehyde solution in phosphate buffer and allow to stand at room temperature for 18 hr.
2- Pass through Sephadex G-25 column (60x1 cm) equilibrated with saline to remove excess glutaralde-hyde.
3- Collect the brown fractions, which contain the activated peroxidase, pool, and concentrate to 1 ml.
4- Add 1 ml of immunoglobulin solution (previously dislyzed against saline) to the peroxidase solution.
5- Add 2 ml of carbonate- bicarbonate buffer and leave for 24 hr at 4°.
6- Add 0.1 ml of lysine solution and leave the mixture at 4° for 2 hr.
7- Dialyze against several changes of PBS at 4°.
8- Add an equal volume of saturated ammonium sulfate to the conjugate and allow standing at 4° for 30 min.
9- Centrifuge for 20 min at 4000 g and discard supernatant.
10- Dissolve precipitate in approximately 1 ml of saline and dialyze extensively against several changes of PBS. (Alternatively, sulfate ions may be removed by gel filtration chromatography on Sephadex G-50).
11- The conjugated may be separate from free antibody by chromatography on sephacry S-300 column (prepared as described in section 3-3-1-2 step 4 A&B).
12- Store conjugated after addition of equal volume of glycerol, and store at 4°.

3-6 Preparation of anti-CEA-Coated polypropylene tubes:

3-6-1 Material, Solution, and Appartus:

1- IgG antibodies to CEA solution 5 mg/ml in 5 mg/ml saline (Guinea pigs Anti-CEA prepared as described in section 3-2).
2- Polypropylene tubes (50x13 mm).
3- Stock solution of glutaraldehyde.
4- Phosphate buffer saline, pH 7.2, (PBS).
5- Carbonate buffer, pH 9.0.
6- Prepare a stock coating solution containing 25 µg/ml anti-CEA in phosphate buffer saline (PBS:10mM phosphate, 150 mM NaCl, pH 7.2).
7- Horizontal tray shaker.

3-6-2 Coating methodologies:

Step 1: Activation of polypropylene tubes (50 x 13 mm)

1- The inner surface of each Polypropylene tubes were treated with 3 ml of 0.1% glutaraldehyde in 0.1M carbonate buffer, pH 9.0 (freshly prepared of stock glutaraldehyde solution) for 3 hr, at 56°C on horizontal tray shaker.
2- AT the end of reaction period (3 hr), the tubes were then cooled to room temperature, and removed the containing fluid by gentle aspiration.
3- The glutaraldehyde treated tubes were washed ten times with distilled water.

Step 2: Binding of anti-CEA to inner surface of Polypropylene tubes.

1- Add 2.5 ml of stock coating solution to each glutaraldehyde treated tubes; the tubes were capped and kept over night at 4°C on horizontal tray shaker.

Chapter Three

2- AT the end of reaction period, remove the fluid by aspiration and save, the tubes were washed three times with phosphate buffer saline.

3- The protein content in the aspirated coating solution and in the pooled washing solution was estimated by Lowry method[172].

4- Finally the tubes were washed with distill water then air drying, storage until use.

3-6-3 Calculation:

The amount of anti-CEA that bound to the inner surface of polypropylene tubes was determined by difference between the initial amount and that found in pooled aspiration solution.

3-7 Binding capacity assessment of anti-CEA to polypropylene tubes:

3-7-1 Material, reagent, and appartus:

1- Glutaraldehyde treated polypropylene tubes (prepared as described in section 3-6-2 step 1).

2- ^{125}I anti –CEA solution about 4000 cpm/100 ml (specific activity 15 mci per microgram of protein from Byk-sangte Diagnostica).

3- LKB gamma count type 1270 Rack.

3-7-2 Assessment Methodology

1- Marked series of glutaraldehyde treated tubes from 1-20 (first set of tubes).

2- 100 µl of ^{125}I- anti –CEA (4000 CPM) was added to each tube. The final volume was complete to 2.5 ml using phosphate buffer saline, pH 7.2, 0.1 M, the tubes were capped and kept over night at 4°C with moderate horizontal shaking.

3- The second set of tubes consist of 100 µl of radioio dinated anti – CEA in order to obtain total count.

Chapter Three

4- AT the end of reaction period, aspiration of the contents of all tubes was then carried out carefully, except those for total count (second set).

5- The empty tube was transferred to gamma counter and the CPM bound is measured.

6- The radioactivity of second set tubes was then measured.

3-7-3 Calculation of binding capacity:

1- The mean net count for each group of tubes was counted in gamma counter for 1.00 min.

2- Correction of the count activity of all tubes from background was carried out. Count activity for empty glutaraldehyde treated tubes.

3- Total binding (TB) represent the amount of ^{125}I- labeled anti bodies bound to the polypropylene tubes (first set tubes).

4- The percent of binding value = The mean of labeled anti–CEA used in the first set of tubes divided by mean of total count (CPM) and multipilled with factor 100 in order obtain the percentage of binding.

$$\% \ Binding \ = \frac{TB \ (CPM \ )corr}{TC \ (CPM \ )} \ X \ 100$$

3-8 Assay conditions for EIA experiments:

All the following experiment in this section were carried out in two sets, the first set to estimate the total binding using guinea pig anti-CEA coated tubes. (The coated tubes utilized in this study were prepared as described in section 3-6). The second sets to determine the non specific binding were performed in untreated polypropylene tubes. Also, all following experiments included two stages. In the first stage, incubation of antigen and antibody and the antigen-antibody complex are separated from free antigen. The second stage the immoboilized antibody-antigen

Chapter Three

complex was incubated with peroxidase0labeled antibody which binds to one or more remaining antigenic sites.

3-8-1 Amount of CEA (Antigen):

First stage Procedure:

Increasing concentration (0.03-1 µg) of purified CEA (the CEA utilized in this study was prepared as described in chapter 2) were added in all tubes (coated and uncoated tubes).

The final volumes were made up to 1 ml with phosphate buffer, pH 7.3, 0.05 M (all tubes).

All tubes were tightly sealed with cellophantap and incubation for 24 hr at $25 \pm 1°C$ with moderate horizontal shaking.

At the end period of incubation the contents of all tubes were discarded by inversion and the tubes were washed 4x with 0.15 M saline containing 0.05% Tween 20 (A four wash cycle was accomp-lished by filling the tubes up to 1 ml volume with Tween-saline, allowing it to sit for 20S, and discarding the contents. After washing the tubes completely emptied by inversion and striking against a paper towel.

Second Stage Procedure:

1. After wash cycle to all tubes (coated & uncoated tubes), two hundred fifty microliter of anti-CEA conjugate with peroxidase (the rabbit anti-CEA (PRA) conjugate with peroxidase utilized in this study was prepared as described in section 3-5-2) were then added.
2. The final volumes were made up to 1 ml with phosphate buffer, pH 7.3, 0.05 M (as described in step 2 of first stage procedure.
3. All tubes were tightly sealed with cellophane tap and incubated at $25 \pm 1°C$ for 24 hr with moderate horizontal shaking.
4. At the end period of incubation, A spiration of the contents of all tubes were then carried out carefully.

Chapter Three

5. Wash cycle as described in step 4 of first stage.
6. 1.5 ml of substrate was then added to each tube and reaction was allowed to proceed for 1 hr in the dark at room temperature. (Substrate of white raddish peroxidase consisted of 0.2 ml of methanolic solution of 0- dianizidine (0.01 gl/ml) and 0.05 ml of 30% hydrogen peroxide added to 20 ml of PBS. The substrate solution should be made immediately before use.)
7. The reaction was terminated by adding 0.1 ml of 2.5 M sulfuric acid to each tube.
8. The absorbance was measured at 436 nm.

Calculation:-

3-8-2 Amount of anti–CEA conjgate peroxidase (rabbit anti-CEA conjugate peroxidase (PRA)).

First stage Procedure:

1- 0.1 µg of CEA were added to two set of polypropylene tubes (coated and uncoated tubes).
2- The steps 2,3 and 4 in first stage of section (3-8-1) were followed exactly.

Second stage procedure:

1- After wash cycle for all tubes as mentioned in procedure of first stage, different volumes of anti-CEA conjugated (PRA) (50,100,1250,150,200,250)µl were added.
2- The steps 2,3,4,5,6,7,and8 in procedure of second stage in section (3-8-1) were followed exactly.

Calculation:-

1- The method of calculation of the experiment (3-8-1) was followed exactly.
2- The SB% was plotted against the amount of PRA conjugate.

3-8-3 Incubation Temperature Effect:

This experiment was performed according to two protocols.

3-8-3-1 The first protocols: Temperature of first incubation:

First Stage:

The steps 1,2,3,and 4 in first stage procedure in section (3-8-2) was repeated at different temperature of incubation (4,10,25,30,35, 40,45)°C.

Second Stage procedure:

1- After wash cycle, two hundred microliter of PRA conjugate was then added to each tube and incubated at 25± 1°C for 24 hr.

2- The steps 2,3,4,5,6,7 and 8 in second stage procedure in section (3-8-1) were followed exactly.

Calculation:-

1. The method of calculation of the experiment(3-8-1) was followed exactly.

2. The SB% was plotted against the temperature of first incubation.

3-8-3-2 The second protocol: second incubation temperature effect:

First stage procedure:

1- 0.1 µg of CEA was added to two set of polypropylene tubes (coated and uncoated tubes).

2- The final volumes were made up to 1 ml as described in step 2 of first stage procedure in section (3-8-1).

3- All tubes were tightly sealed with cellophane tap and incubation for 24 hr at 10 ± °C with moderate horizontal shaking.

4- Step (4) in first stage procedure in section (3-8-1) was followed exactly.

Chapter Three

Second stage procedure:-

1- The first step in second stage procedure of first protocol in this experiment (3-8-3-1) was then repeated at different temperature of incubation (4,10,20,25,30,35,40, 45°C).

2- The step 2,3,4,5,6,7 and 8 in second stage procedure in section (3-8-1) were followed exactly.

Calculation:-

1- The method of calculation of the experiment (3-8-1) was followed exactly.

2- The SB% was plotted against the temperature of second incubation.

3-8-4 Effect of Incubation time

This experiment was performed according to two protocols:

3-8-4-1 The first protocols: time of first incubation.

First Stage:

1- The steps 1,2,3,4 in first stage procedure of second protocol in section (3-8-3-2) were followed except at different time of incubation (0-5,1,2,4,6,8,12,24)hr.

Second stage:

1- After wash cycle, two hundred microliter of PRA conjugate was then added to each tube.

1- The steps 2,3,4,5,6,7 and 8 in the second stage procedure in section (3-8-1) were followed exactly except second incubation were carried out at 10°C ± 1 for 24 hr.

Calculation

1. The method of calculation of the experiment (3-8-1) was followed exactly.

2. The SB% was plotted against the time of first incubation.

3-8-4-2 Second protocol: time effect of second incubation.

First stage procedure

2- The step 1,2,3,4 in first stage procedure of first protocol in this experiment (3-8-4-1) was followed. Just the incubation time was 3 hr and the incubation temperature was 25 ± 1°C.

Second stage procedure:

1- To all tubes two hundred microliter of RAP conjugate was then added to each tube and incubation at 10 ± 1 for certain time intervals (0.5,1,2,3,4,5,6,7,8,9 and 24 hr).

2- The steps 2,3,4,5,6,7 and 8 in second stage procedure in section (3-8-1) were followed exactly.

Calculation:

1- The method of calculation of the experiment (3-8-1) was followed exactly.

2- The SB% was plotted against the time of second incubation.

3-8-5 Effect pf pH:

To demonstrate the effect of pH, the experiment was carried out in two protocols:

3-8-5-1 First protocol: pH effect on binding between guinea pig anti CEA which coated polypropylene tube and CEA molecule:

First stage procedure:

1- 0.1 µg of CEA was added to two set of polypropylene tubes (coated and uncoated).

2- The final volumes were made up to 1 ml with phosphate buffer 0.05 M of differ pH (5.7, 6, 6.5, 7, 7.3, 7.5, and 8).

3- Tubes were tightly sealed, incubated for 2 hr 10 ± 1°C and washed with Tween- saline as described previously.

Chapter Three

Second stage procedure:

1- After wash cycle, to all tubes two hundred microliter of RAP conjugate was then added to each tube and the final volume were made up to 1 ml whit phosphate buffer pH 7.3, 0.05 M.

2- The tubes were sealed, incubated for 3 hr at 10± 1°C, washed with Tween–saline, and then incubated with substrate. The enzyme reaction was terminated by addition 0.4 ml of 2.5 sulfuric acid to each tube. The absorbance was measured at 436 nm.

Calculation:

1- The method of calculation of the experiment (3-5-1) was followed exactly.

2- The SB% was plotted against pH of Ist incubation

3-8-5-2 Second protocol: pH effect on second binding.

First stage procedure:

1- 0.1 µg of CEA was added to two set of polypropylene tubes (coated and uncoated).

2- The final volumes were made up to 1 ml with phosphate buffer 0.05 M, pH 7.3.

3- Steps 3 in section 3-8-5-1 first stage procedure were follow exactly.

Second stage procedure:

1- After wash cycle, two hundred micrliter of PRA conjugate was then added to each tube.

2- The final volumes were made up to 1 ml with phosphate buffer 0.05 M of differ oH (5.7,6,6.5,7,7.3,7.5,8).

3- All tubes were sealed, incubated for 2 hr at 10± 1 °C, washed with Tween-saline, and then incubated with substrate. The enzyme reaction was terminated by addition 0.4 ml of 2.5 ml sulfuric acid to each tube. The absorbance was measured at 436.

The method of calculation of the experiment (3-8-1) was followed exactly.

The SB% was plotted against pH of second incubation

3-8-6 Ionic strength effect:

In order to investigate the effect of ionic strength on condition assay of EIA the experiment was performed according to two protocols.

3-8-6-1 First protocol: Effect of ionic strength during first incubation method.

First stage procedure:

1. 0.1 µg of CEA was added to two set of polypropylene tubes (coated and uncoated).
2. The final volumes were made up to 1 ml with phosphate buffer, pH 7.3, 0.05 m. this experiment was repeated at different concentration of phosphate buffer rang (0.001, 0.01, 0.05, 0.08, 0.1, 0.2, 0.4, 0.6, 0.8, 1 M). Also the experiment was repeated by using distill water. The pH of the buffer solution was fixed at pH 7.3 at all concentration of phosphate buffer.
3. All tubes were tightly sealed, incubated for 2 hr at $10°C \pm 1$ and washed with Tween-saline as described previously.

Second stage procedure:

1- After wash cycle, to all tubes two hundred microliter of PRA conjugate was then added to each tube and the final volume were made up to 1 ml with phosphate buffer, pH 7.3, 0.05M.
2- The tubes were sealed, incubated for 3 h at $10 \pm 1°C$, washed with Tween–saline, and then incubated with substrate. The enzyme reaction was terminated by addition 0.4 ml of 2.5 ml sulfuric acid to each tube. The absorbance was measured at 490 nm.

Chapter Three

Calculation:
1. The method of calculation of the experiment (3-8-1) was followed exactly.
2. The SB% was plotted against the molarity.

3-8-6-2 Second protocol: Effect of ionic strength in second incubation.

First stage procedure:
1- 0.1 µg of CEA was added to two set of polypropylene tubes (coated and uncoated).
2- The final volumes were made up to 1 ml with phosphate buffer, pH 7.3, 0.05M.
3- All tubes were tightly sealed, incubated for 2 hr at 10C± 1°C and washed with Tween-saline as described previously.

Second stage procedure:
1- After wash cycle, to all tube two hundred microliter of RAP conjugate was then added to each tube and the final volume were made up to 1 ml with phosphate buffer pH 7.3, 0.05 M. Also this experiment was repeated at different concentration of phosphate buffer range (0.001,0.01,0.05,0.08,0.1,0. 2,0.4,0.6,0.8,1 M). also the experiment was repeated by using distill water. The pH of the buffer solution was fixed at pH 7.3 at all concentration of phosphate buffer.
2- The step (2) in experiment (3-8-6-1) second stage was preformed as outlined.

The bound CEA was determined as described in section (3-8-1).

The percentage of specific binding (SB%) was calculated the SB% was plotted against the molarity.

3-9 Preparation of standard curves:

3-9-1 Solutions:

1. CEA standards; different concentration of CEA were prepared by serial dilutions for stock purified CEA with phosphate buffer. The working range of the assay was constructed from 0 to 250 ng/ml. All standard solution was conserved by sodium azide (< 0.1 %) and store at 4°C.
2. Antibody –coated tubes:
3. Antibody- peroxidase conjugate (PRA).
4. Diluent: phosphate buffer pH 7.3, 0.05 M.
5. The substrate solution made immediately before use as described previously in section (3-3-2).
6. Untreated polypropylene tubes (13x50 mm).
7. PBS –Tween: 0.88% NaCl, 0.05M sodium phosphate, 0.05% Tween 20, pH, 7.1

3-9-2 Procedure:

1- Number a triplicate series coated and uncoated polypropylene tubes (guinea anti-CEA coated tubes).
2- Sequently, 100 µl of standard CEA (working range of the assay was from 0 to 250 ng /ml).

The final volume was completed to 1 ml using phosphate buffer pH 7.2, 0.05 M.

3- All tubes were tightly sealed with cellophane tap and incubation for 3 hr at 25 ± 1 °C with moderate horizontal shaking.
4- At the end period of incubation the contents of all tubes were discarded by inversion and the tubes were washed 4x with 0.15m saline containing 0.05% Tween 20 as described previously.

Chapter Three

5- Two hundred microliter of PRA conjugate was then to each tube. The final volumes were made up to 1 ml with phosphate buffer 0.05 M, pH 7.3.

6- All tubes were again tightly sealed with cellophane tap and incubated at 25± 1°C 2 hr with moderate horizontal shaking.

7- At the end period of incubation, aspirations of the contents of all tubes were then carried out carefully.

8- Wash cycle as described previously.

9- 1.5 ml of substrate was then added to each tube and reaction was allowed to proceed for 1 hr in the dark at room temperature.

10- The reaction was terminated by adding 0.4 ml of 2.5 M sulfuric acid to each tube.

11- The absorbance of the tangerine colored product was completely soluble measured at 436.

3-9-3 Calculation:

1- In all measurement the spectrophotometer was set to zero with distill water.

2- Correction absorbance for all tubes from nonspecific binding was carried out as described previously.

3- The (B/Bmax)% ratio was computed for each standard as follows:

$$(B/B\,max)\% = \left(\frac{Standard\ absorbance}{Maximum\ absorbance\ (absorbance\ of\ 250\ ng/ml)} \right) \times 100$$

4- The standard curve was drawn by plotting the (B/Bmax) % value for each standard against the corresponding concentration ng. ml^{-1} on log-log graph paper.

5- The resulting concentration of sample and controls can be directly interpolated from the standard curve by the use of their (B/Bmax)% value.

3-10 Result and Discussion

3-10-1 Extraction and purification of peroxidase enzyme: -

The preparation described here, the white radish roots were selected as sources for peroxidase isoenzyme. The results indicated the highest of peroxidase specific activity in the crude extraction (Table 3-1). This result is in agreement with many investigator have observed the highest peroxidase activity in roots of red and white radish among other sources of plant such as turnip, redbeet, and leaves of barley, spinach cauliflower, cress, peanut and seed of soy been[168-171].

The purification procedure included fractionation with ammonium sulfate (35-90% saturation). The purpose of this process to remove debris, most of bulk protein such as proteases and other substance which often interfere with adsorption step, further more, ammonium sulfate fractionation is employed primarily to concentrate the protein and to obtain a solution suitable for chromatography. This step increased the specific activity (7.8) fold with a yield of 67.1% (Table 3-1).

The intermediate step in peroxidase purification protocol is ion exchange when partially purified peroxidase obtained by ammonium sulphate fractionation applied on DEAE-cellulose, the column was wash with starting buffer to elute the unabsorbed protein. These fractions represent protein with no net charge or a net charge of same sign as the DEAE–cellulose pass through the column, unretained at pH 8 (under experimental conditions). The result indicated the highest peroxidase specific activity was in wash fractions. Selected fractions containing most of peroxidase activity were collected pooled, dialyzed against distilled water at 4°C then concentrated.

Reasons for choosing DEAE-cellulose ion exchange chromatography as intermediate purification stage include its:

Chapter Three

1. To isolate basic peroxidase from the acidic peroxidase and other peroxidase form which are absorbed to DEAE-cellulose under experimental conditions.
2. To remove negatively charged contaminating proteins, which are absorbed to DEAE-cellulose under experi-mental conditions.
3. To prepare a suitable solution for next experiment.
4. Further more, the results of many investigation[169] has been shown that basic peroxidase contained 75% of the original peroxidase present in some sources of plant such as root of red and white radish.
5. Ease of performance.

In general the purification of basic peroxidase isoenzyme on DEAE-celluose ion exchange showed 21.7 fold with 51% yield, the purity of isolation peroxidase was analyzed and confirmed by conventional poly acryl amide gel electrophoresis by peroxidase activity assay and coomasie blue stain as marker for detection peroxidase Figure (3-1-B).

The purpose of the final step purification (gel filtration on sephacryl S-300 column) was to remove aggregation, degradation product and prepare purified peroxidase enzyme suitable for direct application.

The elution pattern of this experiment revealed as shown in figure (3-1-A) an asymmetrical peak containing peroxidase activity, represent finally purified peroxidase (basic isoenzyme).

In general this step of purification has shown 28 fold of purification with 44.3% yield. These results of purification protocol were summarized in table (3-1), and indicated that each step in the process contributed significantly to final peroxidase enzyme. The use of gel filtration as final step provided good resolution and yield.

Chapter Three

Generally the purification of white radish peroxidase enzyme by this simple method may lower the cost very significantly. More over, the peroxidase purified in this way will have higher specfic activities than the commercial preparation, which has direct impact on the final enzyme immunoassay.

3-10-2 Antibody productions

During the past two decades there has been a tremendous increase in the realization of utility of antibodies directed against tumor marker as tools in biochemical studies[131,141,146]. Antibodies against tumor marker can be used.

1. To detect and assay quantitatively the concentration of tumor marker.
2. To concentrate and purify tumor marker from dilute solutions and mixtures.
3. To study the multimolecular forms, and conformational structures of tumor marker.
4. To localize tumor marker in sectioned cell.
5. To study the appearance and modification of tumor marker in the course of embryonic and phylogenetic development. Concomitantly in immunology there has been increasing knowledge concerning the many factors that can influence the multifaceted and complex sequence of events of the immune rsponse beginning with the introduction of an antigen into a host to the formation of humoral antibody.

3-10-2-1 The choice of animal species

The more common animals used for immunization are rabbits, goats, sheep, chickens, horses, guinea pigs, and mice[173]. The eventual goals of having antibody against a specific protein or polypeptide may determine the specific species for immunization. Important

Chapter Three

Generally the purification of white radish peroxidase enzyme by this simple method may lower the cost very significantly. More over, the peroxidase purified in this way will have higher specfic activities than the commercial preparation, which has direct impact on the final enzyme immunoassay.

3-10-2 Antibody productions

During the past two decades there has been a tremendous increase in the realization of utility of antibodies directed against tumor marker as tools in biochemical studies[131,141,146]. Antibodies against tumor marker can be used.

1. To detect and assay quantitatively the concentration of tumor marker.
2. To concentrate and purify tumor marker from dilute solutions and mixtures.
3. To study the multimolecular forms, and conformational structures of tumor marker.
4. To localize tumor marker in sectioned cell.
5. To study the appearance and modification of tumor marker in the course of embryonic and phylogenetic development. Concomitantly in immunology three has been increasing knowledge concerning the many factors that can influence the multifaceted and complex sequence of events of the immune rsponse beginning with the introduction of an antigen into a host to the formation of humoral antibody.

3-10-2-1 The choice of animal species

The more common animals used for immunization are rabbits, goats, sheep, chickens, horses, guinea pigs, and mice[173]. The eventual goals of having antibody against a specific protein or polypeptide may determine the specific species for immunization. Important considerations in choosing species are the source and availability of the immunogen. As might be expected the larger animals require more antigen for the production of antibody, but upon respond can yield more serum than others. Ordinarily one cannot obtain large amounts of serum from repeated bleedings of mice. However, there are few instances in which categorical evidence has shown one species of common laboratory animal to give consistently better responses than another to any particular immunogen[170-174].

There is little doubt that rabbits should be the first choice for most purposes unless very large amounts of serum are needed. Rabbits are cheap, easy to care for, robust in the face of quite intensive immunization, and easy to bleed. All animals were remaining under immunization for many months, they were kept clean, healthy and well fed.

3-10-2-2 The route of injection

For soluble immunogens, it is generally believed that the efficiency of stimulation of the immune response is related to the site of inoculation. A probable series, in order of increasing effect, is intravenous < intramuscular < subcutaneous < intraperitoneal < intradermal < intraarticular < intranodal. The principal reasons for the differences in efficiency are the speed with which antigen is lost from the site of injection and the likelihood of it passing through the lymph nodes or other centers of immunological activity on the way. These considerations, however, are radically affected by the use of adjuvants, especially oily adjuvants, which may stimulate a brisk local cellular reaction and release antigen over a period of several weeks or even months.

Using oily adjuvants, then, the injection site can be chosen principally with a view to minimizing discomfort to the animal. Generally

Chapter Three

this means intramuscular injections in rabbits or subcutaneous injections in guinea pigs; note that water in oil emulsions must never be given intravenously because of the virtual certainty of fatal fat embolism. Subcutaneous or intradermal injection of Freund's emulsions almost invariably leads to ulceration, but provided the sites are well chosen rabbits and guinea pigs show no sign of distress or loss of condition.

Difficulties in preparing antisera against some of the antigens of interest in immunoassay have led people to try a wide variety of methods of immunization. Most of these variations have been irrational (which does not mean to say they have not worked on occasion), but two deserve special mention. By injection of immunogen (angiotensin I, adsorbed on carbon black and emulsified in Freund's adjuvant) directly into rabbit lymph nodes and spleen, Boyd and Peart[180] obtained improved results that they believed to be due to more direct stimulation of the immune system. A subsequent comparative trial gave rather equivocal results[181], however, and the method was too difficult to be widely used. Injection into the Peyer's patches (lymphoid patches in the intestinal wall, quite easily visible in the rabbit) is technically much simpler but has proved no more successful in some investigators[170,181].

Much simpler than the intranodal method, and now quite widely used, is the method of multiple intradermal inoculation introduced by Vaitukaitis et al.[182] The immunogen is introduced at 40 or more sites spread widely over the body surface. Antibody response to this primary immunization is much greater than to a first infection given in the usual way, and pore than one booster injection is usually required. Comparison with the usual intramuscular injection schedule showed no great difference in fficiency, although the multiple intradermal technique (with only one booster) required rather less immunogen and yielded effective antisera in shorter period of time.

Chapter Three

Since most sensitive immunoassay techniques of current interest rely on antibody of the highest possible avidity, it is evidently desirable (and economical of immunogen) to use the lowest dose that will be fully effective. This dose is very much smaller than most of the published literature recognizes, and a suitable priming (first) inoculation for rabbits or guinea pigs will generally be of the order of 100 µg. A range of 50-1000 µg should cover all needs, depending on the purity and immunogenicity of the material in question (but it is sensible to start at the lower end, since an animal showing lack of response after a sufficiently long trial can then be given a larger dose, whereas an animal producing poor anti-serum after high dosage is beyond hope of salvage). The dosage required for larger animals does not increase in proportion to body weight: 0.25-5 mg is satisfactory for sheep and 0.5-10 mg for donkeys. For conjugated happens, incidentally, these figures refer to total conjugate weight.

Booster injections are always needed to obtain antisera of the highest titer and avidity. Practical experience suggests that good results will be obtained using a booster dose about half the size of an effective priming dose, given by the same route (not necessarily at the same site) and using Freund's complete adjuvant on each occasion. It is recognized that these recommendations are somewhat at variance both with immunological theory (which would suggest a progressive increase in dose) and with the advice of other authors to avoid repeated use of Freund's complete adjuvant, especially subcutaneously, because of abscess formation and hypersensitivity reactions. There is some documented evidence in support of the suggested reduction in dose,[1] but the repeated use of complete Freund's adjuvant is a recommendation that stems only from satisfactory, albeit uncontrolled, experience.

The repeated booster doses that is usually required for the best antiserum should not be given too frequently. It has been shown[180,181] that no further rise in titer results from a second injection given before the response to the first is reaching its peak. At least 4 weeks should pass between injections of Freund's emulsions. After the first booster, or sometimes after the second, antibody response may be quite prolonged and many people believe that a rest of 3-6 months is desirable before the next injection if antiserum of the highest avidity is required; the evidence in favor of this approach is not strong. Although short immunization courses for particulate antigens are the rule, usually in the belief that antisera will become less specific as immu-proceeds, this is not necessarily the case. Prolonged immunization on may result in more stable IgG antibody of higher titer and, because of repeated bleeding over a period of time, in much greater yield.

3-10-2-3 Collection and storage of immune serum[180-183]

Animals immunized with Freund's emulsions should be bled 7-10 days after booster injections. If the blood is taken from a vein rather than by cardiac puncture, two or three bleeds can be taken on successive days, but the animal should then be rested for 3-4 weeks before further bleeding or before boosting again if the original antiserum was not of satisfactory quality.

Blood should be collected in clean, dry, glass bottles and allowed to clot at room temperature or at 37° until the clot has retracted; it may help to "ring" the clot with a glass rod to promote separation. The sample should then be centrifuged and the serum be separated without undue delay in order to avoid unnecessary hemolysis, which looks unaesthetic

After separation from the clot, antiserum may be stored without significant deterioration for long periods of time with 0.1% sodium azaide

Chapter Three

added as an antibacterial agent

Antisera to be used in capillary precipitin tests must be crystal clear so that the faint ring of precipitation can be easily seen. Untreated sera become turbid on storage, due to precipitation of denatured lipoprotein; such precipitates can be removed by membrane filtration prior to use, but it is usually, better to reduce the severity of the problem by extracting the bluk of the lipoprotein at the time the serum is first prepared.

3-10-2-4 Isolation and characterization of anti –CEA

Antibodies against CEA developed 4 weeks after the strate of rabbits and guinea pig immunization. The simple double- diffusion analysis depicted in figure (3-2) suffice for detection of specific antibodies to CEA in the an antisera. This technique as seen in figure (3-2) serves to detect the presence of precipitating antibodies to CEA.

EIA technique cannot be used with whole antiserum as this markedly inhibits CEA binding in nonspecific way[181]. Consequently specific antibody must be extracted and the method must be suitable for use with relatively large number of samples.

Anti-CEA was isolated and purified from other immunoglobuline subclasses and some serum proteins by ammonium sulfate precipitation at 41% saturation and DEAE- cellulose ion exchange chromatography. This techniques found to be most satisfactory, the anti-CEA was found to be free of high and low molecular weight contaminants and migrate as gamm globulins on cellulose acetate electro-phoresis, as shown in figure (3-3). This material designated pure specific anti-CEA was also found to be free of contaming protein as determined by immunoelectrophoresis figure(3-4)

The main characteristic of immunoelectrophoresis technique is its ability to give a dual characterization of antigenic material that is with regard to both electrophoretic and serological properties as in the double diffusion in gel technique.

During immunoelectrophoresis at pH 8.3 on glass slides, two precipitin arcs formed between the purified CEA and each preparation of anti-CEA figure(3-4), thus indicating that the complex (antigen –antibody) are homogeneous and free of crossreacting.

When the rabbits anti CEA and guinea pig anti-CEA compar by double diffusion technique., as seen in figure (3-5) illustrates that comparison of two anti-CEA with same multideterminanet antigen molecule (CEA molecule) resulted in complete fusion of the precipitate even when the specificity of anti–CEA differ on determinant level., Further more antigenic determinant are small parts of the surface structure of CEA[21,22] the observation of complete fusion even if it is constanitly obtained with many different antisera.

From this study the current information about the biochemical and immunochemical characteristic of CEA is bases on result obtained with anti-CEA material. The results of this also doubt about the use of antiserume to purify CEA for the immunoassay of the human CEA.

3-10-3 Enzyme antibody conjugate

3-10-3-1 Types and Mechanism of coupling

Although a varity of methods can be used for coupling enzyme to antibody[182-185], the conjugated procedures most commonly used with peroxidase were the two-stage glutaraldehyde[185] and periodate oxidation[182] methods. In the former procedure peroxidase was first mixed with an excess of the dialdehyde glutaraldehyde, which reacts with free amino groups of the enzyme via only one of its active aldehyde groups, The second aldehyde was unable to react with the same or other peroxidase molecules. This may be due to blockage of the majority of the amino group of the enzyme by allisothiocyanate which occure in white

Chapter Three

and red radish[186]. After gel filtration chromatography to remove excess glutaral-dehyde, the activated enzyme is mixed with the immuno-globulin preparation to allow the free aldehyde group to combine with an amino group of the immuno globulin. The reaction scheme is illustrated in figure (3-6):

Step one

$$Enzyme - NH_2 + CHO.CH_2.CH_2.CH_2.CHO$$
$$\downarrow$$
$$Enzyme - N + CH.CH_2.CH_2.CH_2.CHO$$

(Remove excess glutaraldehyde)

Step two

$$Enzyme - N + CH.CH_2.CH_2.CH_2.CHO + NH_2 - Antibody$$
$$\downarrow$$
$$Enzyme - N + CH.CH_2.CH_2.CH_2.CH = N - Antibody$$

Figure (3-6): Enzyme-antibody coupling by the two-step glutaraldehyde procedure.

The peroxidase –anti CEA preparation was precipitated at 4° with an equal volume of saturated neutral $(NH_4)_2SO_4$ solution, the purpose of this step is to remove free enzyme.

The conjugated prepared in this way had molecular weight of approximately 210,000 indicating that it was composed of on peroxidase and one antibody molecule[185,186]. Sephacryl S-300 chromatography of the reaction mixture revealed three peaks the largest fraction appears in void volume, and atrail of low molecular weight multimer and free antibody. The void-volume fractions (22-27 in fig 3-7) are pooled, and the preparation was found to exhibt high levels of peroxidase activities. Also, the preparation was appropriate for immunoassay studies.

The limited data available indicate that, the use of labels prepared

Chapter Three

by the two step methods lead to an increase in assay sensitivity over assays using labels prepared by the one step method. The reason was that peroxidase has few free amino groups available for reaction with glutaraldehyde, whereas IgG has many, if peroxidase and IgG are incubated together with glutaraldehyde, IgG will effectively compete with peroxidase for available GDA, leading to extensive intermolecular cross-linking of IgG with little coupling of peroxidase.

Conjugates prepared in two step method have been shown to contain a homogeneous derivative[16,185,186] with a molecular weight of 90,000, but the coupling efficiency is poor at around 25% and 5% for antibody and enzyme, respectively[169,185,186]. The low efficiency in this system appears to be due to the relative paucity of reactive amino groups in peroxidase. In contrast the periodate oxidation method of conjugation[184] is not dependent on the presence of reactive amino groups but relies upon the generation of active aldehyde groups after periodate oxidation of the carbohydrate moiety of peroxidase. These aldehyde groups combine with the amino groups of added immuno-globulin to form Schiff bases, which are subsequently stabilized by reduction with sodium borohydride. Conjugates prepared by this procedure contain high molecular weight derivatives[168,169,185], but the coupling efficiency is increased to approximately 60% for both antibody and enzyme[168,169,184,185].

Recent studies using a modification of the method described by Kato et al.[188] have shown that peroxidase can be satisfactorily coupled to antibody by coupling via sulfhydryl groups introduced into both the immunoglobulin and enzyme structures[186-188]. Conjugates prepared in this way contain active derivatives that are heterogeneous in relation to molecular weight but retain good enzyme and antibody activity[188].

Owing to their simplicity and sensitivity, enzyme-linked

Chapter Three

immunoadsorbent assay (ELISA) type assays are becoming established as the method of choice for screening for antigens derived from, and antibodies directed against, microorganisms. Enzymeantibody conjugates are also used in immunohistochemistry, as cytotoxic agents directed against tumor cells and for the detection of specific antibodies in cell cultures.

The first application of an enzyme-antibody conjugate in an immunoassay was reported in 1972. Since that year additional techniques for conjugating a variety of enzymes to antibodies have been developed. Unfortunately, little attempt has been made to standardize enzyme-antibody conjugates. Very few comparisons have been made of the merits of different enzymes and different cross-linking procedures. The actual composition of most enzyme labels has not been reported. Few authors report the efficiency of the coupling reactions; where they do, the results often vary widely even when the same cross-linking method is used. The ideal conjugation method should be technically undemanding; affect neither the enzyme nor antibody activity; efficiently couple both the enzyme and antibody; minimize competing side reactions leading to the formation of enzyme-enzyme or antibody-antibody conjugates; not polymerize the conjugate; be flexible and controllable, so that the composition of the label can be tailored for each particular application; lead to the formation of a homogeneous conjugate.

3-10-3-2 Choice of enzyme

The criteria governing the choice of enzyme were listed in following

1. Availability of low-cost purified homogeneous enzyme preparations
2. High specific activity or turnover number
3. Presence of reactive residues through which the enzyme can be cross-linked to other molecules with minimal loss of either enzyme

or antibody activity
4. Capability of producing stable conjugates
5. Enzyme absent from biological fluids
6. Assay method that is simple, cheap, sensitive, precise, and not affected by factors present in biological fluids.
7. Enzyme, substrate, cofactors, etc., should not pose a potential health hazard.

Few, if any, enzymes completely meet all these requirements. Alkaline phosphatase, horseradish peroxidase (HRP), and β-D-galactosidase are the most widely used enzymes. This does not imply that these enzymes are ideal, but only that they are the most satisfactory enzymes currently employed. Relatively few enzymes have been evaluated as labels, and it is certainly possible that superior enzymes remain to be utilized.

The data presented indicate that the white and red radish roots can serve as source of peroxidase, which are useful in structural and perhaps functional studies for immunoassay study the choice of peroxidase used in this study, in so far as their source is concerned, was based on availability.

3-10-4 Preparation of antibody coated –polypropylene tubes

Immobilization of antibodies on plastics is primarily of interest because of the usefulness of immunoassays based on agglutination of antibody-coated latex (polystyrene) beads, and because of the observation by Catt and Tregear that antibodies adsorbed to polystyrene or polypropylene tubes could be used for solid-phase radioimmunoassay. The development of solid-phase enzyme immunoassays utilizing antibodies immobilized on plastics has further increased this interest. Antibodies immobilized on plastics have also been used in a variety of ways as immunosorbents. In the broadest definition, plastics could

Chapter Three

include a wide range of polymeric materials; for our purposes here, the discussion will be limited to thermoplastics, molded in the form of beads, plates, or tubes. Although an extensive body of literature has evolved on the practical application of these plastics for use in immunoassays, relatively few quantitative studies have been done on antibody immobilization.

3-10-4-1 Mechanism of antibody coated tube:

Methods for immobilization have been for the most part based on simple adsorption of antibody to plastic surfaces, a phenomenon that most authors attribute to hydrophobic bonding. Immobilization of antibody by covalent linkage to a plastic surface has also been done.

Despite the widespread interest and application of the technique of coating antibodies onto plastic surfaces the mechanism by which this noncovalent attachment occurs has been investigated by only a few workers and is consequently understood best as a phenomenological process proteins in aqueous solution exposed to plastic surfaces tend to adhere to the surface in an extremely tenacious manner and to retain some of their biological activity. Catt's early work examined the effects of temperature, pH, and ionic strength on the coating of antibodies on plastic surfaces but found no dramatic effect on the amount of antibody that could be coated. Mishell et al. examined the effect of various parameters on the coating of antibodies on polypropylene disks and also found relatively little dependence on pH and ionic strength, but noted some dependence on temperature with more and faster coating occurring at higher temperatures.

At Clinical Assays many researcher[189,190] have examined the coating properties of many different antisera. These have shown a similar lack of dramatic effects of pH and ionic strength on antibody coatability. Other researcher[192] have shown, however, that, once an

Chapter Three

antibody is coated on a plastic surface, it is extremely difficult to remove all absorbed protein completely from the surface. Oxidizing agents, reducing agents, chaotropic agents, detergents, alcoholic potassium hydroxide, mineral and organic acids, and some organic solvents may destroy the immunological properties of antibodies coated on a plastic surface, but they will not remove the destroyed protein. The only treatment in our experience capable of totally removing the degraded protein from the plastic surface is boiling in an aqueous solution for at least 15 mim.

The studies of Pesce et al.[195] provided for the first time a quantitative measure of the amount of antibody exposed to a plastic surface that actually became attached to it. It had been recognized for some time that antibody coating solutions could actually be used several times to coat several new plastic surfaces with apparently little or no depletions. Pesce and his co-workers showed that the saturation limit of 1 cm^2 of plastic surface was about 1 µg of protein and that below the saturation limit the amount of antibody adsorbed to the surface was proportional to the amount of protein in the coating solution. Morrisey and his co-workers investigated the general problem of plasma proteins interacting with plastic surfaces by physical means and arrived at the conclusion that most plasma proteins had about the same ability to interact with plastic, except for fibrinogen, which seemed to be unique in its ability to actually displace previously coated proteins. The general mechanism of coating proposed by these authors was the one most often accepted by researchers in the field; that was, the antibodies adhere to the plastic surfaces by nonspecific hydrophobic interactions.

The most recent contribution to our understanding of the interactions of proteins and plastic was provided by Cantarero[197], who studied a series of proteins ranging form lactalbumin to bovine γ-M and found coating behavior to be substantially independent of molecular weight. By a clever combination of radiolabeling experiments and immunoenzymic measurements, he was able to demonstrate that certain proteins can "stack" on top of proteins previously coated on a plastic surface. He was also able to show slight differences between the coating abilities of bovine γ-globulin subclasses 1 and 2. These observations may provide explanations for the variability that sometimes plagues experimenters trying to make reproducible tubes[196,17].

Kato and his worker[188] have developed method of pretreating plastic tubes with glutaraldehude in attempt to bind the antibody covalently to the plastic tube. The purpose of this step was to provide a more controllable and higher capacity coating process than the simple buffer coaing would allow. This technique consists basically of prewashing the plastic tube first with a solution of long-chain aliphatic primary amine or diamine.

The hydrocarbon tail of the plastic surface and provide reactive amino functions for the next reactive step. Also the glutaraldehyde treatment probably does not put more antibodies on the tube, but permits a large proportion of coated antibody molecules to retain their ability to bind antigen despite the effects of powerful interactions with the tube surface.

3-10-4-2 Tube selections

Perhaps the single most critical reagent in the preparation of antibody-coated tubes is the raw plastic tube itself. The safest course for an individual researcher to follow is to deal with a large reputable manufacturer of plastic tubes and to try to stockpile a particular lot of raw plastic tubes that will be large enough to maintain continuity in the assay project. The only guide as to which tubes to select remains at this point a very empirical one. The antiserum to be coated must be tried with the tubes under consideration for selection. That combination of tube and antibody that gives the best curve shape, reproducibility, and stability should be selected. It should be noted that the investigator have occasionally found that while one rabbit antibody coats satisfactorily on a particular lot of plastic tubes, another rabbit antibody may not give satisfactory results under the same conditions. The most conservative approach is to treat tube and antibody as an interactive whole, taking neither reagent for granted.

Polypropylene tubes are most commonly used in commercial coated tube kits. They are favored over polystyrene tubes because they are more easily handled with automatic filling equipment and are less susceptible to breakage in shipping. Experiments in our laboratories have shown little difference in antibody coatability between polypropylene and polystyrene[12]. Similarly extensive attempts to find differences in coatability between uncolored and polypropylene with various color additives have met with no success. Researchers making more than one type of antibody-coated tube may want to consider using different colored tubes to minimize the chance for confusion and wasted experiments.

While most of our experience was with round-bottom 12 x 50 mm tubes, most of what we have found for tubes probably holds true for other types of plastic surfaces. Such diverse have coated commercially available surfaces as round-bottom test tubes, conical centrifuge tubes, microfuge tubes, plastic scintillation vials, and plastic balls of various sizes and materials.

The advantages of the coated-tube immunoassay in general stem from the extreme simplicity of the method. Misclassification errors in separation of bound and free that could arise from tracer breakdown or in vivo use of radiopharmaceuticals have no effect on the system. Only tracer material that is recognizable by the antibody is counted in the bound fraction. Thus, the antibody specificity that generally allows for the assay of specific compounds in complex mixtures also minimizes problems that may be serious in other separation systems.

3-10-5 Nonspecific absorbents measurement and other factors interfering with the binding of CEA to anti-CEA

Nonspecific binding is another problem common to double antibody and nonspecific precipitation separation techniques and arises from entement adsorption of free tracer to the bound fraction. Since the bound fraction in the antibody-coated tube system is probably only one antibody molecule thick, entrapment is not a problem in coated tubes. Adsorptior of tracer to plastic surfaces can occur, but washing the antibody-coated tube prior to use with a buffer containing a protein such as gelatin or bovine serum albumin (BSA) will fill up uncoated plastic sites and render hydrophobic tracer less likely to stick. It is also advisable to add such carrier proteins to tracer solutions to minimize tracer loss to plastic pipette tips and to the surfaces of storage containers.

The measurement of nonspecific binding (NSB) in coated-tube systems can be done in one of two ways. The simplest is to add the tracer in question to a tube coated with antibody to another molecule to which cross-reactivity is less than 0.1%. We have found, for example, that despite the observation that cold T_3 cross-reacts in our T_4 tubes at only 3%, substantial binding of tracer amounts of T_3 tracer occurs in the absence of T_4 to compete for binding sites. Alternatively, a gelatin or BSA-coated tube may be used.

The other method of measuring NSB is to add over-whelming amounts of cold inhibitor into the assay tube. This approach may be simpler for those laboratories that are evaluating commercial coated-tube kits.

The elimination of centrifugation is one of the foremost advantages of using antibody-coated tubes. This results in considerably fewer experimental variables with which the assayist must deal. Variable decanting techniques and carry-over of precipitates are also done away with.

A coated tube separation of bound and free is accomplished by simple aspiration or decantation. For small assays a Pasteur pipette or large plastic pipette tip attached to a trap and water aspirator suffices as an aspiration device. For larger assays and greater throughput we have devised multiheaded aspirators that will aspirate 12-14 tubes at a time. This apparatus usually requires a mechanical vacuum pump system to provide sufficient suction. A repeated attempt to affect tube-to-tube variability by scraping the antibody-coated surface with glass or plastic pipette tips has shown little or no effect. These results suggest the area swept by a pipette tip is too small in comparison to the total area to grossly affect the results.

Caution should be exercised, however, in attempting to wipe an antibody-coated tube with a large surface area material such as a cotton tip applicator or folded filter paper strips. We have observed removal of counts in a highly variable manner when a misguided attempt was made to improve tube-to-tube replication by wiping tubes after aspiration. Subsequent experience has shown that when tubes are uniformly aspirated, no further treatment is required to attain coefficients of variation approaching counting error.

Decanting tubes rather than aspirating has proved to be a popular, low capital investment approach to separating bound and free. Reproducibity is improved if the rim of the tube is blotted on paper toweling prior counting covalent linkage to a plastic surface has also been done.

3-10-6 Maximum binding capacity of antibody to polypropylene tube

A simple method for quantitating antibody immobilized on plastics was to measure removal of protein from the adsorbing or coupling solution. This can be done by determining protein absorption at 280 nm or by the Lowry technique. However, this approach does not allow for desorption of loosely bound antibody and cannot be used to measure immobilization of a given antibody in the presence of other proteins, as would occur if antibody were being immobilized from whole serum. For purified antibodies, the Lowry method of protein determination can be used to measure immobilized antibodies on a plastic surface, as described by Kondorosi et al.[192] for measuring IgG adsorbed to polymethylmetaacrylic beads: following adsorption with antibody, the beads are washed 10 times with 0.05 M sodium phosphate buffer, pH 8.0, to remove unadsorbed protein, the beads are treated with 0.2N NaOH for 15 min to elute bound protein, and the amount eluted is determined by the Lowry method. Measurement of amino acid content after acid hydrolysis has been used to determine antibody bound to agarose and porous glass and could also be used to measure antibody immobilization on some plastics.

Quantitative studies on antibody binding to plastics have been done both with purified antibodies and whole serum. For binding by simple adsorption, all the plastics reported to date show binding, although there were quantitative differences. The data presented in Table (3-2) show that binding of rabbit IgG, after 1 hr at room temperature or 37°C, to all types of plastics occurred, and that the percentage bound decreased with increasing IgG concen-tration. There were some differences in the two studies cited in regard to adsorption of IgG to cellulose nitrate, which may be attributable to different buffers used for adsorption.[9] The polyethylene tubes used (Minisorp, NUNC, Roskilde, Denmark), which have a low surface energy and were designed to prevent blood clot adhesion in serum collection, still showed considerable binding of antibody. Both studies showed approximately the same percentage of binding of rabbit IgG at 100 or 200 µg/ml to polystyrene, the plastic most often used for solid-phase immunoassays, and the percentage of adsorption at 1 and 10 µg/ml was approximately the same as that found by Engvall et al.[198] for adsorption of sheep IgG to polystyrene. The duration of coating also influences the amount of antibody immobilized. Increasing the adsorption time from 1 hr at room temperature Table (3-2) to 18 hr increased the adsorption to polystyrene tubes of rabbit IgG at 100, 10, and 1 µg/ml to 11.7, 65.1, and 91.8%, respectively.

Because most solid-phase immunoassays based on antibody adsorption to plastic use polystyrene as the solid-phase carrier, the majority of quantitative studies have used this plastic. A composite of studies designed to show adsorption of IgG to polystyrene as a function of IgG concentration is illustrated in Figure (3-8) All used polystyrene tubes (Falcon Plastic tubes, 2 mm x 75 mm) except for one study, which used 11 mm x 70 mm NUNC polystyrene tubes, so that the available surface area for adsorption was approximately the same. It can be seen from the figure that the results obtained by different investigators using different immunoglobulins, adsorbing buffers, and incubation temperatures were very similar. It can also be concluded that adsorption of antibody to these tubes is linear wiith concentration up to 1 µg/ml; concentrations of IgG above this level adsorbed to a lesser degree, as was found for other types of plastics as well Table (3-2).

Chapter Three

If IgG is diluted in whole serum, which contains proteins that compete for binding sites on the plastic surface, adsorption still occurs. However, the adsorption is only linear with concentration up to a 100 ng/ml concentration and the percentage bound at high concentrations (≥10 µg/ml) was markedly reduced, giving values of approximately 5% adsorption at IgG input of 10 µg/ml[192-194].

The studies cited above show that there were a limited number of antibody binding sites on polystyrene and other plastics and that increasing the concentration of antibody in adsorbing solutions above 1-10 µg/ml does not give a linear increase in antibody bound. This may be due to saturation of binding sites or limitations in the total surface area available for binding. The maximum amount of immunoglobulin (Ig) that can be bound by adsorption is shown in Table (3-3). The concentration of Ig in the adsorbing solutions was not given in all the references cited, but when given, were at levels of 100 µg/ml or higher. The data presented in the original sources were converted to nanograms of Ig bound per square millimeter of surface area of plastic in order to compare data. It can be seen that the amounts adsorbed to polystyrene, whether in the form of tubes or microspheres (latex particles), were in a similar range; the value for polymethylmetaacrylic beads was lower.

Increasing the amount of antibody bound to a plastic surface should give a corresponding increase in the sensitivity of a solid-phase immunoassay. However, it has been noted in some of the references cited here, and in others as well, that increasing the concentration of antibody in absorbing solutions beyond a level of 10 µg/ml does not give an increase in immunoassay sensitivity. This was apparently due to desorption of antibody from the plastic surface, which is greater at higher antibody concentrations, or it may be due to steric hindrance caused by aggregated or closely packed antibodies. To alleviate this problem, covalent linkage of antibody to polypropylene tube were used to increase the amount of antibody effectively. In the three examples of covalent linkage shown in Table (3-3), the amount of IgG that could be immobilized by covalent coupling to polystyrene or polypropylene was far greater than that which could be obtained by adsorption to polystyrene. The increased level of IgG binding on polypropylene was also reflected in the sensitivity of an immunoassay done with these beads, but the increase was not proportional to the amount bound: approximately 30 times as much antibody could be immobilized on nylon beads as on polystyrene beads of the same diameter (3.2 mm), which resulted in a 10-fold increase in sensitivity for detection of serum IgG by an enzyme-linked immunoassay.

It can be concluded from the studies presented here that IgG from a variety of species can be immobilized on several types of plastics, and that the amount of antibody that can be adsorbed to polypropylene is not highly dependent on the antibody source, the conditions used for adsorption, or the form of polypropylene used. An increase in the amount of antibody bound per unit surface area of plastic can be achieved by covalent linkage, but further studies are needed to determine whether this increase results in increased sensitivity of immunoassay for various antigens.

3-10-7 Assay condition results:

A schematic representation of non competitive method was shown in figure (3-9) as seen in that figure, immobilized antibody in excess was incubated with standard or test antigen after washing, the immobilized antibody- antigen complex was incubated with an excess of enzyme- labeled antibody which bind to one or more remaining antigen sites[106,187]. The concentration of the product from the enzyme reaction was directly proportional to the concentration of stander or test antigen.

Chapter Three

To design an assay with optimal sensitivity, it was essential to:

a. Choose an antiserum of highest possible affinity.

b. Use incubation times that allow equilibrium between antigen and antibody.

c. Use lower concentrations of antigen and antibody and longer time for color development.

d. Determination of nonspecific binding.

It is desirable to include a set of blank tubes in each assay; containing antigen and buffer (dilute in same way as in sample) these tubes are processed just as if antibody were present and provide a measure of the nonspecific binding blank. It should be kept in mind that nonspecific sticking may be different in buffer than it was tissue or native serum.

3-10-7-1 Effect of CEA concentration:

Different concentrations of CEA were used for binding to polypropylene coated tubes. In figure (3-10-a) the result obtained using 0.03-1 µg of CEA depicted. A suitable binding capacity was obtained when 0.1 µg or more of CEA were present. Also figure (3-9-a) shows that any CEA concen-tration below 100 ng/ml was given a measurable response. Since it was likely that 100 ng/ml or more was sufficient to saturate all antibody site.

The adsorption process, unlike antigenantibody interaction, is non specific, thus, during the first incubation of immobilized antibody (coated tube) with antigen and with enzyme labeled antibody in second incubation, the latter binds specifically to immobilized immune reactant, but may also be adsorbed directly on to the solid phase. This nonspecific adsorption of enzyme activity can be minimized by inclusion of a nonionic detergent such as Tween-20. This did not interfere with antigen–antibody reaction but prevent formation of new hydrophobic interaction between added proteins and solid phase without disrupting to any appreciable extent the hydrophobic bond already formed between the previously adsorbed protein and plastic surface. Nonspecific of peroxidase label to rabbit anti CEA was very low, usually < 3% of maximum activity bound (100 %) as determined by a blank tube (uncoated tube) as shown in figure (3-10-a).

In all subsequent experiment, 0.1 µg of CEA in the incubation mixture was used. This is minimal quantity of CEA giving the desired level of binding.

3-10-7-2 Effect of rabbit anti- CEA conjugate peroxides (PRA)

The effect of different volume of anti- CEA labeled with peroxides (50-250 µl / tube, keeping the incubation volume constant) on the assay procedure for the assay of CEA was investigated. A volume of 200 µl was found to be convenient, as it gives sufficient binding even with very short binding time as shown in figure (3-10-B).

Also figure (3-10-b) reveals that PRA binding capacity is very high. This means that with the specific assay condition, the PRA binds to antigen binding site.

The advantage of this techniques is the possibility of binding several enzyme labeled antibody molecules to a single polyvalent antigen molecule (CEA), thus providing an element of amplification. This may be an advantage in procedures in which the spectrophotometeric system for assay of lower concentration of antigen.

For further assays, (PRA) a conjugate of 200 µl was chosen.

3-10-7-3 Effect of temperature:

The influence of temperature on the antige- antibody reaction varies with the antibody and incubation condition. In general, the K_a increases as the temperature was lowered, and antigen binding was maximal at or near 4C, provided that equilibrium is reached figure (3-10-c).

The relationship between K_a and temperature can be described mathematically by equation

$$\Delta F° = \Delta H° - T\Delta S°$$

Where $\Delta H°$ and $\Delta S°$ represent the enthalpy and entropy contribute contributions to binding, respectively, T is the absolute temperature, and $\Delta F°$ is the standard free energy of binding. ΔH was usually negative, a reflection of decreased binding at increased temperature. The effect of temperature on the specific binding was given in figure (3-10-c) the binding, of antigen (CEA) by antibody was maximal at 4°C and at other temperature lower than 30°C the binding of CEA by anti-CEA antibody is normally improved at low temperature, but only under equilibrium condition. The approach to equilibrium was slowed because of the decreased frequency of collision between CEA and anti CEA, for this reason, many immunoassays utilize a preliemnary incubation at ambient temperature, follow by longer period of incubation at low temperature in immunoassays involving large molecular weight protein antigen, an initial 60- minute incubation at 37°C may shorten the overall time requirement in the assay by as 24 to 48 hours. The use of incubation temperature above 37°C is undesirable because of the danger of protein denaturation. In view of these results the optimal temperature incubation in all experiment were adjusted at 10°C.

3-10-7-4 Effect of time:

The time required for the first and the second incubation has to be established. The first incubation is run for 0.25-24 hr, and keeping the second incubation constant (24 hr). As can be seen in figure (3-10-d-1), the reaction is very fast, and plateau values were reached within 2-3 hr at all CEA level tested.

Chapter Three

The first incubation period can now be kept constant (2 hr) and the second on varied. During the first 3 hr three was a rapid increase in specific binding, there after a slower increase take place figure (3-10-d-2). This slow increase is still observable after 24 hr. 3 hr incubation, is selected as a suitable time for the second incubation step. This suggests that shorter incubation times improve assay sensitivity, longer period of incubation were unsuitable because of the danger of antibody or enzyme denaturation and irreversible dissociation of antibody-antigen complex.

3-10-7-5 Effect of pH:

The analysis of the influence of pH on the specific binding of CEA molecule is illustrated in figure (3-10-e). The pH has little effect on CEA binding over a wide range (pH 5.7 -8) tested. This result was consistent with the idea that CEA interaction with antibody was hydrophobic interaction.

3-10-7-6 Influence of ionic strength:

The specific binding of CEA to antibody were reported to be enhanced when the ionic strength of the assay condition were reduced (3-10-f). Suggesting that the bonds primarily involved in the binding reaction were ionic in nature. However, specific binding were measured with virtually unaffected sensitivity when different concentration of phosphate buffer range(0.001-1 M) and distilled water, no significant difference in specific binding was observed between the estimates obtained from the different dilutions, as shown in figure (3-10-f). In view of these results, the phosphate buffer concentration in all experiments was adjusted at 0.05 M.

3-10-8 The standard curve:

A standard curve was included in every assay. It helps provide for the spontaneous variations seen in the assay from day to day. It was also a means of detecting deterioration of the stander antigen and

Chapter Three

labeled enzyme. Ideally, incubation mixtures containing standard and unknown antigen should be identical in every respect.

The standard curve should cover a broad range of antigen concentration, extending from minimal to maximal specific binding. While two fold dilutions are normally used in the working part of standard curve, a narrower dilution span may be desirable, particularly when standard curves are nonlinear since dilutions of standard antigen are generally very dilute, the dilutions must be made accurately, since there is no way of directly verifying the antigen concentration once the dilution have been made. The instability of highly diluted standard solutions can also be a problem, and as noted, the inclusion of protein in the medium is sometimes desirable so as to minimize denaturation obvious problem in terpretation arise when the standard antigen itself is inpure or was obtained from a heterologus species.

A number of ways of handling the experimental data have been recommended, and there is no general agreement as to what is truly optimal.

When serial concentration of CEA solution were assay by EIA techniques, a sigmoidal curve relating precent of B/Bmax (ordinate) versus actual concentration could drawn through the data figure(3-11) and determine the antigen content of tissue sample where they fall on the standard CEA curve. There was no real advantage in correcting each sample from nonspecific binding, since the blank was already built in to the standard curve. Since the graph of ratio B/Bmax (%) versus of CEA concentration is sigmoidal in character figure (3-11-a), a sigmoidal transformation results in further lineari-zation of the curve. Logit, probit, or arcsine transformations may be used and of them the logit is the simplest in terms of the actual mechanics of the calculation. If the percentage of ratio of B/Bmax (%) is designed as y, then

Chapter Three

$$\text{Logit}(y) = \ln[y/(100-y)] \quad \text{------------------} \quad (1)$$

Where y is the percentage response, in this equation y is define a

$$y = 100[Ab_i / Ab_{max}] \quad \text{---------------------------} \quad (2)$$

Where Ab_i= the sample absorbance at concentration i

Ab_{max}= the absorbance of maximal antigen concentration.

The ratio of logit y is then poltted against the log antigen concentration. The advantage of the logit transformation is that it lends itself to computerized programs for calculating the data. Logit log paper suitable for manual computation is also available. Atypical logit versus log plot of data from figure (3-11-a) was shown in figure (3-11-c).

Chapter Three

TABLES

TABLE (3-1): Purification steps of peroxidase Isoenzyme from white radish roots

Purification step	Volume (ml)	Protein mg/ml	Activity (units/ml)	Total activity (units)	Specific activity (units/mg)	Purification fold	Yield %
Crude extract	95	1.95	82.1	7799.5	42.1	1	100
$(NH_4)_2SO_4$ fraction 35-90% saturation	25	0.67	221.4	5535	330.4	7.8	67.1
DEAE - cellulose ion exchange wash-fraction	27	0.16	146.4	3952.8	915.0	21.7	50.66
Sephacryl S-300 gel filtration	24	0.12	142.5	3420	1187.5	28.2	43.84

*one peroxidase unit (IU) is define as amount of enzyme which catalyze the oxidation of micromolar (µ mole) of substrate(O-dianisidine) per minute under the standard assay condition

TABLE (3-2): Adsorption of ^{125}I-LABELED rabbit IgG to plastics

IgG added (µg/ml)	Radioactivity adsorbed (%)					
	Polystyrene	Polyvinyl	Cellulose nitrate	Polyallomer[a]	Polyethylene	Reference
2200	4.4	-	6.0	-	3.8	190
200	12.2	-	12.3	-	4.5	190
100	10.0	7.4	6.0	11.8	-	189
10	46.4	39.8	18.2	46.9	-	189
1	47.6	69.4	37.1	55.8	-	190
3	-	-	-	52.1	-	our result

[a] copolymer of ethylene and propylene.

TABLE (3-3): Quantitation OF immunoglobulin immobilization ON plastics

Immunoglobulin (Ig) bound	Solid-phase support	Immobilization technique	Maximum Ig bound (ng/mm^2)	Reference
Guinea-pig IgG	Polypropylene tubes	Covalent linkage	1000	Our result
Sheep IgG	Polypropylene (latex)	Covalent linkage	100	191
Rabbit IgG	Nylon beads	Covalent linkage	590	190
Rabbit IgG	Polypropylene (latex)	Adsorption	5.7	189
Rat Ig	Polymethylmetaacrylic beads	Adsorption	0.9	192
Bovine IgG	Polypropylene tubes	Adsorption	3.2	193
Bovine IgG	Polypropylene tubes	Adsorption	2.9	193
Human IgG	Polypropylene (latex)	Adsorption	3.6	194

FIGURES

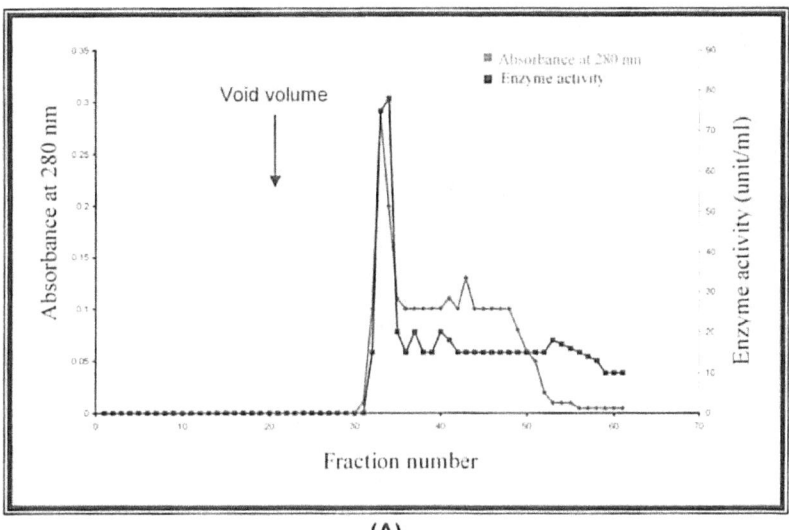

(A)

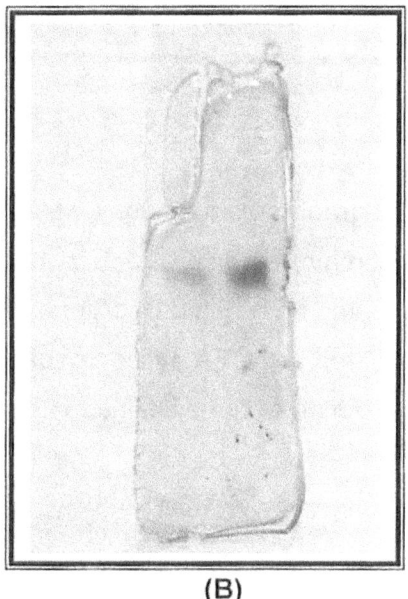

(B)

Figure (3-1):

(A) Gel filtration profile of peroxidase on sephacryl S-300 column.

(B) PAGE slab electrophoresis illustrates the protein present in pooled fractions peak on sephacryl S-300 column.

(All details are explained in the text)

Chapter Three

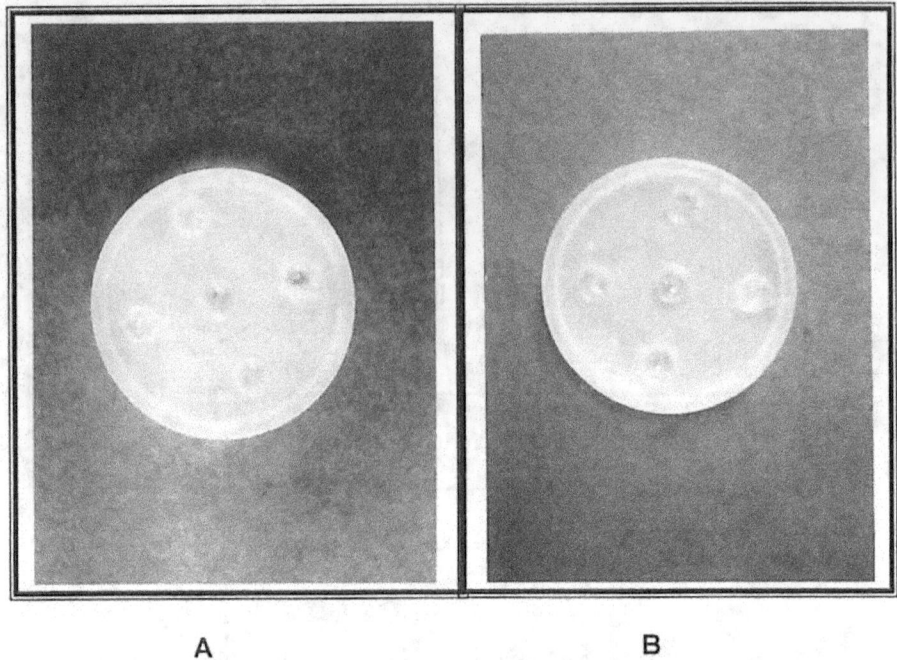

Figure (3-2): Photograph of Ouchterlony Agrarose gel double diffusion. Plate central well contains purified CEA. The peripheral wells of
(A) Contain untreated anti-CEA antiserum of rabbits.
(B) Contain untreated anti-CEA antiserum of guinea-pig.
(All detail are explained in the text)

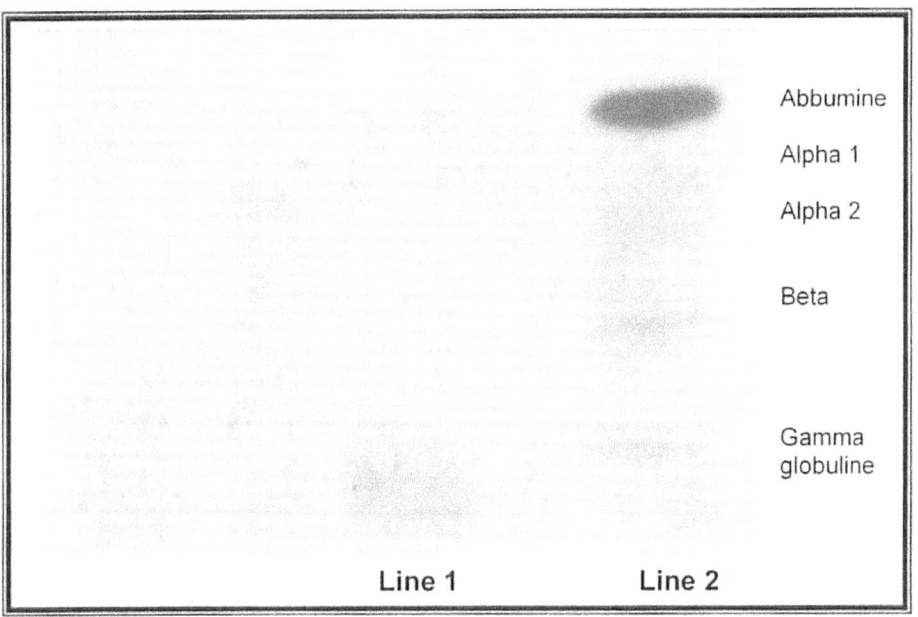

Figure (3-3): Cellulose acetate electrophoresis of anti-CEA antiserum.
Line 1: finally purified IgG anti-CEA.
Line 2: Immunized rabbit serum.
(All detail are explained in the text)

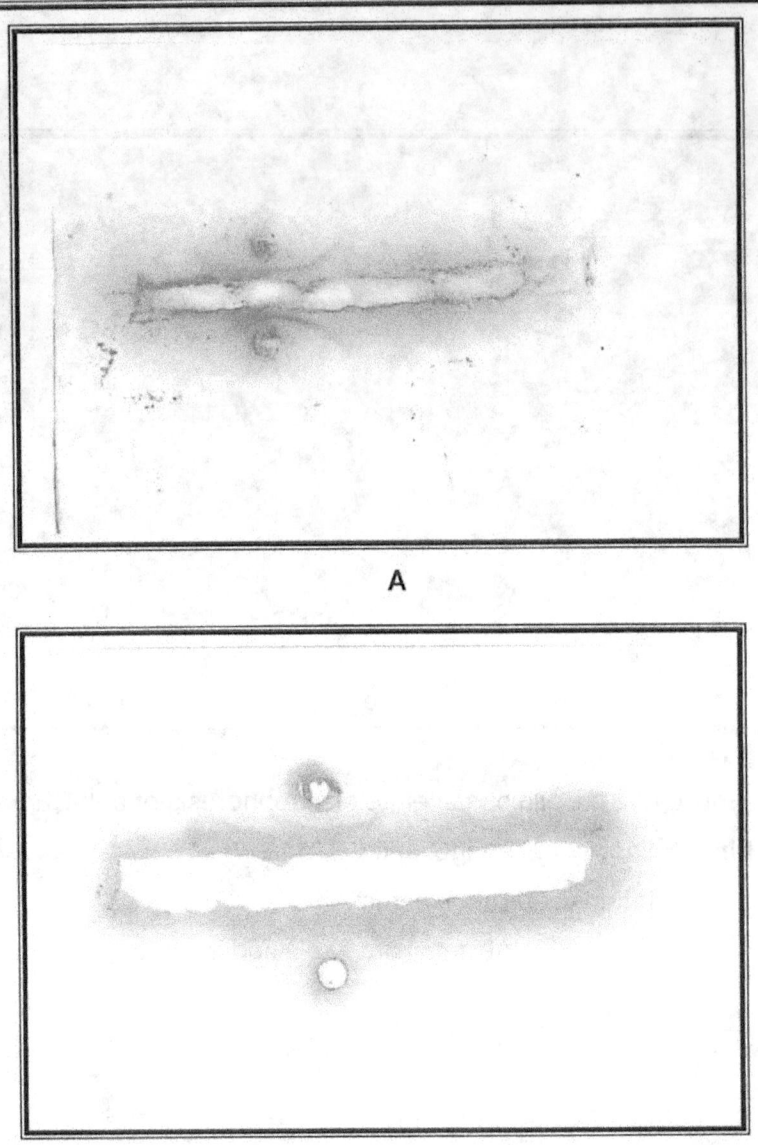

Figure (3-4): Immunoelectrophoretic pattern of purified CEA against purified IgG beta-globulin region:
    (A) Contained rabbit purified anti-CEA (IgG).
    (B) Contained guinea-pig anti-CEA (IgG).
        (All detail are explained in the text)

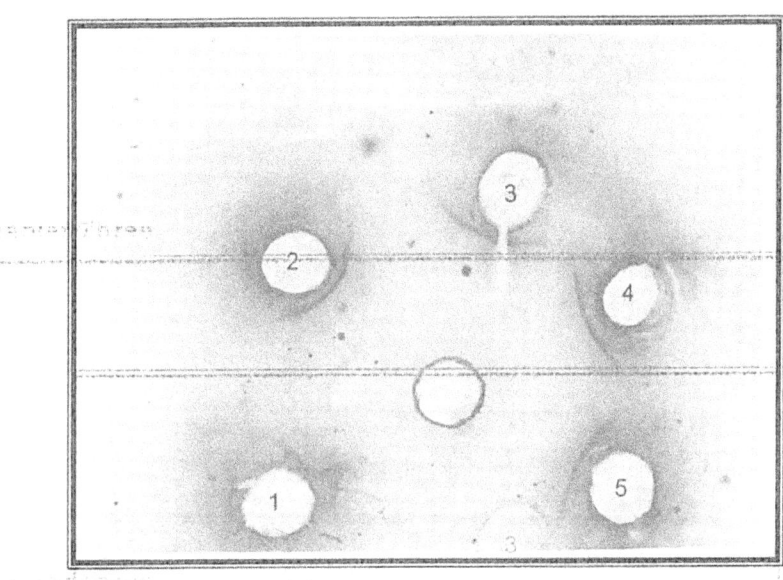

Figure (3-5): Photograph of oucterlony agraose gel diffusion. Plate central well contain purified CEA. The peripheral wells 1,2= guinea pig purified anti-CEA, (IgG) 3,4,5 well rabbit purified anti-CEA (IgG).

(All detail are explained in the text)

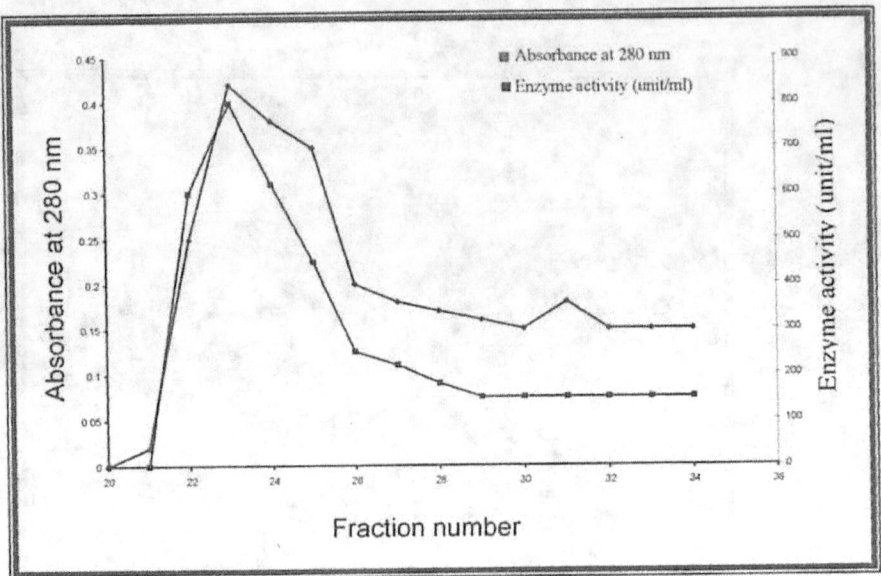

Figure (3-7): Gel filtration profile of peroxidase anti-CEA preparation on sephacryl S-300 column.
(All detail are explain in the text)

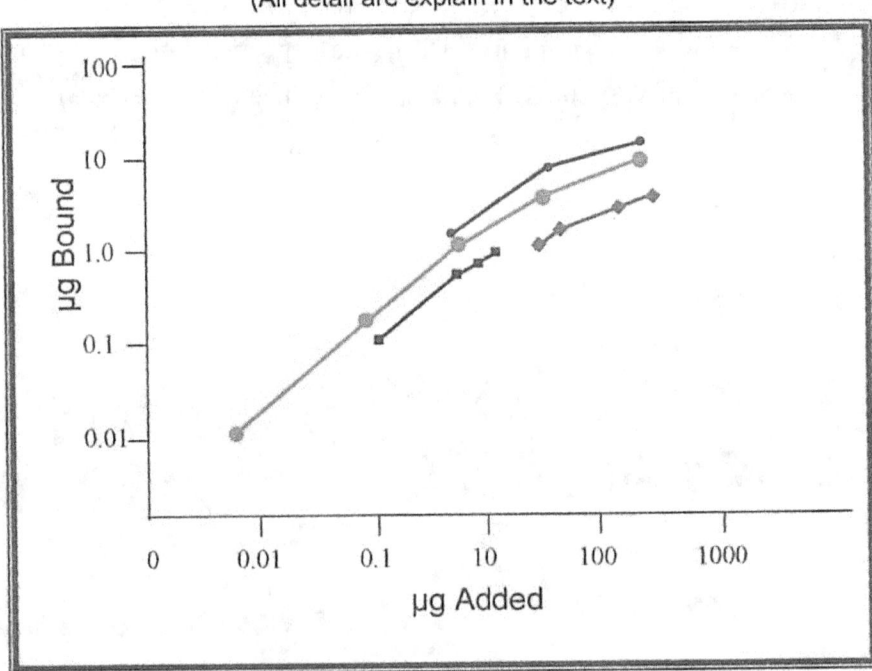

Figure (3-8): effect of immunoglobulin (IgG) concentration on adsorption of IgG to polystyrene •——•, Rabbit IgG, adsorbed for 18 hr at room temperature, [189] •——•, Rabbit IgG and sorbed overnight at room temperature, [195] •——•, Bovine IgG adsorbed for 3 hr at 37°, [173] •——•, Human IgG adsorbed for 1 hr at 37°(190).

SANDWICH EIA

1- Attach antibody to solid phase

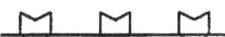

2- Incubate with sample

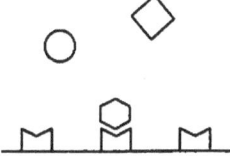

3- Incubate with enzyme-labeled antibody

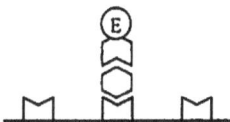

Figure (3-9): Schematic for a noncompetitive solid phase enzyme immunoassay.

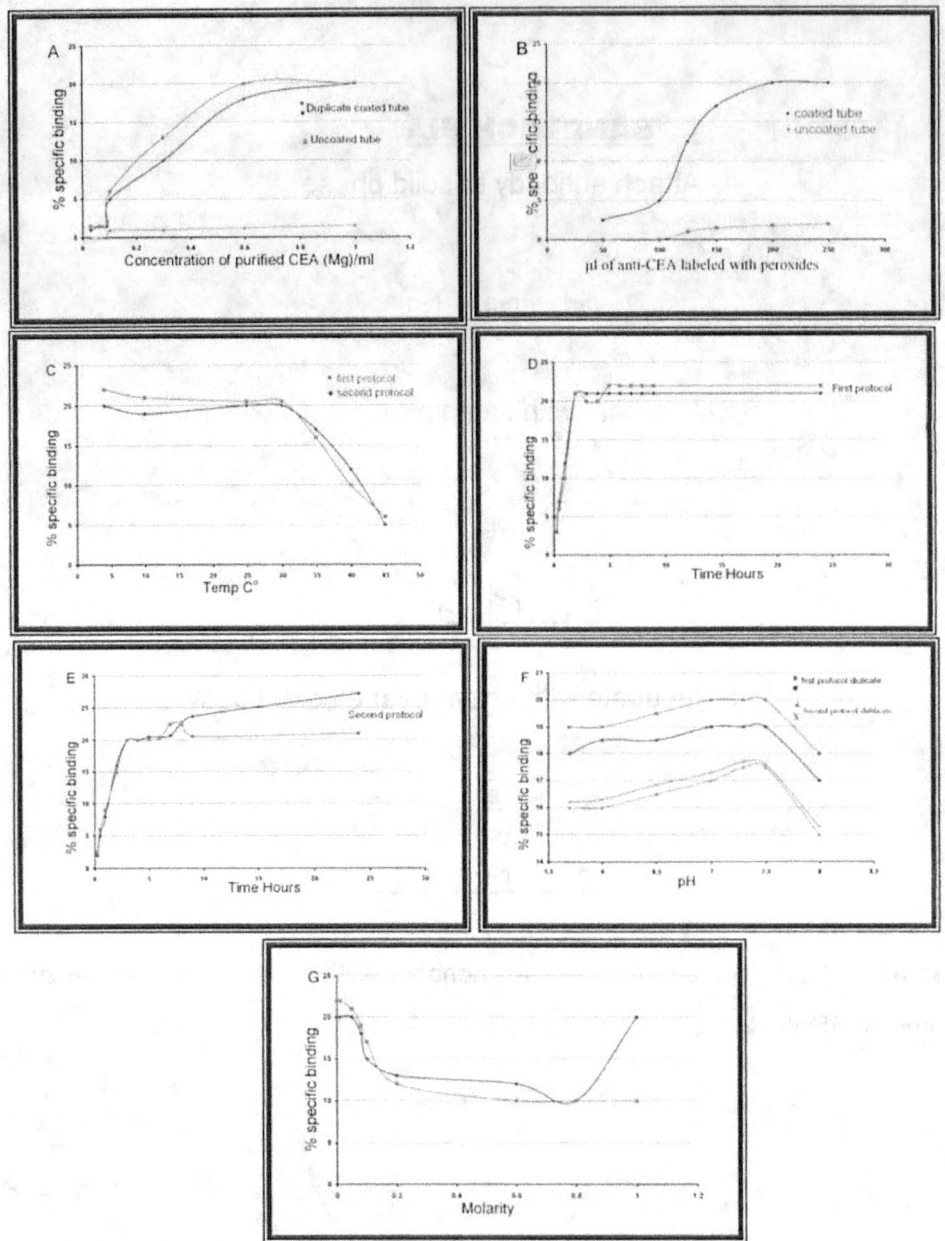

Figure (3-10): A-G; Assay condition of EIA binding of anti-CEA coated polypropylene tube to CEA:
A: Concentration of CEA any= concentration below long.
B: PRA =200 µl
C: Temperazure= 10°C
D: First incubation time= 2hr
E: Second incubation time=3hr
P: pH=7.2
G: Ionic strength=0.05M phosphate buffer
(All detail are explained in the text)

Chapter Three

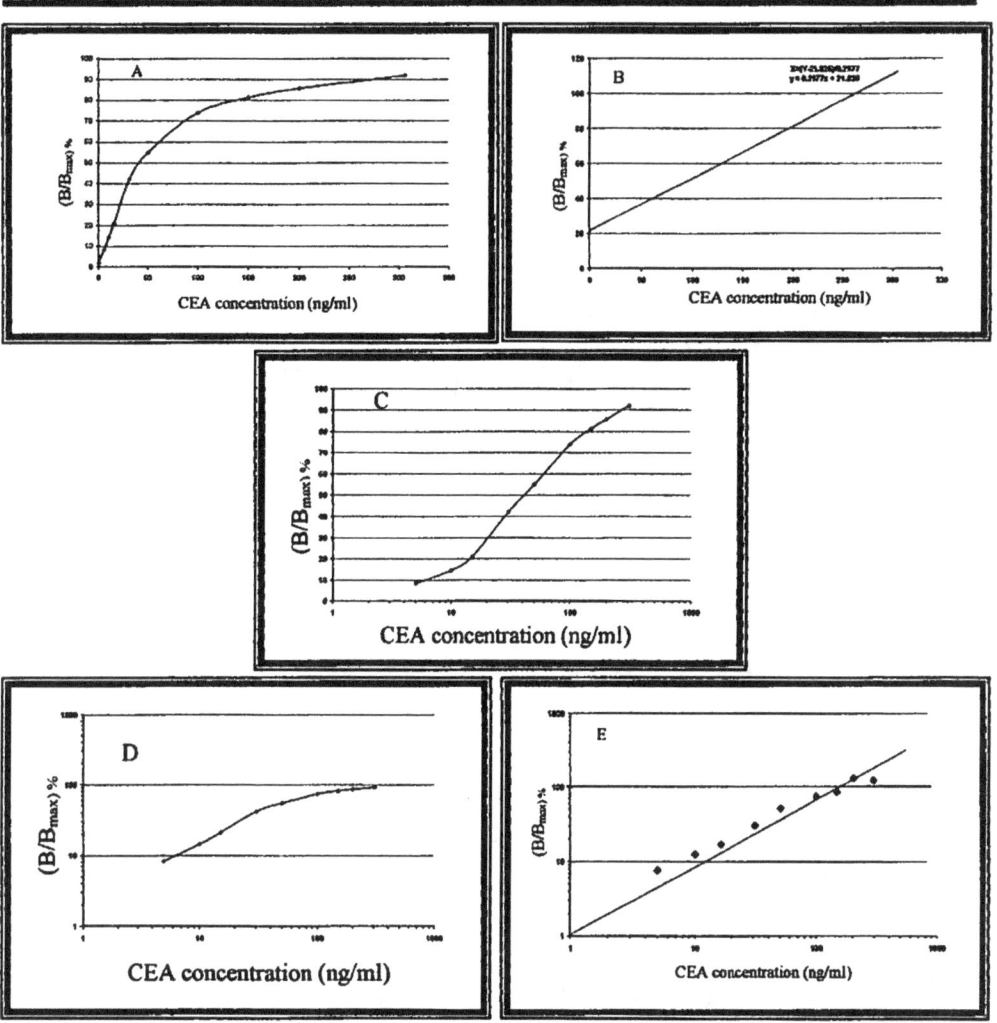

Figure (3-11): Standard curve of EIA for CEA assay. Each points represent the mean of triplicate determination:

- A- Arithmetic plot.
- B- Linear regression analysis by using a least square linear regression method for arithmetic plot.
- C- Semi logarithmic plot (logarithm of concentration) this curve is sigmoid.
- D- Logarithmic plot (logit-log representation).
- E- Best-fit linear-regression has been drawn through each set data of logarithmic plot.

(All detail are explained in the text)

Chapter Four

Evaluation

&

Clinical Application

of

EIA Kit

Chapter Four

Abstract

The aim of this study was to evaluate enzyme immunoassay technique for measuring the levels of CEA in sera, fluid and tissue exctracte of adenocaricnoma digestive organs and normal individuals. The assay employs enzymatic activities for determination. The level of CEA were investigated in sera of two groups of malignant human colorectal tumors, and one group of benign CR tumors as well as normal healthy groups as reference control. Results of this study revealed that serum CEA was significantly elevated in the cancer group (9.75 ± 4.77 ng/ml) when compared with benign and healthy control groups (2.73 ± 1.32 ng/ml) and 0.710 ± 0.30 ng/ml) respectively.

The comparative study was carried out between EIA and RIA technique in attempt to overcome the limitation of specificity, sensitivity and accuracy. The result of that indicated that there was good correlation between two system and comparable sensitivity.

The data presented show that the EIA techniques offers a very rapid and extremely sensitive method for routine testing and can be easily done on a large number of sample appear to be as good a diagnostic aid for cancer.

Chapter Four

Introduction

In recent years a number of immunoassays have been developed for the determination of circulating levels of CEA. The original CEA immunoassay, a radioimmunoassay (RIA), based on competitive inhibition described by Thomson et al[18,109,167]. It used ^{125}I – labeled CEA (^{125}I-CEA) and the Farr method of 50% ammonium sulfate precipitation to separate free from antibody bound ^{125}I-CEA. Other widely used radioimmunoassay use ^{125}I-CEA. Sample preparations also differ in that some methods require precipitation with perchloric acid (PCA) and subsequent dialysis of PCA, while others use sera or plasma directly.

The enzyme-immunoassay (EIA) combines both the high specificity of an immunological method with the great sensitivity of a method used for the determination of enzymatic activities. The EIA is a useful alternative method to RIA; it has the advantage of not using isotopes. In general the EIA is solid phase immunoassay based on the sandwish principle.

Several RIA kits for CEA have become commercially available, but to our knowledge no EIA kit available and no comparative evaluation has yet been made on the measurement of CEA.

The objective of this study to report the comparative quality and performance of EIA and RIA assay.

Chapter Four

Materials and methods

4-1 Chemicals:

All chemicals and reagents used in this study were of analytical grade, they were obtained from the following companies.

TABLE (4-1): The chemicals used and the companies that supplied them

	Chemicals	Company
1-	Immunoradiometric assay kit for CEA level.	Diasorin Inc. (USA)
2-	Tris(hydroxymethyl) amino methane, Bovine-serum albumine(BSA), $MgCl_2$, urea, $ZnCl_2$ and $CaCl_2$.	Fluka: (Switzerland)
3-	Glycine, NaOH, HCL, $HClO_4$, Na_2CO_3, NaCl, PEG-3300, $NaHPO_4$, NaH_2PO_4.	BDH, limited, Poole (UK)

4-2 Instrument:

TABLE (4-2): Instruments used and companies that supplied them.

	Instruments	Company
1-	Gamma counter type 1270-rack Gamma II,	LKB
2-	Spectrophotometer ultraspec type 4050	
3-	UV-210 a double beam spectrophotometer	Shimadzu
4-	PH-meter	Pye-Unicam
5-	Cooling centrifuge; with a maximum speed 5000 r.p.m.	Hettich
6-	Cooling centrifuge type 202-MK; with a maxmum speed 13.500 r.p.m.	Sigma
7-	Memmert water bath, memmert incubator	West Germany
	SM-shaker	England

4-3 Solutions:

Tris/HCl buffer (0.01M, pH 7.4): it's prepared by dissolving 1.2114 gm of tris (hydroxyl methyl) amino methane in 900ml de-ionized distilled water. Then the pH was adjusted to 7.4 using HCl (0.1M) the volume was made up to 1 liter with de-ionized distilled water.

Other buffer solutions were prepared by dissolving the appropriate amount of salt in distilled water and the required pH was adjusted. Other solutions used are indicated in each experiment.

4-4 Patients:

The study was carried out on one hundred seventy-six colorectal patients with benign, pre-malignant and malignant tumors (122 males) whom subjected to curative surgery. Their age mean was 44 (range 3.5-85 years).

Four groups of CRC patients, one group with benign colorectal tumors and one group with ulcerative colitis used as a pre-malignant were included in this study.

According to the histopathological examination of the resected pieces. The patients were grouped into the following.

- ❖ Group 1: contained of 16 patients with benign colorectal tumor.
- ❖ Group 2: consisted of 26 patients with ulcerative colitis disease.
- ❖ Group 3: contained of 42 patients with colon cancer stage-B.
- ❖ Group 4: included of 25 patients with colon cancer stage-C.
- ❖ Group 5: consisted of 43 patients with rectal cancer stage-B.
- ❖ Group 6: contained of 24 patients with rectal cancer stage-C_3-D.

The patients were admitted for treatment to: (Baghdad Hospital), (University Hospital, Al-Nahrane College of Medicine), (Al-Mustansiryah Privet Hospital), (Al-Yarmook Teaching University Hospital), (Nursing Home Privet Hospital), (Al-Shaheed Hospital) and (Al-Hussany Hospital). Patients suffered from any disease that may interfere with this study were excluded. All surgical operation of colorectal tumors were down under the super vision of surgeons: Dr. Zuhair Al-bahrani, Dr. Hassan Al-Sakafi, Dr. Saaeb Sedeq, Dr. Faleh Al-Aubaidy, Dr. Azam Qanbar Agha,

Dr. Abd Al-Salam Al-Tai, Dr. Dhiaa Al-Kinani, Dr. Najeeb Sulaiwah, Dr. Hekmet Abd Al-Rasool and Dr. Nazar Taha Makky.

4-5 Blood Sampling:

Blood samples (5-7)ml were collected from patients mentioned above, left for 15-30 minutes at room temperature; blood clots were separated at 3000 r.p.m. for 10 minutes using centrifuge. Sera were aspirated and stored at -20°C until time of analysis. The samples were not thawed and refrozen before testing.

TABLE (4-3): The host information of patients which were used in this study

Patients	Number	Type of tumor	Metastases	Age rang (Years)
Group I	16	Benign tumor (polyps)		35-21
Group II	26	Pre-malignant (ulcerative colitis U.C.)		37-45
Group III	42	Colon cancer stage-B		54-70
Group IV	25	Colon cancer stage-C	Liver and lymph node	50-58
Group V	43	Rectal cancer stage-B		40-85
Group VI	24	Rectal cancer stage-C_3-D	Liver and lymph node	37-56

The weight of respected tissue samples ranged between (0.65-19.55)gm.

4-6 Collection of specimens and preparation of tissue homogenate:

The source of tissue in this series of experiments was human colon tissue. The specimens removed surgically for primary adenocarcinoma of the colon were taken only the central, obviously cancerous portion was used as tumor tissue for extraction.

Normal tissue extract was prepared from section of colon more than 7cm distant from the visible edges of the tumor. In this way the

Chapter Four

problem of individual-specific antigenic differences between normal and tumor tissue was overcome. All tissues were placed in labeled clean polystyrene container in normal saline and kept at-20°C until use; some times the specimens were processed immediately. Only pathologically confirmed benign and tumor tissue specimens were taken into the study.

4-6-1 Tissue preparation:

Samples were trimned of fat, weight, minced, in four volumes of homogenization buffer, (10% glycerol, 10-mM dithiotheritol, 10 mM Tries, 1.5 mM EDTA). The homogen-ization was done in an ice bath.

The homogenate was filtered through a nylon mesh sieve to eliminate fibbers of connective tissues then centri-fuged at 2000 xg for 10 min at 4°C.

After removing the upper layer of fat, an appropriate volume of tissue homogenate (500-µl) was dilute to 2.5 ml with homogenization buffer and treated with an equal volume of 1.2 mole/liter perchloric acid. After 30 min, the mixture centrifuge at 2000 xg for 10 min and the supernatant was dialyzed for 12 hours against distilled water.

CEA was determined in an aliquot of perchloric acid extract by the soild phase sandwich (EIA) as described in section (2.4.2).

4-7 Protein Assay:

The total protein in the tissue homogenate was measured by the method of Lowry.

Aliquots were taken from the cytosol for each test.

4-8 Estimation of CEA by IRMA method:

The assay protocol was described in chapter two section (2-8-6) were followed exactly to estimate the level of CEA in the specimen.

4-9 Determination of CEA by EIA Method.

The CEA-EIA method used in this study was a soild phase enzyme-immunoassay based on the sandwich principle.

Chapter Four

The CEA-EIA kit utilized in this study was prepared as described in chapter 3-section(3-8).

The same assay protocol was described in chapter three, in section (3-8) were followed to estimate the level of CEA in the specimen.

The resulting concentration of the patient samples and control can be directly interpolate from the standard curve by the use of their $(B/B_{max})\%$ values as described in chapter three in section (3-9), figure (3-11).

4-10 Statistical Analysis

The result of serum and tissues determination of CEA was analyzed statistically and the values were expressed as mean ±SD. The levels of significance were determined by analysis of variance (ANOVA).

4-11 Results and discussion

Enzyme immunoassay are now firmly established as precise quantitative method for the determination of various antigenic substances and antibodies[106,129]. There are few reports describing an enzyme-linked immunoassay for CEA[106]. This method was developing for the detection of CEA in human serum, human fluide and carcinoma tissue.

In order to fully evaluate EIA kit which was prepared as described in chapter (3), as a pontential kit rapid routine testing of human serum samples and other fluide sample in research or clinical diagnostic. The present study was primarily designed to evaluate the following factors:

1- Determination of the reference range.
2- Measuring range.
3- RepRoducibility.
4- Correlation between RIA and EIA.
5- Sensitivity, specificity, accuracy and Efficiency of EIA kit.
6- Recover assay.

7- Determination of CEA in carcinoma colon tissue.

4-11-1 Reference and measuring range:

The reference range was calculated from CEA concentrations in 144 of healthy persons. Concentrations between 0.3 and 3.0 ng/ml were found. The value did not follow a normal distribution; the median value was 0.9 ng/ml figure (4-1).

Measuring range: with the EIA concentration of 0.5-60 ng/ml can be measured directly. Most serum sample analysed showed a CEA-concentration within this range. If the concentration exceeds 60 ng/ml the sample has to be diluted with a diluent (bovine serum albumine in phosphate buffer).

4-11-2 Reproducibility:

In order to study the reproducibility, 3 types of evaluations were done. In the 1st type known amounts of CEA in the range of 0.5 to 10.0 ng/ml were add either to buffer or to normal human serum, and replicate assaye were done on each sample on the same day, in the 2nd type of experiments, CEA sample prepared as above were assay on differ day, over a period of 42 days. The samples were stored frozen during this period. Results of these 2 sets of experiment presented in tables (4-5) and (4-6) show the reproducibility and accuracy of EIA assay method. In the 3rd type of experiments, 8 sera with different concentration were measured on 5 different days; the result of this experiment was shown in table (4-7). It can be seen that the CEA-EIA kit was highly reproducible. The CEA-EIA method can be preformed equally well with sera as well as with other fluide or carcinoma tissue speciment.

4-11-3 Correlation of RIA and EIA

Determination of CEA values on serum sample of 15 patients was done by RIA method; as well as the EIA-method. The result presented in table (4-8) indicated that the RIA result were slightly elevated to those of

Chapter Four

EIA, but there is good correlation between two systems (correlation factor r=0.967, n=15).

A series of determination of CEA values was made on 118 human serum samples by the RIA an EIA method. The results presented in chart (4-2) show the correlation coefficient r=0.927, n=118).

There is reasonable correlation between RIA and EIA if only samples with concentration below 20 ng/ml are analysed. The values obtained by RIA are on average 1 ng/ml lower than corresponding value obtained by EIA.

Single values, however, may show considerable differences. In some samples higher concentrations (above 5 ng/ml) were measured by RIA while the EIA show values within the normal range (below 2 ng/ml). in other samples a reverse behaviour was found for the assays for value above 20 ng/ml the linear relationship for data sets was poor. These variations in the upper range of assay-system were of little clinical significance.

From these data the conclusion came that some tumors may be diagnosed with one of the two methods because of differences in the specificity of the antibodies used.

4-11-4 Sensitivity, specificity, accuracy, and efficiency of EIA kit.

The present study was primary designed to evaluate specificity and sensitivity of a double antibody CEA EIA. The results in table (4-9) demonstrate the comparative analysis of the sensitivity, specificity, accuracy and efficiency. The EIA techniques were most useful in separating cancer from non cancer patients. The advantages of the enzyme-immun-ological method are the high sensitivity and specificity within a broad measuring range. In general, the results in table (4-10) indicate that the enzymatic CEA assay method measures the CEA level

Chapter Four

in sample with sensitivity and specificity comparable to common RIA method.

It should be noted however that some specimens exhibit markedly different CEA values when assay by the two methods. Differences in specificities of the anti CEA antibodies employed by the two methods might have caused the different results. Evidence for multiple antigenic have cause the different and iso antigens has already been given by many of investigator[17,18,109,167].

In general, to design an assay with optimal sensitivity, it was essential to (a-)choose an antiserum of highest possible affinity, (b-)use incubation times that allow an equilibrium between antigen and antibody, (c-) use lower concentration of antigen and antibody and longer times for color development.

With these factors taken in a count, the sensitivity of EIA assay was comparable of that of radiommunoassay or other techniques.

4-11-5 Recovery assay:

To three sera containing low CEA concentrations were added known amount of standard CEA and assay according the assay procedure of the kit (described previously in chapter 3). The CEA values abtained were compared to expected values, the CEA recovery for all samples experiment showed a range of 85-103%, average 94 %(table 4-10).

4-11-6 Result of Tissue Determination of CEA in Colorectal tumors Cancer and Normal Specimens:

4-11-6-1 Normal Specimens:

Tissue CEA was assayed in 32 specimens of normal Fig(4-3) the normal level of this glycoprotein is presented in table (4-11) indicating a mean value of 2.2 ± 0.81 ng/mg cytosol protein (cp) and range of 0-3.7 ng CEA/mg protein. The specificity of CEA in tissue homogenate for

Chapter Four

excluding normal individuals was 93%, by regarding the normal-/abnormal cutoff value of 3.0 ng/mg cytosol protein. At present no report was available in the literature on the cutoff value of CEA was tissue homogenate.

4-11-6-2 Benign colorectal Tumor:

When the assay was performed on 16 patients with benign colon tumors, supernormal levels (concentration> 3ng/mg cytosol protein) of CEA were observed in 4 of these patients, suggesting a specificity of 75% table (4-12) and mean value of 2.8 ± 0.05 ng/mg cytosol protein. Table (4-11) which was not significantly different from that of normal ($p>0.05$). There have been no previous reports on the CEA level in cytosol with tissue benign tumors.

4-11-6-3 Colorectal Cancer Tissue:

The distribution of CEA in colorectal carcinoma tissue is shown in fig (4-3). CEA concentration > 3 ng/mg protein was found in 51/62 primary carcinoma. The percentage sensitivity of CEA for cancer specimens was about 82% table (4-11), compared with 6% for normal specimens. The mean value of CEA in cancer specimens is 17.25 ± 3.4 which is significantly higher ($p>0.05$) than in benign and normal (table 4-11). One male case that shows very high levels of CEA (117 ng/mg protein) died within 3 month after surgery.

Most research on CEA has concentrated on measure-ment of this glycoprotein in sera from patients with cancer. However, a logical first step in the study of tumor markers would be examination of the tumor tissue for the presence of particular marker of interest. Primary colorectal carcinoma in contrast to metastatic disease rarely causes elevation of circulating levels of CEA. Our work shows that this was not due to the absence of CEA from primary tumors. It could however relate to the tumor bulk which may not be sufficiently large to produce elevate serum level at the localized stage, the prognostic value of CEA in the tissue is not yet defined. Some authors reported a correlation between presence of CEA in the tissue and a worse prognosis[146,147]; authors found such a relationship only in tumors of 3 cm or smaller[150,175]; others deny any relation between CEA and prognosis[11,13,167] or do not take into account this problem[146]. Furthermore, CEA in the tissue does not appear to be related to the degree of differentiation of tissue[146].

Analysis of CEA in the tissue may prove to be helpful in evaluating plasma CEA as marker for recurrence. Subsequently in tumors with low CEA tissue values must produce bulky metastases before blood CEA concentration increases measurably. Also, the clinical utility of the tests may lie in providing additional information on the tumor proliferation rate in term of planning the treatment for patient with early stage colon cancer.

4-12 General Discussion

A more serious problem in the application of the competitive EIA relates to the difficulties caused by the need to incubate enzyme-labeled antigen or antibodies with biological fluids such as serum, urine, or tissue extract. These fluids contain proteases, and noncompetitive enzyme inhibitors may also be present. Such substances, when present, may alter the activity of the enzyme used as label. This difficulty was avoided in the noncompetitive EIA. Techniques in which the incubation with test samples was carried out separately from the incubation with enzyme-labeled antibody.

The noncompetitive EIA offers additional advantages. Since most of such assays employ enzyme-labeled antibodies, the purification and specific enzyme-labeling of individual antigens is not necessary. Thus, the same enzyme-labeling procedure and solid phase attachment method can be used for different antibodies. Another advantage of the noncompetitive EIA was the possibility of binding several enzyme-labeled antibody melcule to single polyvalent antigen molecule, thus providing an element of amplification.

This may be an advantage in procedure in which the ultimate sensitivity has not attained, i.e., the sensitivity limit is not set by the affinity between the antigen and antibody.

The EIA assay can be easily done on a large number of patient samples with a minimum of equipment and this technique appear to be as good a diagnostic aid for cancer.

The EIA system described here should provide the basis for developing an attractive alternative to traditional CEA assay procedure.

TABLES

TABLE (4-4): Within assay variability of CEA values in buffer and in normal human serum as determined by EIA method

Assay day	No. replicate assays	CEA (ng/100 µl test sample)						
		A"	B	C	D	E	F	G
1	1	11.0	2.3	0.6	0.59	6.1	1.5	1.17
	2	11.3	2.6	0.5	0.50	6.2	1.3	1.13
	3	10.9	2.3	0.5	0.57	6.3	1.3	0.91
	4	10.8	2.5	0.6	0.56	5.9	1.4	1.05
	5	10.8	2.5	0.6	0.60	6.2	1.4	0.96
	6				0.54	5.9	1.5	0.97
	Mean	10.96	2.44	0.56	0.57	6.1	1.4	1.03
	S.D.	± 0.21	± 0.13	± 0.06	± 0.022	± 0.17	0.09	± 0.10
16	1		2.5	0.58	0.58		1.3	0.98
	2		2.4	0.58	0.60		1.5	0.92
	3		2.6	0.54	0.54		1.4	0.95
	4		2.4	0.57	0.57		1.6	1.10
	5		2.5	0.55				
	Mean		2.48	0.56	0.57		1.45	0.99
	S.D.		± 0.08	± 0.03	± 0.025		± 0.13	± 0.079

" Test sample A; approximately 100 ng CEA per ml of 0.01 M sodium acetate-0.065 M NaCl-0.001 M disodium EDTA buffer, pH 6.1, containing 20% BSA; B, 1:4 dilution of A in same buffer; C, 1:20 dilution of A in same buffer; D, NHS; E, approximately 50 ng CEA per ml were added to D; F, 1:5 diltuion of E using D as dilutent; G, 1:10 dilution of E using D as diluent.

TABLE (4-5): Interassay variability of CEA values in buffer and in NHS as determined by EIA method

Assay day	CEA (ng / 100 μl test sample)					
	A"	B	C	D	E	F
1	10.99	2.44	0.58	0.56	1.40	1.03
3	10.51	2.56	0.54			
8				0.58	1.53	1.10
14	10.2	2.7	0.53			
16		2.5	0.55			
21	10.6	2.62	0.47	0.56	1.46	0.99
31	1056	2.50	0.53	0.47		
42				0.60		1.15
Mean	10.57	2.55	0.53	0.55	1.46	1.06
S.D.	± 0.28	± 0.094	± 0.036	± 0.065	± 0.065	± 0.07

" Test sample A; approximately 100 ng CEA per ml of 0.01 M sodium acetate-0.065 M NaCl-0.001 M disodium EDTA buffer, pH 6.1, containing 20% BSA; B, 1:4 dilution of A in same buffer; C, 1:20 dilution of A in same buffer; D, NHS; E, approximately 10 ng CEA per ml ; F, NHS containing approximately 5 ng CEA per ml.

TABLE (4-6): Reproducibility of the abbott CEA-EIA test : Plasma CEA Measurments (ng / ml)

Serum No.	1	2	3	4	5	6	7	8
Assay day :1	2.4	20.7	96.0	4.2	2.1	5.1	19.0	43.0
2	1.5	20.1	90.0	4.6	2.5	4.2	21.6	48.0
3	2.4	21.9	88.0	5.4	2.7	5.7	20.0	49.5
4	2.1	24.0	94.0	5.3	5.2	4.8	20.9	58.0
5	2.4	24.0	90.0	5.1	1.9	4.8	20.8	57.0

TABLE (4-7): Comparison Between EIA-and RIA- method serum CEA Measurements (ng/ml)

EIA	25.0	1.0	4.5	1.2	3.0	5.8	4.2	1.3	1.2	7.0	2.8	9.7	5.5	1.0	3.0
RIA	46.0	2.2	7.1	6.3	6.3	9.9	5.0	8.4	1.2	9.0	3.0	10.6	6.0	1.0	12.3

FIGURES

Figure (4-1): Frequency-distribution histogram for CEA by EIA in serum from healthy adults

N	140
Median	0.90
97.5% Percentile	3.00
2.5% Percentile	0.30
Mean Value	1.24
Standard Deviation	0.73

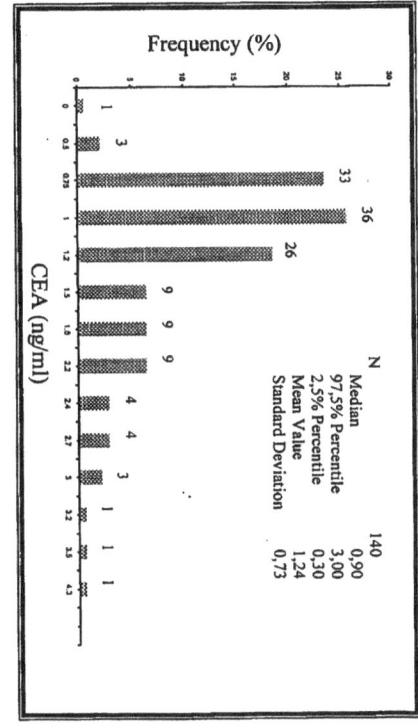

Figure (4-2): Correlation diagram between RIA(x) and EIA (Y)

Chapter Four

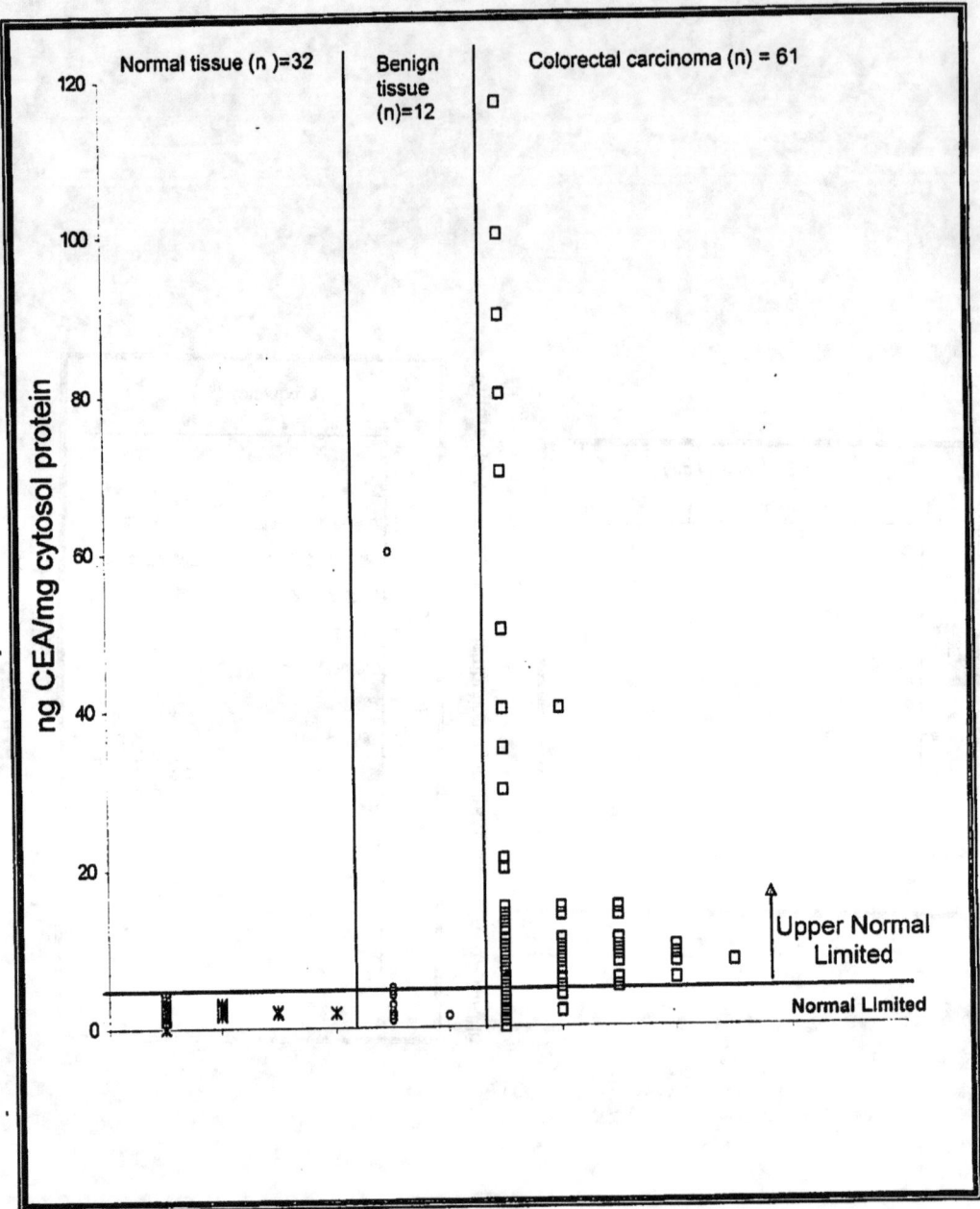

Figure (4-3): Distribution of CEA value in human colorectal carcinomas, benign colorectal tumors, and normal breast tissues. (n)=Number of patients

References

1- Gold, P.; Freeman, S.O.; (1965). J. Exp. Med., 121; 439.

2- Burtis, C.A.; Edward, R.; Ashwood E. R.; (1999). "Tetiz Text Book of Clinical Chemistry" 3rd. ed., Philadelphia, W.B., Saunders Co. chap. 23.pp 722-748.

3- Hall, M.J., Jakson, M., Johson, J. T., Schultz, H., Fortenberry, D., Bright, C., Hua. H., Ying. J., Sykes, P.A.; (1999), clin. Chem., 45 (6): Allo.

4- Nakagoe, T., Nanashima, A., Sawai, T., Tuji, T., Yamaguchi, E., Jibiki, M., Yamaguchi, H., Yasutake, T., Ayabe, H.,Matuo, T., Tagawa, Y.; (2000) Oncology, 59:131-138.

5- Hannarstoms, S.; Shively, J.F.; Paxron, R.J.; Beatty, B.G.; Larsson, A.;et al.,(1989). Cancer Res., 49.4852.

6- Ayude, D., Fernandez-Rodriguez J., Rodriguez Berrocal, F.J., Martinez zorzano, V.S., de-carlos, A., Gil E., paez-de-la-caden, M.; (2000), oncology, 59(4): 310-316.

7- Harnmarstorm, S.; (1999). Semin. Cancer Biol., 9(2): 67.

8- Herlyn, M., Sears, H.F., Steplewskiz., Koprowski, H.; (1982), J.Clin. Immunol.; 2(2): 135-140.

9- Zhou, D., Henion.T., Jungalwals, F.B., Berger, E.G., and Hennet, T.J.;(2000),J.Biol chem.,275,22631-22634.

10- Zhou, D., Berger, E.G., and Hennet, T.J, (1999), Eur.J. Biochem. 263,571-576.

11- Al-Kazzaz, F.F.; (2000), "Biochemical characterization of carcinoembronic Antigen in some colorectal Tumor"ph.D. Thesis, supervised by Al-Mudhaffar S.A., College of Science, Al-Mustansiriyah University.

12- Al-Atrackchi, S.A.M; (2002), "Protein Engineering of carcinoembryonic Antigen and their Receptors Located in

References

Mulignant Mammry tissues" ph.D. Thesis Supervised by Al-Mudhaffar S.A. College of Science, Baghdad University.

13- Eaman A. s; (2001) " Biochemical studies on some Tumor markers in oral cancer " PH.D Thesis, supervised by Al – Mudhaffar S. A., college of science, Baghdad University – Iraq.

14- Huodo, I., Doi To, Endo, H., Hosokawa, Y., Nishikaw, Y., Tanimizu, M., Jinno, k., Kotani, Y.; (1998), Eur. J. Cancer, 34 (13): 2041–2045.

15- Renehan, A. G., Painter, J. E., Atkin, W. S., potten, C. S., Shalet, S. M., O'Dwyer, S. T.; (2001), Br. J. caner.; 88(1); 107–113.

16- Araki, T., Miki, C., Kusunoki, M.; (2001), scand. J. Gastroenterol; 36 (4): 399–404.

17- Kirkham, K. E.; Hunter, W. M.; (1971), "Radioimmunoassay Methods " London, LongMan group Lom, chap 1,6,15p8,p46, pp142–144.

18- Kin, J. C. Cong, G, Roh, S. A, and part, K. C., (1999). Mol. Cells, 9 (138): 133–137.

19- Maha, D., Fischer, N., Decimo, D., and Fuchs, J. (2000) Beochim Biophys. Act, 1492, 414–424.

20- Schullery, D. S., Ostrowski, J., Denisenko, O. N., stempka, I., shnurevs, M., Suzuki, H., Gschwendt, M. and Bomszty, K., (1999) .J. Biol, Chem. 274, 15101- 15109.

21- Boer, U., Neuschafer-Robe, F., Moller, U., and puschel, G.P. (2000) Biochem, J. 15,839-847.

22- Fierro–Monti, Mathews and I. M.B., (2000). Trends Biochem sci. 25,241–246.

23- Chudchia, C., Jones, E. Y., (1997) Annu, Rev. Biochem, 66, 823–862.

24- Holmes, E. H., (1999) Arch. Biochem. Biophys. 270, 630–646.

References

25- Kolbinger, .F., streff. M. B., and katopodis .A. G., (1998) J. Biol. Chem. 273, 433-440.

26- Holmes, E. H.; Hakomori, .S. Ostrander and I. G.K. (1987) J..Biol. Chem. 262, 15646–15658.

27- Dennis, J.W., Granovsky, M., and Warren, C. E., (1999) Beochem. Biophys Acta 1473, 24–341.

28- Nishinars, S., Hirags, T., Ikehara, Y., Kudo, T., Iwasaki, H., Morozumi, K., Akamatu, S., Tachikawa, T., Narimatsu, H., (1999) Glycobiology 9, 607–616.

29- Wojciechowicz, D.C., Park, P.Y., Datta, R.V., and paty, P.B. (2000) Biochem. Biophys. Res. Commun. 273, 147-153.

30- Zhou, D., Henion, T.J., (2000) J. Biol. Chem. 275, 22631–22634.

31- Ujita, M., Mc Auliffe, J., Hindsgaul, O., and Fukuda, M. (1999), J. Biol. Chem 274, 16717–16726.

32- Ujita, M., Misra, A. K., Mc Auliffe, J., Hindsgaul, O. and Fujud, M.; (2000); J. Biol, chem.. 275, 15868 – 15875.

33- Kafasla, P., Patrinous–Georgoula, M., and Guialis, A.; (2000) Biochem, J. 338, 350, 495-503.

34- Huang, S.; (2000) .J. Struct. Biol. 129, 233 – 240.

35- Tolnay, M., Vereshchagina, L.A., and Tsokos, G.C.; (1999) Biochem, J. 338, 417–425.

36- Rudd, P. M., Wermald, M.R., and Dwek, R. A.; (1999), J. Mol. Biol. 239, 351 – 366.

37- Leverroer, S., Cinato, E., Paul, C., Derancourt, J., Demark, M., Leanderson, T., and Legraverend, C.; (2000) .J. Biol. Chem. 381, 1031–1040.

38- Witte, M.M, and scott, r. E; (1997) proc. Natl. Acad. Sci U.S.A. qu, 1212-1217.

References

39- Faure, E., Equils, O., sieling, P.A., Thomas, L., Zhang, F. X., Kirschning, C. J., Polintarutti, N., Mizio, M., and Arditi, M.; (2000) J. Biol. Chem. 275, 11058–11063.

40- Nanjo, C., Gold, P., Freeman, S. O., and Kvupey, J., (1972) Nature 238, 183–185.

41- Kupchik, H. Z., Zamcheck, N., and Saravis, C. A., (1972) J. Natl. cancer Inst. 51, 1741–1749.

42- Coligan, J. E., Lauen chleger, J.T., Egan, M.I. and Todd, C. W., (1972) Immunochemistry 9, 377–386.

43- Terry, W.D., Henkart, P.A., coligan, J.E., and Todd, C.W. (1972); J. Exp. Med. 136, 200–204.

44- Westwood, J.H., Thomass, P. and Foster, A.B.; (1974) Biochem. Soci. Trans 2, 1250–1251.

45- Thomas, P., Westwood, J.H., and Foster, A. B.; (1974) Biochem. Soc. Trans. 2, 1248–1249.

46- Leahy, D.J.; (1997) Annu. Rev. cell. Biol. 13, 363 – 393.

47- Huang, J., Hardy, J.D., Sun, Y., and Shively, J.E.; (1999) J. cell sci 112, 4193–4205.

48- Oikaw, S., Nakazato, H., Kosaki, G.; (1987). Biochem. Biophys. Res. Commun. 142–511.

49- Saragoui, H.U., Greene, M.I., chrusciel, R.A., and kahn, M.; (1992) Biol Technolhy 10, 773–778.

50- Maryam, T., Uri, S., Abraham, F., Joe. M, John. M, and Clifford, P.S.; (2000) .J. Biol. Chem. 275, 35, 26935-26945.

51- Bates, P.A., Luo. J, and Sternberg, M.J.; (1999) Mol. Biol. 259, 718–736.

52- Stroop, C.J. M, Weber, W., Nimtz, M., Gutierrez Gallego, R., Kamerling, J.P., and Vliegenthart, J.F.; (2000) Arch. Biochem. Biophys 374, 42–51.

References

53- Bierhuzen, M. F. A., Maemura, K., and Fukudn, M., (1994) J. Biol. Chem. 269, 4473–4479.

54- Wojciechowicz, D.C., Park, P.K., Datta, R.V., and Paty, P.B.; (2000) Biochem Biophys. Res commun 273, 147– 153.

55- Valli, M., Bardoni, A., and Trinchera, M.; (1999) Glycobiology 9, 83–91.

56- Tapping, R.L., Akashi S. Miyake K. Godowski, P.J., and Tobias, P.S., (2000) J. Immunol., 165, 5780–5787.

57- Yamanaka, T., Kuroki, M., Kinugasa, T., and et .al; (1996), protein Exp. Purfi, (4): 438–442.

58- Magdelenat, .H.; (1992) J. Immunol. Meth., 150, 133-139.

59- Patel, P. S., Adhvaryu, S. G., Balar, D. B., et al (1994) Anticancer Res., 14: 747-752.

60- Leconte, A., Carambois, V., Ychou, M., Robert, B., Pourqier, D., Terkikh, A., Mach, J.P., and Pelegrin, A.; (1999) Br. J. cancer 9, 1373–1379.

61- Zimmer, R. and Thomas, P. (2001) cancer Res. 61, 2822–2826.

62- Jang, M., Shyu, S. K, Wilkinson, M.F.; (2000) cell, 102, 135–138.

63- Nakagoe, T., Sawai, T., Tsuji, T., Jibiki, M., Ohbatake, M., Nanashina, A., Yamaguchi, H., Yasutake, T., Ayabe, H., Arisawa, K.; (2001) Tumor Biol; 22, 115–122.

64- Edlund, M., Blikstad, I., and Obrink, B., (1996) J. Biol. Chem. 271: 1393–1399.

65- Lorenzen, D.R, Dux, F., Wolk, U., Tsirpouchtsi, Haas .G., and Meyer, T.F., (1999) J. Exp Med, 190, 1049 –1058.

66- Benchemol, S., Fuks, A., Joth, S., Beauchemin, N., Shirota, K., stannes, C.P.; (1989) cell, 57, 327-332.

67- Lesk, A.M., and Chothia, C. (1982) J. Mol. Biol. 13, 363–393.

68- Leahy, D. J.; (1997), Annu Rev. cell Dev. Biol. 13, 363 – 393.

References

69- Jones, E.Y., Davis, S. J.; Williams, A.F.; Harlose, K., and stuart, D.I. (1992), Nature 360, 232–239.

70- Rao, Y., Wu. X. F, Yip. P, Gariepy, J. and siu C.H; (1993) J. Biol chem. 268, 20630–20638.

71- Zhou, H., Fuks, A., Alcaraz, G., Bolling, T.J., and stanners, C.P., (1993) J. cell Biol. 122, 951–960.

72- Jessup, J. M., and Thomas, P.; (1998) "in cell Adhesion and communication Mediated by the CEA Family; Basic and clinical perspectives (stanners, C.P., ed) PP 195-222, Harwood Academic Publishers, Amsterdam, Netherlands.

73- Keesee, S.K., Briggman, J.V., Thill, G., and Wu. Y.J; (1996) crit. Rev. Eukaryotic Gene Exp., 6, 189–214.

74- Wagner, H, E., Toth, C.A., steele, G. D., and Thomas, P.; (1992) Clin. Exp Metastasis 10, 25–31.

75- Hashino, J., Fukada, Y., Oikawa, S., Nakazato, H., and Nakanishi, T.; (1994), clin Exp metastasis 12, 324-328.

76- Thomas, p., Gangopadhyay, A., steele. G, Andrew C., Nakazato, H., Oikawa, S. and Jessup, J. M.; (1995) cancer lett 25, 59-66.

77- Leconte, A., Garambois, V., Ychou, M., Robert, B., Pourquier, D., Terskikh, A., Mach, T. P., and Pelegrin, A., (1999) Br. J. cancer 9, 1373-1379.

78- Hostetter, R. B., Augustus, L. B., mankarious, R., chi. K, Fan. D., Toth. C. A., Thomas, P., and Jessup, J. M.; (1990) J. Natl. cancer Inst. 82, 380-385.

79- Gangopadhyay, A., Lazure, D. A., and Thomas, P. (1997) Cancer Lett. 1818, 1-6.

80- Gangopadhyay, A., Bajenova, O., Kelly, T. M., and Thomas, P. (1996) Cancer Res. 56, 4805-4810.

References

81- Toth, C. A., Thomas, P., Broitman, S. A., and Zamcheck, N. (1982) Biochem, J. 204, 377-381.

82- Gangopadhyay, A., and Thomas, P. (1996) Arch. Biochem. Biophys. 334, 151-157.

83- Zimmer, R., and Thomas, P. (2001) Cancer Res. 61, 2822-2826.

84- Gangopadhyay, A., Lazure, D. A., Kelly, T. M., and Thomas, P. (1996) Arch. Biochem. Biophys. 328, 151-157.

85- Olga, V., Bajenova, Regis, Z., Eugenia, S., John, S., Rowswell, A., Nanji and Peter, T.; (2001). J. Biol. Chem. 276, 33, 31067-31073.

86- Kenan, D. J., Query, C. C., and Keene, J. D.; (1991) Tren ds Biochem. Sci 16, 214-220.

87- Hammarstrom, S., Engvall, E., Johanson, B. G., Svenson, S., Sundblad, G., and Goldstein, I. J.; (1995) proc. Natil- acad Sci. US 72, 1528-1532.

88- Colign, J. E., and todd, C. W., (1975) Biochemistry 14, 805-810.

89- Westwood, J. H., and Thomas, P.; (1995) Br. J. Cancer 32, 708-719.

90- Fuks, A., Banjo, C., Shuster, J., Freem, S. O., and Golg, p.; (1974) Biochem Biophys Acta 417, 123-152.

91- Uriel, J., Trojan, J., Moro, R., and etal; (1983) Acad, Sci 417, 321-325.

92- Naval, J., Villacamp, M. J., Goguel, A. F., and etal; (1985) proc. Natl. Acad Sci. USA 82, 3301-3316.

93- Sunil, M., Salil, D.; (1997) "Molecular Biotechnology". 2nd ed. Wiley-Liss publication. New York. P 109-120.

94- Blundell, T. L.; (1994). Trends in Biotechnolog 12 (s), 145-155.

95- Underhill, D. M., Ozinsky, A., Hajjar, A. M., Stevens, A., Wilson, C. B., and Bassetti, M., and Aderem, A., (1999) Nature 401, 811-815.

96- Gold, P., and Freeman, S. O., (1965) J. Exp. Med 122, 467-481.

References

97- Luow., Wood, C. G., Earley, K., Hung, M. C., and Lin, S. H., (1997) Oncogene 14, 1697-1704.

98- Togayachi, A., Kudo, T., Ikehara, Y., Iwasaki, H., Nishihara, S., Andoh, T., Higashiyama, M., Kodama, K., Nakamori, S., and Narimatsu, H.; (1999) Int. J. Cancer 83, 70-79.

99- Okajima, T., Nakamura, Y., Uchikawa, M., Haslam, D. B., Numata, S. I., Furukawa, K., Urano, T., and Furukaws, K.; (2000) J. Biol. Chem. 10, 1074-

100- Gallouzi, I. E., Brennan, C. M., Stenberg, M. G., Swanson, M. S., Eversole, A., Maizels, N., and steitz, J. A.; (2000) proc Natl. Acad. Sci. USA 97, 3073-3078.

101- Gold, P., Krupay, J., and Ansari, H., (1970) J. Natil. Cancer Inst, 45, 219-222.

102- Tanaka, K., Nagura, H., Hamada, Y., Yamaura, M., Hioki, K., Watanable, K., Yamamoto, M.; (1990). J. Surg. Oncol., 34, 106.

103- Hamada, Y., Yamam, M., Hioki, K., Yamamoto, M., Nagura, H., Walanabe, K.; (1985. Cancer 55, 136.

104- Kammerer, R., Hahn, S., Singer, B. B., Luo, J. S., and Von Kleist, s.; (1998). Eur. J. Immunol. 28, 3664-3674.

105- Hauck, C. R., Lorenzen, D., Saas, J., and Meyer, T. F.; (1997) Infect Immun 65, 1863-1869.

106- Lindhorst, E.; (2000). Tumor Biol; 21, 116-122.

107- Costanza, M. E., Pinn, V., Schwartz. R. S., and Nathanson, L.; (1993) New Engl. J. Med. 289, 520-522.

108- Hellstrom, I., and Shepard, T. H.; (2000); Int. J. Cancer 6, 336-351.

109- Obrinl, B.,; (1991) BioEassays 13, 227-234.

110- Lindblom, A., Liliegren, a.; (2000) Br. Med. J. 320, 424-427.

111- Kos, J., Werle, B., Lah, T., Brunner, N.; (2000), Int. J. Biol. Marker, 15(1): 84-89.

References

112- Tanimizu, T., Ishihara, H., hattori, H., Hamada, S., Hirayama, R.; (1998) Cancer, 83(4): 660-665.

113- Ekins, R. P.; (1994) Br. Med. Bull 30, 3-11.

114- Altrakchi, S. A.; (2004) accepted for puplication in Al-Taqani Journal, No 868 in 20/9/2004.

115- Tomita, T. T., Safford, J. W., and Hirata, A. A., (1974) Immunology 26, 291-298.

116- Nakagoe, T., Fukushima, K., Nanashina, A., Sawa, T., Tsuji, T., Jibiki, M., Yamaguchi, H., Yasutake, T., Ayabe, H., Matuo, T., Tagawa, Y.; (2001), J. Gastroenterol. Hepato 16, 176-183.

117- Thomson, D. M., Krupey, J., Freedman, S. O., and Gold, p., (1969) proc. Natl acad, Sci US 64, 161-167.

118- Logerfo. P., Krupey, J., Hansen, H. J., (1971) New Engl. J. Med. 285, 138-141.

119- Go, V. L. W., Schutt, C. G., Moertel, C. G., Summerskill, W. H. J., and Butt, H. R., (1972) Gastroenterology 62, 754.

120- Egan, M. L., Lautenschleger, J. T., Coligan, J. E., and Todd, C. W., (1972) Immunochemistry 9, 289-299.

121- Macsween, J. M., Warner, N. L., Bankhurst, A. D., and Mackay, I. R.; (1972) Br. J. cancer 26, 356-360.

122- Mcpherson, T. A., Band, P. R., Grace, M., Hyde, H. A., Patwardhan, C. W.; (1973) Int. J. Cancer 12, 42-54.

123- Coller, J. A., Crichow, R. W., and Yin, Y. K.;(1973) Cancer Res 33, 1684-1688.

124- Gebauer, G., Muller-Ruchhoiltz, W.; (2001) Cancer Dete-prev., 25(4), 344-351.

125- Huang, J., Hardy, J. D., Sun, Y., and Shively, J. E.; (1999) J. cell Sci. 112, 4193-4205.

References

126- Huang, J., Simpson, J. F., Glackin, C., Riethorf, L., Wagener, C., and Shively, J. E.; (1998) Anticancer Res 18, 3203-3212.

127- Gold, P., (1967) Cancer 20, 1663-1667.

128- Gold, J. M., Banjo, C., Freeman, S. O., and Krupey, J.; (1973) Fed proc. 32, 4444.

129- Murata, K., Miyoshi, E., Kameyama, M., Ishikawa, O., Kabuto, T., Sasoki, Y., Hiratsuka, M., Ohigashi, H., Ishiguro, S., Honda, H., Takemura, F., Taniguchi, N., and Imaoka, S., (2000) Clin cancer Res 6, 1772-1777.

130- Holbarn, A. M., Mach, J. P., Macdonald, D., and Newlands, M.; (1994) Immunolog 26, 831-843.

131- Hirchfeld, M., Kirschning, C. J., Schwandner, R., Wesche, H., Weis, J. H., Wooten, R. M., and Weis, J. J.; (1999) J. Immunol 163, 2382-2386.

132- Bald win, A. S. J., (1996) Ann, U., Rev. Immuno., 14, 649-683.

133- Koda, Y., Kimura, H., Mekdad, E., (1993) Blood, 82, 2915-2919.

134- Bishayee, S., Dorai, D. T., (1980). Biochem. Biophys Acta, 623; 89-97.

135- Mizuno, Y., Kozutsumi, Y., Kawasaki, T., Yamashida, I., J. Biol. Chim., 256, (9): 4247-4252.

136- Miller, R. L., Collawn, J. F., Fich, W. W., (1992) J. Biol. Chem., 257,(13): 7574-7580.

137- Kjemtrup, S., Borkhsenious, O., and Raikhel, N., (1995), Plant. Physiol. 109(2) 603-610.

138- Kino. M., Yamaguchi, K., Umeka, H., and Furiatsu, G., (1996) Biosci. Biotechnol-Biochem 59(4); 683-688.

139- Banjo, C., Gold, P., Gehrke, C. W., Freeman, S. O., and Krupey, J.; (1974) Int. J. Cancer 13, 151-163.

References

140- Nakagoe, T., Sawai, T., Yuji, T., Jibiki, M., Nanashima, A., Yamaguchi, H., Yasutake, T., Ayabe, H., Matuo, T., Tagawa, Y.; (2002), Dig. Dise. Sci; 47, 322-330.

141- Mach, J. P., and Pusztaszer, G.; (1992) Immuno-chemistry 9, 1031-1034.

142- Nakago, T., Fukushima, K., Itoyanagi, N., Ikuta, Y., Oka, T., Nagayasu, T., Ayabe, H., Hara, S., Ishikawa, H., Minami, H., (2002) J. cancer Res. Clin oncol., 128, 257-264.

143- Darcy, D. A., Turberville, C., and James, R., (1973) Br. J. Cancer 28, 147-160.

144- Turberville, c., Darcy, D. a., Laurence, D. J. R., Johns, E. W., Neville, A. m., (1973) Immunochemistry 10, 841-843.

145- Baxi, B. R., Patel, P. S., Adhvaryu, S. G., and Payal, P.; (1991) Cancer 67, 135-140.

146- Nakagoe, T., Sawai, T., Tsuji, T., Jibiki, M., Nanashima, A., Yamaguchi, H., Kurosaki, N., Yasutake, T., Ayabe, H.; (2001) J. Gastroenterol, 36, 166-172.

147- Fornes, N. M., Tanka, M., Matos, D.; (2001) Int. J. Biol Markers 16(1), 27-30.

148- Mach, J. P., Carrel, S., Merenda, C., Sordat, B., and Cerottin, J. C.; (1974) Nature 248, 704-706.

149- Khoo, S. K., Hunt, P. S., and Mackay, I. R.; (1973), Am. J. Dig. Dis. 16, 1-7.

150- Gold, P., Wilson, T., Romero, R., Shuster, J., Shuster, J., and Freeman, S. O.; (1973) Dis. Colon Rect. 16, 258-265.

151- Ona, F. V., Zamcheck, N., Dhar, P., Moore, T. L., and Kupchik, H. Z.; (1973) cancer 31, 324-331.

152- Mccarney W. H., and Hoffer, P. B.; (1994) Radiology.

References

153- Dhar, P., Moore, T., Zamcheck, N., and Kupchik, H., (1992) J. Am. Med. Assoc. 221, 31-35.

154- Khoo, S. K., (1974) Med. J. Austral. 1, 1025-1029.

155- Wechsler, M., Logerfo, P., Feminella, J., and Lattimer, J. K.; (1993) J. urol. 109, 669-701.

156- Khoo, S. K., and Mackay, E. V., (1974) cancer 34, 542-548.

157- Laurence, D. J. R., Neville, A. M., (1972) Br. J. cancer 26, 335-355.

158- Hansen, H. J., Snyder, J. J., Miller, E., Vandevoorde, J. P., Neal Miller, O., Hines, L. R., and Burns, J. J., (1994) Human pathol 5, 139-147.

159- Delwiche, R., Zamcheck, N., and Marcon, N., (1993) cancer 31, 328-330.

160- Laurence, D. J., Stevens, U., Bettelheim, R., Darcy, D., Leese, C., Turbervill, C., Alexander, P., Johns, E. W., Neville, A. M., (1972) Br. Med. J. iii, 605-609.

161- Scope, R., (1992)," Protein purification principle practice" New York; Velag P. 162-200.

162- Janson, J. C., Ryden, L.; (1998)," Protein purification" 2nd. Ed., New York; A John Wiley & Sons, Inc. Chap. 1 & 14.

163- Chamberlain, J., Jargarinec, N., Ofher, P., (1996) Biochem. J., 99, 610-615.

164- Rogers, G. T., Searle, F., and Bagshawe, K. D.; (1994) Nature 251, 519-521.

165- Aberman, L. E., Pettychna, L. I., and Lutsyk, M. D.; (1991). Biochem. J. 63(3), 70-76.

166- Avellana, A. V., Joubert, R. and Bladier, D.; (1990). Anal Bi. Chem.. 190(1), 26-31.

167- Bucdon, R. H.; (1985) Enzyme for Immunoassay practice theory of enzyme Immunoassay p. 178.

References

168- Edward, F., Rossomando, (1990)," Measurment of enzyme activity Method in Enzymology" 182, 42.

169- Schmander, H. P., (1997) Peroxidase Methods in Biotechnology, Taylor and Francis. London.

170- Sadasivam, S., and Manickam., (1996) peroxidase Biochemical Method, P., 108. New age international (P) limited publisher.

171- Shannon, and Kay., (1966). J. Biol. Chem.. 241(a), 2166-2172.

172- Lowry, O. H., Rosebrough, N. J., Farr, L., Randell, R., (1951). J. Biol. Chem.. 193, 265.

173- Parker, W. C., (1967),"Hand book of Experiment Immunology" Backwell. Scientific publication oxford P. 423-450.

174- Shvari, F., and Morell, A., (1970). J. Immunol. 104, 1310-1318.

175- Wassan, A. A., (2000),"Biochemical studies on alphafeto-protein and some tumor in Gastric Cancer" ph.D Thesis supervised by Al-Mudaffer, S. A., College of Science, Baghdad University.

176- May soon, K. H., (2001),"Molecular characterization of testostrone receptor in Mammary Tissues effected by tumors". M.Sc. Thesis supervised by Al-Mudaffar, S. A., college of Science Baghdad University.

177- Wester, Meier, (1996)," Electrophoresis in practice" New York, Springer. Verlage P. 162-200.

178- Nis, H., Axelsen, (1983)," Hand book of immunoprecipitation in Gel Techniques" (3rd .ed) W. A. Banjamin. Inc. London.

179- Sternberger, P. H., Hardy, J. J., Cuculis, and Meyer, H. G., (1970). J. Histochem. Cytochem 18, 315-320.

180- Boyd, G. W., and Pear, W. S., (1988), Lancer, 2, 129.

181- Hurn, B. A., and London, J.,"Radioimmunoassay Methods" (1990) churechill Livingston, Edinburgh, P. 121.

References

182- Vaitukaitis, J. B., Robbins, E., Nieschlag, and G. T., Ross, (1991) J. clin. Endocrinol 33, 988.

183- Mcfarlane, A. S., (1972) Nature 149, 439-452.

184- Boorsma, D. M., and Streefkerk, J. K., (1976) J. Histochem Cytochem 24, 481.

185- Mannick, M., and Downey, W., (1993) J. Immunol. Methods 3, 233.

186- Nakane, P. K., Ram, J. S., and Pierce, G. B., (1996) J. Histochem. Cytochem 14, 789.

187- Nakane, P.," Immunoassays in the clinical Laboratory" (1979) New York.

188- Kato, K., Fukui, H., Hamaguchi, and Ishikawa, E., J. Immunol. (1996) 116, 1554-1563.

189- Herrmann, J. E., Collins, M. F., (1976) J. Immunol. Methods 10, 363.

190- Christensen, P., Johansson, A., and Nielsen, V., (1978), J. Immunol. Method. 23, 23.

191- Quash, G., Roch, A., Niveleav, J., Grange, T., Keolouangkhot, and Huppert, J., (1978). J. Immunol. Method 22, 165.

192- Kondorosi, E., Nagy, J., and Denes, D., (1977) J. Immunol. Method.

193- Cantaero, L. A., Butler, J. E., and Osborne, J. W., (1990) Anal. Biochem. 105, 375.

194- Kochwa, S., Brownell, M., Rosen field, R. E., and Wasserman, L. R., (1967), J. Immunol. 99, 981.

195- Pesce, A. J., Ford, D. J., Gaizutis, M., and Polak, V. E., Biochim. Biophys (1997) Acta. 492, 399.

196- Morrisey, B. W., and Fenstermaker, C. A., (1976) Trans. Am. Soc. Artif. Oragan 22, 383.

References

197- Cantarero, L. A., Butler, E. L., and Osborne, J. W., (1990) Anal. Biochem. 105, 375.

198- Engvall, E., Jonsson, K., and Per/monn, P., (1991) Biochim., Biophys. Acta. 251, 427.